T0073698

The Power of BDSM

SEXUALITY, IDENTITY, AND SOCIETY SERIES

Series Editor
Phillip L. Hammack

The Power of BDSM

Play, Communities, and Consent in the 21st Century

Edited by

BRANDY L. SIMULA
ROBIN BAUER
LIAM WIGNALL

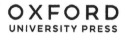

OXFORD
UNIVERSITY PRESS

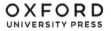

Oxford University Press is a department of the University of Oxford. It furthers
the University's objective of excellence in research, scholarship, and education
by publishing worldwide. Oxford is a registered trade mark of Oxford University
Press in the UK and certain other countries.

Published in the United States of America by Oxford University Press
198 Madison Avenue, New York, NY 10016, United States of America.

CIP data is on file at the Library of Congress

ISBN 978–0–19–765859–8

DOI: 10.1093/oso/9780197658598.001.0001

Printed by Integrated Books International, United States of America

Contents

PART I INTRODUCING BDSM

PART II PLAY AND PRACTICES

Series Foreword

The Oxford Series on Sexuality, Identity, and Society provides a space for scholarly inquiry that situates sexuality in historical time and place. Since 2009, entries in the series have documented the distinctiveness of sexuality in the 21st century. As we enter the third decade of the century, the story of sexual identity becomes clearer: It is a story about the rise of cultural and scientific understanding of sexual diversity, a story about the reclamation of stigma through new narratives that situate diverse practices and identities as legitimate, meaningful, and healthy. It is a story about the gradual erosion of (or at least formidable challenge to) normative thinking about sexuality. Resistance to normative thinking has come from everyday acts of visibility and social movements working for justice for those who hold minoritized sexual identities or engage in practices once denigrated. Resistance has also come from the scientific activism of sophisticated interdisciplinary and cross-national scholarship. This volume represents one example of such scholarship.

Among the forms of sexual diversity that have flourished in the 21st century, kink/BDSM continues to be among the most culturally misunderstood and least studied in sufficient depth and breadth. Most who come to me seeking information and guidance bring stereotypes and discomfort toward the way in which, at a distance, kink dynamics appear to violate a cardinal rule of human intimacy that has (thankfully) become the norm: the rule of symmetry between partners. And yet there is excitement, the thrill of an adrenaline rush, when novices—be they curious students or journalists or budding practitioners—discover the psychological and interpersonal potentials of kink. Foremost, kink is playful. The power asymmetry that defines kink dynamics is not meant to actually subordinate the will of another; it is meant to psychologically liberate the individual from established scripts and to empower them. As has been well documented in social scientific inquiry, the play that constitutes kink is both fun and serious. As such, it necessitates a collaboratively developed script. This script, whether written or verbalized among partners, forms the second defining feature of kink: it is consensual, its power play never forced upon someone (for that constitutes abuse). In forcing its practitioners to develop intentionality and mutuality to their dynamics and in blending both the pleasure of role play and the seriousness of taboo, kink creates a uniquely empowering and liberating psychological and intimate experience.

As kink has come out of the shadows in this century, so too have social science theory and research shifted their paradigmatic gaze from one of pathology to one of diversity. This volume, edited by leaders in the field Brandy Simula, Robin Bauer, and Liam Wignall, represents an important and distinctive contribution to this growing body of work. The start of the volume is particularly fitting of this historical moment, with a chapter by Thomas Weinberg, a key intellectual architect of the paradigm shift in the social sciences which began in earnest in the 1970s and ultimately came to document kink practitioners and communities through a non-pathologizing lens. A chapter by Liam Wignall on the role of the internet in kink research then immediately reminds us that we are no longer in the 20th century, with its top-down approach to information and its decidedly inaccessible context for most forms of sexual diversity. The expansive possibilities afforded for the relationship between individuals and information, as well as for sociality in general, makes our century decidedly unique.

The chapters in this volume are noteworthy for their international scope and the breadth of perspectives on kink they assume. With topics ranging from community, identity, desire, relationships, representations, and specific practices (e.g., rope bondage, pup play, age play), contributors cover an impressive terrain. The volume is especially to be lauded for its attention to intersectionality and to such issues as ethics and politics. These areas have often been lacking in kink/BDSM research, and it is refreshing to see them prominently addressed in the volume.

When I started teaching my students about kink in seminars on intimate diversity, only a brave few would admit they had kinky desires or had engaged in kinky practices. In less than a decade, the pattern has shifted, with many students comfortable not just sharing that they are kinky but proudly explaining their practices and the value they have for their psychological and intimate lives. With visibility and a willingness to be authentic about one's desires and experiences, we come to a place of ever-expanding support for autonomy in our intimate lives. This book represents an important piece of scholarship in the social scientific documentation of kink in our century, and I trust its value will be apparent to those whose curiosities have led them here.

Phillip L. Hammack
Santa Cruz, California
September, 2022

Foreword

We congratulate the editors and authors of *The Power of BDSM: Play, Communities, and Consent in the 21st Century* for creating this new ground-breaking volume. Researchers in the area of BDSM (bondage and discipline, dominance and submission, sadism and masochism), colloquially called *kink*, have often had to contend with clueless and often hostile institutional review boards. We salute the contributors to this book for their fine achievement as well as for what the nature, tone, and focus reveal about the current state of BDSM/kink research.

There is a matter-of-fact, almost ordinary tone in describing the kinds of inclinations, behaviors, interactions, and identities that would have been considered bizarre even in the professional literature 10 or 20 years ago. Scholarly writing on BDSM/kink used to be almost conspicuous in its clinical tone, as if to ward off the possibility that the research enterprise could be perceived as salacious. Paradoxically, although this volume incorporates appropriate attention to stigma and its consequences, that stigma is now clearly less than universal. There is remarkably less here about external obstacles, such as being pathologized, subject to legal penalties, ostracized by friends and family, than in previous research volumes. Correspondingly, there is minimal emphasis on the importance of advocacy for BDSM communities. The focus of this book, ostensibly on what were previously seen as unusual or even deviant sexual proclivities, could very well be on other leisure activities/hobbyists, such as stamp or coin collectors.

Whereas previous books on BDSM/kink tended to have a heavy emphasis on psychopathology among practitioners—or, more correctly, attempts to correct and demonstrate the lack of evidence for the assumption that psychopathology is rampant among practitioners—there is no longer a need to devote space and energy to such archaic debates. Similarly, we are relieved to see that there is no discussion of the origins, let alone "etiology," of BDSM interests. In this volume, it is as nonsensical to discuss the reasons for enjoying rope bondage or pup play as to explain why people like to play hockey, listen to music, or engage in oral sex.

This book takes an international focus, often in areas and countries that have previously been neglected by researchers. To their credit, the editors have curated a volume that is geographically and methodologically diverse. Contributors come from Portugal, Australia, Sweden, Germany, the United States, and South Africa. Rather commonly, research participants were recruited via the internet. The role of the web in both the research and the formation of online communities warranted its own chapter (see Chapter 2).

Many of the contributors mention that future research should include the participants who are hardest for scholars to identify and access, that is, those who are referred to, sometimes derisively, as "bedroom players." Indeed, there is understandably minimal attention to those who practice in private, outside the organized world of BDSM communities. Sometimes that is related to monetary considerations and the need for professional privacy. It is also true that some practitioners still think they "invented" and do not participate in the larger BDSM community or smaller special interest groups. In addition, some individuals must still stay in the "closet" rather than risk exposure to licensing boards, family, or social sanctions.

In keeping with a reduced need for explanatory theory and research, the contributors are less likely to be mental health professionals (i.e., clinical psychologists and psychiatrists) and more likely to be using descriptive, sociological, or psychological lenses. Research into BDSM presents some special methodological problems, and this volume seeks to identify those problems and present some solutions. There is a nice array of ethnographic research including the participant-observer stance and an entire chapter devoted to consideration of the position of the BDSM researcher in fieldwork (see Chapter 15). There is substantial attention to the personal perceptions and experiences of the researchers. The ethnographic contributors all went through ethics or internal review boards before undertaking their endeavors, with informed consent; although such a statement would be boilerplate in all human research domains, it remains noteworthy that the participant-observer stance has been normalized in the study of BDSM.

Interestingly—and perhaps correspondingly—this volume is less concerned with the sexual aspects of BDSM desires and activities than one might expect. Kink is depicted as distinct from sexuality, sexually arousing inclinations/fantasies, practices, or identities. On the contrary, there is a striking emphasis on kink as leisure and sheer, delightful play, even in such formerly controversial areas as age play.

Simultaneously, the editors and authors have begun to tackle academically a phenomenon that has been somewhat shrouded historically: the use of BDSM to heal the trauma of prior sexual violence. Courageously, the contributors describe this taboo endeavor and its transformative effects. To be clear, no one is suggesting that clinicians should recommend BDSM as therapy for such trauma, but they acknowledge that engaging in BDSM can be therapeutic for some patients. A sympathetic therapist may be able to use these experiences, and the emotions they generate, as part of the client's healing process from sexual trauma.

The field of BDSM studies has expanded and is growing. This book also looks at the romantic aspects of BDSM and the critical issue of consent and how it is obtained. The authors also discuss how BDSM is integrated into the expression of other diverse sexualities.

The editors have encouraged the contributors to write from intersectional perspectives, and they have succeeded admirably. The chapters are cutting edge as they discuss the effects of and how racism, sexism, and violence permeate and influence the mores of the BDSM community. We are all products of our societies, and these issues affect how BDSM is practiced and understood within communities. BDSM practitioners are now keenly aware of how power differentials in BDSM scenes and relationships can be subverted and how to guard against such abuse, beyond simple consent.

Excitingly, this book is populated by new ideas, contributed by a crop of new, young researchers. This book is an important next step in the quest to understand BDSM. We cannot wait to see what these editors and authors contribute to the burgeoning field of BDSM/kink studies in the years ahead!

Charles Moser

Peggy J. Kleinplatz

Preface

We are delighted to present the first interdisciplinary collection of original research on BDSM in over a decade. At the same time, we also want to acknowledge the particularly challenging context in which this project was undertaken, as well as the impact that the twin pandemics of COVID-19 and systemic anti-Black racism have had on the volume.

The global COVID-19 pandemic created a particularly challenging context for this project, and we are grateful to the many contributors who completed their contributions in the pandemic context. We also think it is important to acknowledge that several contributors whose work we hoped to include in the volume had to withdraw from the volume. The impact of the pandemic on women scholars, scholars of color, and scholars with caregiving responsibilities is having a chilling effect on publication and scholarly writing across the globe; and, like many others, we are concerned about how the impact of the pandemic will exacerbate existing inequities in academia.

The twin pandemics of COVID-19 and systemic anti-Black racism in the United States, including the murder of George Floyd just weeks before the original deadline for contributions to the volume, have also had a particularly pernicious impact on the well-being, career trajectories, and scholarly productivity of Black scholars in the United States. Black scholars across the United States—already subject to the identity tax, tokenism, microaggressions, and myriad other effects of systemic racism—were also repeatedly called upon in the aftermath of the police murder of George Floyd and the resulting protests against police brutality and anti-Black racism to step into diversity, equity, and inclusion conversations and take on a wide variety of additional, nearly always uncompensated activist and service labor. Several prominent US-based scholars of color withdrew from the edited volume in the summer of 2020. Their chapters would have considerably strengthened the volume and made important contributions to the field of BDSM studies.

The volume is prepared according to the American Psychological Association's (APA's) seventh edition stylistic guidelines. We diverge from APA style guidelines, however, in how we capitalize racial and ethnic terminology. The racial identity *Black* reflects a shared sense of social and political identity and community for many people. The term *white* carries a different set of meanings and does not represent a shared culture and history in the way that *Black* does. Additionally, capitalization of the term *white* is often used in contexts that support white supremacist ideology, and capitalization of the term risks conveying legitimacy to white supremacist beliefs. Therefore, throughout the volume, contributors diverge from APA stylistic guidelines around the capitalization of racial and ethnic terms.

Brandy L. Simula

Acknowledgments

As coeditors of this project, we wish to express our gratitude to each of the contributors to the volume for their thorough engagement with our feedback and especially for their work on this project, which has unfolded on the same timeline as the global pandemic.

We are also grateful to Phillip Hammack, Abby Gross, Katharine Pratt, Nadina Persaud, and everyone else at Oxford University Press who supported and helped make this project possible.

Brandy Simula extends her warmest gratitude to her coeditors, Robin Bauer and Liam Wignall, whose expertise, deeply insightful engagement, patience, and good-humored camaraderie throughout the project made it possible to complete this project during a global pandemic. She thanks especially her family of choice, whose support, generosity, humor, and encouragement have helped her think, write, and exist as a full human. She is grateful, as always, to all of the BDSMers who have generously allowed her to learn about their lives, tell their stories, and marvel at the myriad vibrant ways that humans create interactions, communities, and identities that allow for such diverse and beautiful modes of joy, flourishing, connection, and meaning.

Robin Bauer wants to thank Emmanuel and the Knuffels for carrying him through the epidemic. He also wants to thank his coeditors for inspiration and mutual support in finishing this project in challenging times.

Liam Wignall would like to thank the coeditors for providing constant support and guidance throughout the project, particularly during the challenging circumstances. He'd also like to thank the contributors to this edited collection who have engaged substantially with our comments and helped create a book consisting of research across the spectrum of BDSM. Finally, he'd like to thank his partner, Mark McCormack, for his continual support on all the projects he undertakes.

Contributors

Robin Bauer, PhD
Faculty of Social Science
Baden-Württemberg Cooperative State
University
Stuttgart, Germany

Theodore Bennett, PhD
Law School
University of Western Australia
Perth, Australia

Dana Berkowitz, PhD
Department of Sociology
Louisiana State University
Baton Rouge, LA, USA

Daniel Cardoso, PhD
Department of Sociology
Manchester Metropolitan University
Manchester, UK
CICANT, LUSOFONA University
Lisbon, Portugal

Charlotta Carlström, PhD
Department of Social Work
Malmö University
Malmö, Sweden

Angela Cooke-Jackson, PhD, MPH
College of Arts and Letters
California State University, Los Angeles
Los Angeles, CA, USA

Jessica A. Fox, MA
Counseling, Therapy, and School
Psychology
Lewis and Clark College
Portland, OR, USA

Benjamin C. Graham, PhD
Department of Psychology
Cal Poly Humboldt
Arcata, CA, USA

Phillip L. Hammack, PhD
Professor of Psychology and Director
of the Sexual and Gender Diversity
Laboratory
University of California, Santa Cruz

Karen Holt, PhD
School of Criminal Justice
Michigan State University
East Lansing, MI, USA

Zoey Jones, PhD
Department of Law and Legal Studies
Carleton University
Ottawa, ON, Canada

Tsolak M. Kirakosyan, MA
School of Nursing
California State University—Los
Angeles
Los Angeles, CA, USA

Peggy J. Kleinplatz, PhD
Department of Family Medicine, School
of Epidemiology & Public Health
University of Ottawa
Ottawa, ON, Canada

Robert M. Matchett, MA
Department of Sociology
Louisiana State University
Baton Rouge, LA, USA

Tracey L. McCormick, PhD
Department of Languages, Cultural
Studies, and Applied Linguistics
University of Johannesburg
Johannesburg, South Africa

Charles Moser, PhD, MD
Diverse Sexualities Research and
Education Institute
San Francisco, CA, USA

Amber R. Norman, PhD
Department of Counseling
Prescott College
Tallahassee, FL, USA

Patrícia M. Pascoal, PhD
HEI-Lab
Lusófona University
Lisbon, Portugal
CICPSI
Faculty of Psychology
University of Lisbon
Lisbon, Portugal

Rita Quaresma, MA
School of Psychology and Life Sciences
Lusófona University
Lisbon, Portugal

Alejandre Rodriguez, MA
College of Arts and Letters
California State University, Los Angeles
Los Angeles, CA, USA

Valerie Rubinsky, PhD
Department of Communication
University of Maine at Augusta
Augusta, ME, USA

Miles Ruvabalca, BA
Independent Scholar
Arcata, CA, USA

Sinclair Sexsmith, BA
Independent Scholar
Seattle, WA, USA

Brandy L. Simula, PhD
Independent Scholar
Atlanta, GA, USA

Marla Renee Stewart, MA
Independent Scholar
Atlanta, GA, USA

Thomas S. Weinberg, PhD
Department of Sociology
SUNY Buffalo State
Buffalo, NY, USA

Liam Wignall, PhD
Department of Psychology
University of Brighton
Brighton, UK

PART I
INTRODUCING BDSM

Introduction

Understanding BDSM

Brandy L. Simula

Introduction to *The Power of BDSM*

The Power of BDSM: Play, Communities, and Consent in the 21st Century features cutting-edge empirical research by scholars working from a wide range of disciplinary approaches and in diverse national contexts, along with personal reflections from community educators, activists, and practitioners. Designed to be of interest to scholars working in sexuality studies and re-lated fields, teachers of graduate courses focused on sexualities, identities, communities, inequalities, and a broader, non-specialist audience inter-ested in sexualities, society, and identity, *The Power of BDSM* engages per-sistent questions about the relationships among sexualities, identities, and communities: What role do communities play in shaping BDSM identities? How are BDSM communities similar to and different from other kinds of sexuality- and identity-based communities? What are the ethics involved in researching marginalized and stigmatized communities? How do cultural representations shape lived experiences? What are the relationships between structural and personal power?

Chapters in the volume represent a diverse range of disciplinary, method-ological, and theoretical approaches, paralleling the spread of BDSM studies into a wide swath of disciplines. Throughout the volume, contributors high-light the intersections of BDSM with other identities, including gender, race, age, sexual orientation, class, and nationality. In engaging with communities and identities across specific local and national contexts, the volume highlights the commonalities in kink communities and identities across settings. At the same time, in its deep attention to the specificity of local communities across regions and nations, the volume also shows how local

Brandy L. Simula, *Introduction* In: *The Power of BDSM*. Edited by: Brandy L. Simula, Robin Bauer, and Liam Wignall, Oxford University Press. © Oxford University Press 2023. DOI: 10.1093/oso/9780197658598.003.0001 communities can and do develop along different trajectories, influenced deeply by their unique social, legal, political, and economic contexts.

The Present and Future of BDSM Studies

As BDSM studies has proliferated across the last several decades, research on BDSM has continued to expand across the disciplines, with work on BDSM appearing in fields from game studies (Sihvonen & Tuomas Harviainen, 2020) to theology (Henderson-Espinoza, 2018; LeFranc, 2018; Mechelke, 2019) to neuroscience (Luo & Zhang, 2018a, 2018b) to legal studies (Bennett, 2015; Beresford, 2016; Cowan, 2012; Khan, 2014) to biology (De Neef et al., 2019) to tourism studies (Tomazos et al., 2017) and many others, alongside longer-standing traditions of work on BDSM in sociology, anthropology, psychology, cultural studies, and literary studies. Once focused on under-standing the "causes" of pathology or deviant sexuality (for discussion, see Kleinplatz & Moser, 2005; Wright, 2018), BDSM studies now explores myriad questions in relation to BDSM, such as identity development (e.g., Buchanan, 2004; Chaline, 2010; Coppens et al., 2020; Damm et al., 2018; M. Graham, 1998; Highleyman, 1997; Hughes & Hammack, 2019; Langdridge & Butt, 2004; Mosher et al., 2006; Rambukkana, 2004; Sprott & Hadcock, 2018; Wilson, 2005; Zambelli, 2017), the intersections of BDSM with other important identities (Damm et al., 2018) including race (Cruz, 2016a, 2016b, 2020; Liang, 2020; Martinez, 2020), gender (Alvarado et al., 2018; Bauer, 2007, 2008, 2018a, 2018b; Botta et al., 2019; Puig-Rodas, 2019; Simula, 2012, 2013; Simula & Sumerau, 2017), disability (Reynolds, 2007; Sheppard, 2018; Tellier, 2017), and sexual orientation (Better & Simula, 2015; Simula, 2014; Sprott & Hadcock, 2018; Sprott et al., 2020; Sprott & Williams, 2019), how BDSM communities are organized and what role they play in BDSM experiences (e.g., Bauer, 2008, 2018a, 2018b; Dale, 1991; B. Graham et al., 2016; M. Graham, 1998; Harmon, 1997; Holt, 2016; Ortmann & Sprott, 2013; Rubin, 1997; Sharma & Ghupta, 2011; Zamboni, 2018), and better understanding the diverse range of meanings and experiences involved in BDSM (for a review of recent work in BDSM studies, see Simula, 2019b).

While research on BDSM has long centered the voices of white participants, urgently needed research—particularly in the last few decades—has ex-panded the range of individuals participating in research on BDSM to in-clude stronger inclusion of participants of color and to critically interrogate the whiteness and racism of BDSM communities. This work demonstrates the ways that the whiteness of BDSM communities and the white privilege held by many participants shape community norms and interactions so as to exclude and marginalize participants of color (Bauer, 2008; Martinez, 2020; Sheff & Hammers, 2011; Weiss, 2011). At the same time, work in this line of research also documents the ways that participants of color are forming communities and spaces that center participants of color, resisting the racism and whiteness of many BDSM spaces, and using BDSM to explore pleasure (Cruz, 2016a, 2016b, 2020; Liang, 2020).

Additionally, while research on BDSM published in English-language outlets has historically been undertaken primarily in US, Canadian, and UK communities, studies of BDSM are increasingly being conducted in other cultural and national contexts as well, including recent work in Australia (Bennett, 2013; Steinmetz & Maginn, 2015), Belgium (Coppens et al., 2020; Holvoet et al., 2017; Wuyts et al., 2020), China (Luo & Zhang, 2018a, 2018b), the Czech Republic (Drdova & Saxonberg, 2021; Jozifkova & Kolackova, 2017), Finland (Sandnabba et al., 1999, 2002; Santtila et al., 2002), Germany (Bauer, 2014; Cerwenka et al., 2020; Spengler, 1977; Woltersdorff, 2011), Israel (Haviv, 2016), Italy (Faccio et al., 2020; Lasala et al., 2020), the Netherlands (Wismeijer & van Assen, 2013), Poland (Sendler & Lew-Starowicz, 2019), Portugal (Pascoal et al., 2015), South Africa (McCormick, 2018a, 2018b), Spain (Puig-Rodas, 2019), and Sweden (Carlström, 2019), as well as other national contexts. Research on how BDSM communities and practices develop and are carried out in different cultural contexts reveals that while there are a number of commonalities across cultural contexts (e.g., emphasis on consent, specific public or private places where BDSM scenes or play happen), local cultural contexts (e.g., cultural beliefs about BDSM and sexuality, the legal status of BDSM) can contribute to important differences in experiences of BDSM.

With the rise of the internet, dedicated web-based BDSM community sites and social media have expanded access to information about BDSM, providing new narratives that explore BDSM interests (e.g., Hughes & Hammack, 2019; Wignall, 2020) as well as creating opportunities for connection with BDSM participants for those who live in places without BDSM communities and/or who choose not to participate in physical BDSM communities. Research since the early 2010s has explored how virtual spaces and social media are used by BDSM participants (Rambukkana, 2004; Rubinsky, 2018; Wignall, 2017, 2022). This research documents how integral online spaces have become to BDSM communities and shows how—increasingly—access to physical BDSM spaces, events, and communities is mediated through online and virtual communities and networks. In addition to the ways that the rise of the internet has expanded access to BDSM education and events for participants, it has allowed research on BDSM to rapidly expand and made the identification of participants—through online BDSM social networking spaces like FetLife, bondage.com, and others—much easier than in previous decades (see Chapter 2, for a fuller discussion).

BDSM studies has historically been situated primarily in the broader field of sexuality studies, and sexuality studies remains an important and fruitful analytic lens for investigating BDSM. However, a growing body of scholarship troubles the long-standing assumption within BDSM studies that BDSM is always, inherently, or necessarily a sexual identity or practice, critically interrogating the complexity of the relationship of BDSM to sex, sexuality, and the erotic (Faccio et al., 2020; Sagarin et al., 2019; Simula, 2019a, 2019b; Sprott et al., 2020; Turley et al., 2018). Recent work on the experiences of asexual BDSM participants further troubles the long-standing assumption that BDSM is inherently a sexual practice (Sloan, 2015; Winter-Gray & Hayfield, 2019; Zamboni & Madero, 2018).

A growing line of research examines how BDSM participants use BDSM for therapeutic, spiritual, and healing purposes (Baker, 2018; Barker, Gupta, & Iantaffi, 2007; Carlström, 2020; Lindemann, 2011; Sprott, 2020), including in relation to past trauma and/or abuse (Hammers, 2014, 2019; Thomas, 2020). Work in this line of literature also informs a growing body of research on and guidelines for kink-aware counseling and therapy (Ansara, 2019; Barker, Iantaffi, & Gupta, 2007; Dunkley & Brotto, 2018; Kolmes, 2003; Kolmes et al., 2006; Lawrence & Love-Crowell, 2008). Importantly, a large number of studies show that—contrary to stereotypes often perpetuated by popular culture representations of BDSM—psychopathological understandings of BDSM as being correlated with mental illness, pathology, and/or abuse are not more common in the BDSM population in comparison with the general population (Brown et al., 2020; Connolly, 2006; Wismeijer & van Assen, 2013).

In addition to the previously described frameworks through which scholars have studied BDSM, researchers have used a leisure studies framework, investigating how the concept of leisure sheds light on BDSM practices and experiences (Newmahr, 2010b; Prior & Williams, 2015; Sprott & Williams, 2019; Weiss, 2011; Williams et al., 2016). Work that examines BDSM as leisure documents that while many participants describe BDSM as "play," a significant investment of time and resources along with an emphasis on education and developing BDSM-related skills make BDSM in many ways similar to other forms of serious leisure. The leisure studies approach has illuminated the diverse benefits that participants report from BDSM, including pleasure, arousal, fun, psychological benefits, sense of freedom, personal growth, transcendence, and others (Sprott & Williams, 2019).

While the field of BDSM studies has long axiomatically defined BDSM as consensual, studies since the early 2000s have shed light on the complexities of consent in BDSM contexts as well as explored how participants construct, understand, and negotiate context in relation to BDSM practices and relationships (e.g., Barker, 2013; Bauer, 2014, 2021; Cascalheira et al., 2022; Dunkley & Brotto, 2020; Fanghanel, 2020; Holt, 2016, 2018; Kaak, 2016; Sheff, 2021). This work demonstrates the complexities of negotiating consent, emphasizing that structural and interpersonal differences in power and status influence the positions from which participants negotiate BDSM interactions. Research in this area also documents the complex—and not always successful—ways that BDSM communities create guidelines intended to protect participants and respond to reports of consent violations.

In recent years, BDSM studies has also begun the critically important work of disaggregating the diverse practices and identities subsumed under the very broad BDSM umbrella, helping to better understand the diverse motivations and experiences of participants. Work on practices and identities investigates the meanings and experiences of domestic discipline (Carmack et al., 2015; DeGroot et al., 2015), spanking (Labrecque et al., 2021; Plante, 2006), pup play (Langdridge & Lawson, 2019; Lawson & Langdridge, 2020; Puppy Sharon & Toushin, 2004; Wignall, 2017, 2022; Wignall & McCormack, 2017), age play (Bauer, 2018a; Hawkinson & Zamboni, 2014; Lasala et al., 2020; Zamboni, 2018, 2019; Zamboni & Madero, 2018), 24/7 power exchange relationships (Cascalheira et al., 2022; Dancer et al., 2006; Kondakov, 2017), gender play (Bauer, 2007, 2018aa, 2018b; Simula, 2013), race play (Cruz, 2016a, 2020; Kuzmanovic, 2018; Liang, 2020; Musser, 2014; Smith & Luykx, 2017), sensation and pain play (Dunkley et al., 2020; Newmahr, 2010a; Sharma & Ghupta, 2011; Williams, 2006; Wuyts et al., 2020), professional BDSM (Cowan, 2012; Levey & Pinsky, 2015; Lindemann, 2010, 2011, 2012; Pinsky & Levey, 2015; Wilson, 2005), and many others. Understanding the ways that these diverse communities, identities, and practices intersect, overlap, and are distinct is vital to helping us develop a better understanding of the diverse experiences that fall under the broad umbrella of BDSM.

Terminology

One of the challenges of studying BDSM is the fluid and evolving nature of BDSM terminology in both BDSM communities and the scholarship on BDSM. For readers less familiar with BDSM and BDSM terminology, I provide here a brief overview of key terminology, recognizing both that this list is necessarily partial and that the nuances of the usage of these terms both within the academic literature and among BDSM participants themselves are not fully captured here. Indeed, within BDSM communities, the nature of distinctions and overlaps between many of these terms is hotly contested. Throughout the volume, contributors provide definitions of less common terms as they are relevant.

BDSM is an umbrella term that encompasses a variety of terms used interchangeably both in the literature and by participants to refer to a range of consensual practices/activities, desires, communities/subcultures, identities/roles, and meanings. While these terms often overlap in participants' everyday lives, distinctions among them are conceptually important because these terms do not simply indicate differences in preferences for particular activities; they identify different aspects of BDSM. While in academic work we often make important analytical distinctions among identity, community, affiliation, preferences, practices, and relationships, within BDSM communities, many of the terms introduced here and used by contributors throughout the volume are used by participants to refer to multiple levels: For instance, *dominance and submission (D/s)* can be a relationship preference and/or actual practice, an identity (dominant or submissive), and an affiliation (e.g., many communities have groups and events focused specifically on D/s).

Kink is a general term for non-normative sexuality. Like BDSM, it is often used as an umbrella term, but kink is a much broader category than BDSM and includes sexual interests like fetishes, cross-dressing, strap-on sex, voyeurism, etc.[1] *D/s*[2] refers to practices involving exchanges of power and/or to a dominant/submissive relationship. *Sadomasochism* (variously *S/m, s/m, s&m, SM*) refers to practices that involve impact, sensation, pain, and/or a sadist/masochist relationship. Many roles, identities, and practices exist beyond D/s and SM, of course; and chapters in this volume take up many of the diverse ways that participants identify themselves and describe their practices.

The variation in uses and meanings of BDSM terminology extends to the roles and/or identities participants take or identify with. Terms that are used to describe roles or identities are sometimes used synonymously yet are often used to mark significant differences among roles and identities. While I attempt here to provide a concise, general overview of terminology for readers less familiar with BDSM, the definitions are necessarily incomplete and cannot capture the complex, highly nuanced ways participants use these terms to convey their identities and interests. For example, the terms *top*, *dominant*, *master*, and *sadist* can have significantly different meanings for some participants and in some contexts yet are also sometimes used in relatively interchangeable fashion, as are the corresponding terms *bottom*, *submissive*, *slave*, and *masochist*. Importantly, many participants identify with multiple, but not all, of these roles or identities. For example, someone might identify as a submissive (someone who enjoys consensual submission and power exchange) but not as a masochist (someone who enjoys receiving pain). Yet many participants do identify with multiple roles described here (e.g., identifying as both a submissive and a masochist), along with myriad more specific roles and identities that appear throughout the book (e.g., daddy, boi, girl, pup).

A *top* is someone who leads in a given interaction, while a *bottom* is someone who follows in that interaction, and a *switch* is someone who takes different roles either at different times or with different partners (for an in-depth analysis of these roles and identities, see Martinez, 2018). Topping and bottoming may or may not involve power exchange or pain play/SM. For example, rope bondage may or may not involve power exchange, and a D/s relationship may or may not involve SM. *Dominant* generally refers to someone who enjoys exercising power in BDSM contexts, while *submissive* generally refers to someone who enjoys giving up power in BDSM contexts; *switch* can also refer to someone who takes different roles in a D/s context. A *sadist* is someone who enjoys inflicting pain in a BDSM context, and a *masochist* is someone who enjoys receiving pain in a BDSM context.

Participants describe BDSM activities that take place in a particular time-bound space as *scenes*, *sessions*, and/or *play*. The term *scene* has multiple meanings: (a) a noun that refers to the BDSM social scene, either generally or in a specific locale (e.g., "The Houston scene is really happening"); (b) a noun that refers to one or more temporally and/or spatially bounded consensual interactions (e.g., "We were in the middle of a cutting scene"); and (c) a verb that refers to engaging in BDSM activities (e.g., "I'm going to scene with her tomorrow" or "we were scening last night").

Across the wide range of practices, identities, and communities that fall under the umbrella of BDSM, one of the points of commonality is an emphasis on consent. While *safe, sane, and consensual* (SSC) was long the primary framework used by community members for evaluating practices, community members themselves have critiqued the SSC model on the grounds that what is safe varies across individual experiences, abilities, and risk profiles; that few activities humans engage in (BDSM or otherwise) are completely safe; and that the term *sane* both is subjective and contributes to pathologizing understandings of BDSM. Community members have developed alternative frameworks to SSC, including *risk-aware consensual kink* and *personally responsible, informed, consensual kink*, to emphasize individual agency and recognize variability across individual backgrounds, experiences, and desires. Across all of these models, consent is central. Yet, as a growing body of research shows, while consent is foregrounded in definitions of BDSM, in actual practice establishing and containing consent is an ongoing, often murky process, and consent violations do occur (Bauer, 2014, 2021; Beres & MacDonald, 2015; Dunkley & Brotto, 2020; Fanghanel, 2020; Sharma & Ghupta, 2011; Wignall, 2020; Williams et al., 2014).

Structure of the Book

The book is organized in five parts. In Part I, "Introducing BDSM," contributors introduce the field of BDSM studies. In Chapter 1, Weinberg, who has provided a seminal review of the state of scholarship on BDSM every decade since the 1970s, reviews research published in the last decade, reflects on how the field has developed in the last four decades and provides suggestions for future research. In Chapter 2, Wignall provides an overview of how the rise of the internet has shaped both BDSM communities and research on BDSM, calling for future research to engage more thoroughly with the role of the internet in BDSM communities and experiences.

In Part II, "Play and Practices," contributors focus on specific types of BDSM play and practices that fall under the broad umbrella of BDSM, doing the important work of examining the specificities of the practices, forms of play, identities, and interactions involved in specific subcultures of BDSM. In Chapter 3, Jones explores the social world of rope bondage, using an intersectional lens to investigate the embodied experiences of practitioners of rope bondage. In Chapter 4, examining the pup subculture, Matchett and Berkowitz examine identity development processes among pups, demonstrating the importance of social networking and digital communities in the creation of the pup subculture. In Chapter 5, focusing on age play practices, Bauer interrogates how innocence, transgression, and childhood are constructed and deconstructed within age play practices.

In Part III, "Relationships and Communities," contributors focus on the role of relationships and communities in the experiences of BDSMers. In Chapter 6, investigating the experience of kinksters living in Portugal, Cardoso, Pascoal, and Quaresma examine the challenges that kinksters face in their relationships and identities and the strategies they use to navigate those challenges, showing that individual, interpersonal, and societal aspects of relationships are inextricably linked among kinksters. In Chapter 7, focusing on BDSM in South Africa, McCormick traces the development and evolution of BDSM communities in Johannesburg, demonstrating how whiteness and racism have shaped the Johannesburg scene. In Chapter 8, examining the intersections of kink, BDSM, and non-monogamous subcultures in the American South, Stewart shows how BDSM has influenced the evolution of the swingers and non-monogamous communities.

In Part IV, "Representations and Personal Reflections," contributors reflect critically on how BDSM is represented in a variety of spaces and share personal reflections on BDSM participation. In Chapter 9, Graham, Kirakosyan, Fox, and Ruvabalca examine how BDSM is represented in human sexuality textbooks, showing that how BDSM is represented in human sexuality textbooks often diverges significantly from how BDSM participants themselves understand their experiences. In Chapter 10, Bennett focuses on how BDSM is represented and defined in Western common law, interrogating how *violence* is deployed in legal discourse in ways that prevent decriminalization. In Chapter 11, a personal reflection piece, Sexsmith reflects on the role of power and power dynamics in their BDSM experiences, using an intersectional lens to explore power dynamics.

In Part V, "Ethics and Consent in the Scene and in BDSM Studies," contributors examine how consent and ethics are constructed and deployed in both BDSM practices and scholarship on BDSM. In Chapter 12, Norman examines the impact of structural inequalities and racial power dynamics on the negotiation of consent and on BDSM participation and experiences, centering the experience of Black BDSM practitioners. In Chapter 13, Holt explores how histories of sexual victimization affect BDSM play and how participants use BDSM play in therapeutic ways. In Chapter 14, Rubinsky, Cooke-Jackson, and Rodriquez explore trauma play among BDSM participants who have experienced sexual trauma, showing how participants communicate in ways that facilitate a sense of safety in BDSM play. In Chapter 15, Carlström engages in a critical reflection on the role of ethnographic fieldwork in BDSM research, exploring the complex relationships between the field, participants, and the ethnographer.

Notes

1. See (Wignall, 2022) for an extended discussion of terminology.
2. Distinctive capitalization, particularly in names, titles, and roles, is one way that BDSM participants convey the meaning of their relationships and identities in writing (the capital letter marks the top/dominant/sadist/master/mistress role, while the non-capitalized letter marks the bottom/submissive/masochist/slave role; BDSM participants often use differentiated capitalization in scene names to indicate role/identity and to signal the nature of their relationship—Chris and ben, for example).

References

Alvarado, T., Prior, E. E., Thomas, J. N., & Williams, D. J. (2018). Gender effects of BDSM participation on self-reported psychological distress levels. *Journal of Positive Sexuality*, 4(2), 56–60.

Ansara, Y. G. (2019). Trauma psychotherapy with people involved in BDSM/kink: Five common misconceptions and five essential clinical skills. *Psychotherapy and Counselling Journal of Australia*, 7(2). https://pacja.org.au/2019/12/trauma-psychotherapy-with-people-involved-in-bdsm-kink-five-common-misconceptions-and-five-essential-clinical-skills-2/

Baker, A. C. (2018). Sacred kink: Finding psychological meaning at the intersection of BDSM and spiritual experience. *Sexual and Relationship Therapy*, 33(4), 440–453. https://doi.org/10.1080/14681994.2016.1205185

Barker, M. (2013). Consent is a grey area? A comparison of understandings of consent in *Fifty Shades of Grey* and on the BDSM blogosphere. *Sexualities*, 16(8), 896–914. https://doi.org/10.1177/1363460713508881

Barker, M., Gupta, C., & Iantaffi, A. (2007). The power of play: The potentials and pitfalls in healing narratives of BDSM. In D. Langdridge & M. Barker (Eds.), *Safe, sane, and consensual: Contemporary perspectives on sadomasochism* (pp. 203–222). Palgrave Macmillan.

Barker, M., Iantaffi, A., & Gupta, C. (2007). Kinky clients, kinky counseling? The challenges and potentials of BDSM. In L. Moon (Ed.), *Feeling queer or queer feelings? Counseling and sexual cultures* (pp. 106–124). Routledge.

Bauer, R. (2007). Playgrounds and new territories: The potential of BDSM practices to queer genders. In D. Langdridge & M. Barker (Eds.), *Safe, sane, and consensual: Contemporary perspectives on sadomasochism* (pp. 177–193). Palgrave MacMillan.

Bauer, R. (2008). Transgressive and transformative gendered sexual practices and white privileges: The case of the dyke/trans BDSM community. *Women's Studies Quarterly*, *36*(3/4), 233–253. https://doi.org/10.1353/wsq.0.0100

Bauer, R. (2014). *Queer BDSM intimacies: Critical consent and pushing boundaries.* Palgrave Macmillan.

Bauer, R. (2018a). Bois and grrrls meet their daddies and mommies on gender playgrounds: Gendered age play in the les-bi-trans-queer BDSM communities. *Sexualities*, *21*(1–2), 139–155. https://doi.org/10.1177/1363460716676987

Bauer, R. (2018b). Cybercocks and holodicks: Renegotiating the boundaries of material embodiment in les-bi-trans-queer BDSM practices. *Graduate Journal of Social Science*, *14*(2), 58–82.

Bauer, R. (2021). Queering consent: Negotiating critical consent in les-bi-trans-queer BDSM contexts. *Sexualities*, *24*(5–6), Article 1363460720973902. https://doi.org/10.1177/1363460720973902

Bennett, T. (2013). Sadomasochism under the Human Rights (Sexual Conduct) Act 1994. *Sydney Law Review*, *35*(3), 541–564.

Bennett, T. (2015). Persecution or play? Law and the ethical significance of sadomasochism. *Social & Legal Studies*, *24*(1), 89–112. https://doi.org/10.1177/0964663914549760

Beres, M. A., & MacDonald, J. E. C. (2015). Talking about sexual consent: Heterosexual women and BDSM. *Australian Feminist Studies*, *30*(86), 418–432. https://doi.org/10.1080/08164649.2016.1158692

Beresford, S. (2016). Lesbian spanners: A re-appraisal of UK consensual sadomasochism laws. *Liverpool Law Review*, *37*(1–2), 63–80. https://doi.org/10.1007/s10991-016-9182-2

Better, A., & Simula, B. (2015). How and for whom does gender matter? Rethinking the concept of sexual orientation. *Sexualities*, *18*(5/6), 665–680. https://doi.org/10.1177/1363460714561716

Botta, D., Nimbi, F. M., Tripodi, F., Silvaggi, M., & Simonelli, C. (2019). Are role and gender related to sexual function and satisfaction in men and women practicing BDSM? *The Journal of Sexual Medicine*, *16*(3), 463–473. https://doi.org/10.1016/j.jsxm.2019.01.001

Brown, A., Barker, E. D., & Rahman, Q. (2020). A systematic scoping review of the prevalence, etiological, psychological, and interpersonal factors associated with BDSM. *The Journal of Sex Research*, *57*(6), 781–811. https://doi.org/10.1080/00224499.2019.1665619

Buchanan, M. (2004). *Leather is thicker than blood: Identity formation among organized SM practitioners in New York City* [Doctoral dissertation, New School University]. ProQuest. http://proquest.umi.com/pqdweb?did=765271181&Fmt=7&clientId=1917&RQT=309&VName=PQD

Carlström, C. (2019). BDSM—The antithesis of good Swedish sex? *Sexualities*, *22*(7–8), 1164–1181. https://doi.org/10.1177/1363460718769648

Carlström, C. (2020). Spiritual experiences and altered states of consciousness—Parallels between BDSM and Christianity. *Sexualities, 24*(5–6), Article 1363460720964035. https://doi.org/10.1177/1363460720964035

Carmack, H. J., DeGroot, J. M., & Quinlan, M. M. (2015). "A view from the top": Crafting the male "domdentity" in domestic discipline relationships. *Journal of Men's Studies, 23*(1), 63–78. https://doi.org/10.1177/1060826514561976

Cascalheira, C. J., Thomson, A., & Wignall, L. (2022). "A certain evolution": A phenomenological study of 24/7 BDSM and negotiating consent. *Psychology & Sexuality, 13*(3), 628–639. https://doi.org/10.1080/19419899.2021.1901771

Cerwenka, S., Matthiesen, S., Briken, P., & Dekker, A. (2020). Heterosexual practices in different generations—Findings of a Pilot Study for "Gesid Gesundheit Und Sexualitat in Deutschland (Health and Sexuality in Germany)." *Psychotherapie Psychosomatik Medizinische Psychologie, 70*(12), 499–508. https://doi.org/10.1055/a-1129-7318

Chaline, E. R. (2010). The construction, maintenance, and evolution of gay SM sexualities and sexual identities: A preliminary description of gay SM sexual identity practices. *Sexualities, 13*(3), 338–356. https://doi.org/10.1177/1363460709363323

Connolly, P. H. (2006). Psychological functioning of bondage/domination/sadomasochism (BDSM) practitioners. *Journal of Psychology & Human Sexuality, 18*(1), 79–120. https://doi.org/10.1300/J056v18n01_05

Coppens, V., Ten Brink, S., Huys, W., Fransen, E., & Morrens, M. (2020). A survey on BDSM-related activities: BDSM experience correlates with age of first exposure, interest profile, and role identity. *Journal of Sex Research, 57*(1), 129–136. https://doi.org/10.1080/00224499.2018.1558437

Cowan, S. (2012). To buy or not to buy? Vulnerability and the criminalisation of commercial BDSM. *Feminist Legal Studies, 20*(3), 263–279. https://doi.org/10.1007/s10691-012-9209-6

Cruz, A. (2016a). *The color of kink: Black women, BDSM, and pornography*. New York University Press.

Cruz, A. (2016b). Playing with the politics of perversion: Policing BDSM, pornography, and Black female sexuality. *Souls, 18*(2–4), 379–407. https://doi.org/10.1080/10999949.2016.1230817

Cruz, A. (2020). Not a moment too soon: A juncture of BDSM and race. *Sexualities, 24*(5–6), Article 1363460720979309. https://doi.org/10.1177/1363460720979309

Dale, J. (1991). Leather utopia: The normative impulse of S-M communities. *Michigan Feminist Studies, 6*, 177–185.

Damm, C., Dentato, M. P., & Busch, N. (2018). Unravelling intersecting identities: Understanding the lives of people who practice BDSM. *Psychology & Sexuality, 9*(1), 21–37. https://doi.org/10.1080/19419899.2017.1410854

Dancer, P. L., Kleinplatz, P. J., & Moser, C. (2006). 24/7 SM slavery. *Journal of Homosexuality, 50*(2–3), 81–101. https://doi.org/10.1300/J082v50n02_05

DeGroot, J. M., Carmack, H. J., & Quinlan, M. M. (2015). "Topping from the bottom": Relational convergence of meaning in domestic discipline relationships. *Sexuality & Culture, 19*, 85–102. https://doi.org/10.1007/s12119-014-9247-0

De Neef, N., Coppens, V., Huys, W., & Morrens, M. (2019). Bondage–discipline, dominance–submission and sadomasochism (BDSM) from an integrative biopsychosocial perspective: A systematic review. *Sexual Medicine, 7*(2), 129–144. https://doi.org/10.1016/j.esxm.2019.02.002

Drdova, L., & Saxonberg, S. (2021). Generations of BDSM Czech style: The elimination of roles in role-playing? *Sexualities*, *25*(7), Article 13634607211000200. https://doi.org/10.1177/13634607211000200

Dunkley, C. R., & Brotto, L. A. (2018). Clinical considerations in treating BDSM practitioners: A review. *Journal of Sex & Marital Therapy*, *44*(7), 701–712. https://doi.org/10.1080/0092623x.2018.1451792

Dunkley, C. R., & Brotto, L. A. (2020). The role of consent in the context of BDSM. *Sexual Abuse*, *32*(6), 657–678. https://doi.org/10.1177/1079063219842847

Dunkley, C. R., Henshaw, C. D., Henshaw, S. K., & Brotto, L. A. (2020). Physical pain as pleasure: A theoretical perspective. *The Journal of Sex Research*, *57*(4), 421–437. https://doi.org/10.1080/00224499.2019.1605328

Faccio, E., Sarigu, D., & Iudici, A. (2020). What is it like to be a BDSM player? The role of sexuality and erotization of power in the BDSM experience. *Sexuality & Culture*, *24*(5), 1641–1652. https://doi.org/10.1007/s12119-020-09703-x

Fanghanel, A. (2020). Asking for it: BDSM sexual practice and the trouble of consent. *Sexualities*, *23*(3), 269–286. https://doi.org/10.1177/1363460719828933

Graham, B., Butler, S., McGraw, R., Cannes, S. M., & Smith, J. (2016). Member perspectives on the role of BDSM communities. *The Journal of Sex Research*, *53*(8), 895–909. https://doi.org/10.1080/00224499.2015.1067758

Graham, M. (1998). Identity, place, and erotic community within gay leather culture in Stockholm. *Journal of Homosexuality*, *35*(3–4), 163–183.

Hammers, C. (2014). Corporeality, sadomasochism, and sexual trauma. *Body & Society*, *20*(2), 68–90. https://doi.org/10.1177/1357034X13477159

Hammers, C. (2019). Reworking trauma through BDSM. *Signs*, *44*(2), 491–514. https://doi.org/10.1086/699370

Harmon, L. A. (1997). *Thursdays at the torch: The negotiation of non-monogamous relationships among members of a lesbian S/M community* [Unpublished master's thesis]. Loyola University Chicago.

Haviv, N. (2016). Reporting sexual assaults to the police: The Israeli BDSM community. *Sexuality Research and Social Policy*, *13*(3), 276–287. https://doi.org/10.1007/s13178-016-0222-4

Hawkinson, K., & Zamboni, B. D. (2014). Adult baby/diaper lovers: An exploratory study of an online community sample. *Archives of Sexual Behavior*, *43*(5), 863–877. https://doi.org/10.1007/s10508-013-0241-7

Henderson-Espinoza, R. (2018). Decolonial erotics: Power bottoms, topping from bottom space, and the emergence of a queer sexual theology. *Feminist Theology*, *26*(3), 286–296. https://doi.org/10.1177/0966735018756255

Highleyman, L. (1997). Professional dominance: Power, money, and identity. In J. Nagle (Ed.), *Whores and other feminists* (pp. 145–155). Routledge.

Holt, K. (2016). Blacklisted: Boundaries, violations, and retaliatory behavior in the BDSM community. *Deviant Behavior*, *37*(8), 917–930. https://doi.org/10.1080/01639625.2016.1156982

Holt, K. (2018). An exploration of the experience of harm in the bondage/discipline/sado-masochism community. *Violence and Victims*, *33*(4), 663–685. https://doi.org/10.1891/0886-6708.Vv-d-16-00194

Holvoet, L., Huys, W., Coppens, V., Seeuws, J., Goethals, K., & Morrens, M. (2017). Fifty shades of Belgian gray: The prevalence of BDSM-related fantasies and activities in the general population. *The Journal of Sexual Medicine, 14*(9), 1152–1159. https://doi.org/10.1016/j.jsxm.2017.07.003

Hughes, S. D., & Hammack, P. L. (2019). Affirmation, compartmentalization, and isolation: Narratives of identity sentiment among kinky people. *Psychology & Sexuality, 10*(2), 149–168. https://doi.org/10.1080/19419899.2019.1575896

Jozifkova, E., & Kolackova, M. (2017). Sexual arousal by dominance and submission in relation to increased reproductive success in the general population. *Neuroendocrinology Letters, 38*(5), 381–387.

Kaak, A. (2016). Conversational phases in BDSM pre-scene negotiations. *Journal of Positive Sexuality, 2*, 47–52.

Khan, U. (2014). *Vicarious kinks: S/M in the socio-legal imaginary.* University of Toronto Press.

Kleinplatz, P., & Moser, C. (2005). Is S/M pathological. *Lesbian and Gay Psychology Review, 6*(3), 255–260.

Kolmes, K. (2003). *BDSM consumers of mental health services: The need for culturally sensitive care* [Doctoral dissertation, Alliant International University]. ProQuest. http://proquest.umi.com/pqdweb?did=765903391&Fmt=7&clientId=1917&RQT=309&VName=PQD

Kolmes, K., Stock, W., & Moser, C. (2006). Investigating bias in psychotherapy with BDSM clients. *Journal of Homosexuality, 50*(2/3), 301–324.

Kondakov, A. (2017). Master and slave as a collaborative relationship: An analysis of contractual relationships in BDSM. *Novoe Literaturnoe Obozrenie, 147*, 170–183.

Kuzmanovic, D. (2018). Queer race play: Kinky sex and the trauma of racism. In K. Wright (Ed.), *Disgust and desire: The paradox of the monster* (pp. 71–88). Brill.

Labrecque, F., Potz, A., Larouche, E., & Joyal, C. C. (2021). What is so appealing about being spanked, flogged, dominated, or restrained? Answers from practitioners of sexual masochism/submission. *Journal of Sex Research, 58*(4), 409–423. https://doi.org/10.1080/00224499.2020.1767025

Langdridge, D., & Butt, T. (2004). A hermeneutic phenomenological investigation of the construction of sadomasochistic identities. *Sexualities, 7*(1), 31–53. https://doi.org/10.1177/1363460704040137

Langdridge, D., & Lawson, J. (2019). The psychology of puppy play: A phenomenological investigation. *Archives of Sexual Behavior, 48*(7), 2201–2215. https://doi.org/10.1007/s10508-019-01476-1

Lasala, A., Paparo, F., Senese, V. P., & Perrella, R. (2020). An exploratory study of adult baby-diaper lovers' characteristics in an Italian online sample. *International Journal of Environmental Research and Public Health, 17*(4), Article 1371. https://doi.org/10.3390/ijerph17041371

Lawrence, A., & Love-Crowell, J. (2008). Psychotherapists' experience with clients who engage in consensual sadomasochism: A qualitative study. *Journal of Sex and Marital Therapy, 34*(1), 67–85. https://doi.org/10.1080/00926230701620936

Lawson, J., & Langdridge, D. (2020). History, culture and practice of puppy play. *Sexualities, 23*(4), 574–591. https://doi.org/10.1177/1363460719839914

LeFranc, K. M. (2018). Kinky hermeneutics: Resisting homonormativity in queer theology. *Feminist Theology, 26*(3), 241–254. https://doi.org/10.1177/0966735018759451

Levey, T. G., & Pinsky, D. (2015). A constellation of stigmas: Intersectional stigma management and the professional dominatrix. *Deviant Behavior, 36*(5), 347–367. https://doi.org/10.1080/01639625.2014.935658

Liang, M. (2020). Playing with power: Kink, race, and desire. *Sexualities*, *25*(4), 381–405. https://doi.org/10.1177/1363460720964063

Lindemann, D. (2010). Will the real dominatrix please stand up: Artistic purity and professionalism in the S&M dungeon. *Sociological Forum*, *25*(3), 588–606. https://doi.org/10.1111/j.1573-7861.2010.01197.x

Lindemann, D. (2011). BDSM as therapy? *Sexualities*, *14*(2), 151–172. https://doi.org/10.1177/1363460711399038

Lindemann, D. (2012). *Dominatrix: Gender, eroticism, and control in the dungeon*. University of Chicago Press.

Luo, S. Y., & Zhang, X. (2018a). Embodiment and humiliation moderation of neural responses to others' suffering in female submissive BDSM practitioners. *Frontiers in Neuroscience*, *12*, Article 463. https://doi.org/10.3389/fnins.2018.00463

Luo, S. Y., & Zhang, X. (2018b). Empathy in female submissive BDSM practitioners. *Neuropsychologia*, *116*, 44–51. https://doi.org/10.1016/j.neuropsychologia.2017.01.027

Martinez, K. (2018). BDSM role fluidity: A mixed-methods approach to investigating switches within dominant/submissive binaries. *Journal of Homosexuality*, *65*(10), 1299–1324. https://doi.org/10.1080/00918369.2017.1374062

Martinez, K. (2020). Overwhelming whiteness of BDSM: A critical discourse analysis of racialization in BDSM. *Sexualities*, *24*(5–6), Article 1363460720932389. https://doi.org/10.1177/1363460720932389

McCormick, T. L. (2018a). Gay leathermen in South Africa: An exploratory study. *Agenda-Empowering Women for Gender Equity*, *32*(3), 74–86. https://doi.org/10.1080/10130950.2018.1498238

McCormick, T. L. (2018b). Yes master! Multimodal representations of BDSM bodies on a South African website. *Southern African Linguistics and Applied Language Studies*, *36*(2), 147–160. https://doi.org/10.2989/16073614.2018.1476161

Mechelke, J. D. R. (2019). A kinky doctrine of sin. *Theology & Sexuality*, *25*(1–2), 21–44. https://doi.org/10.1080/13558358.2019.1611727

Mosher, C., Levitt, H., & Manley, E. (2006). Layers of leather: The identity formation of leathermen as a process of transforming meanings of masculinity. *Journal of Homosexuality*, *51*(3), 93–123. https://doi.org/10.1300/J082v51n03_06

Musser, A. J. (2014). *Sensational flesh: Race, power, and masochism*. New York University Press.

Newmahr, S. (2010a). Power struggles: Pain and authenticity in SM play. *Symbolic Interaction*, *33*(3), 389–411. https://doi.org/10.1525/si.2010.33.3.389

Newmahr, S. (2010b). Rethinking kink: Sadomasochism as serious leisure. *Qualitative Sociology*, *33*, 313–331. https://doi.org/10.1007/s11133-010-9158-9

Ortmann, D. M., & Sprott, R. A. (2013). *Sexual outsiders: Understanding BDSM sexualities and communities*. Rowman & Littlefield.

Pascoal, P. M., Cardoso, D., & Henriques, R. (2015). Sexual satisfaction and distress in sexual functioning in a sample of the BDSM community: A comparison study between BDSM and non-BDSM contexts. *The Journal of Sexual Medicine*, *12*(4), 1052–1061. https://doi.org/10.1111/jsm.12835

Pinsky, D., & Levey, T. G. (2015). "A world turned upside down": Emotional labour and the professional dominatrix. *Sexualities*, *18*(4), 438–458. https://doi.org/10.1177/1363460714550904

Plante, R. (2006). Sexual spanking, the self, and the construction of deviance. *Journal of Homosexuality*, *50*(2/3), 59–79. https://doi.org/10.1300/J082v50n02_04

Prior, E. E., & Williams, D. J. (2015). Does BDSM power exchange among women reflect casual leisure? An exploratory qualitative study. *Journal of Positive Sexuality*, *1*, 12–15.

Puig-Rodas, I. (2019). Gender differences in Spanish BDSM practitioners [Meeting abstract]. *International Journal of Sexual Health*, *31*, A312–A313. https://doi.org/10.1016/j.jsxm.2017.04.546

Puppy Sharon, & Toushin, S. (2004). *The Puppy Papers: A Woman's Life and Journey into BDSM*. Wells Street.

Rambukkana, N. (2004). Taking the leather out of leathersex: The internet, identity, and the sadomasochistic public sphere. In K. O'Riordan & D. J. Phillips (Eds.), *Queer online: Media, technology, and sexuality* (pp. 67–80). Peter Lang.

Reynolds, D. (2007). Disability and BDSM: Bob Flanagan and the case for sexual rights. *Sexuality Research and Social Policy*, *4*(1), 40–52. https://doi.org/10.1525/srsp.2007.4.1.40

Rubin, G. (1997). Elegy for the valley of the kings: Aids and the leather community in San Francisco, 1981–1996. In M. Levine, P. Nardi, & J. Gagnon (Eds.), *Changing times: Gay men and lesbians encounter HIV/AIDS* (pp. 101–144). University of Chicago Press.

Rubinsky, V. (2018). "Sometimes it's easier to type things than to say them": Technology in BDSM sexual partner communication. *Sexuality & Culture*, *22*(4), 1412–1431. https://doi.org/10.1007/s12119-018-9534-2

Sagarin, B. J., Lee, E. M., Erickson, J. M., Casey, K. G., & Pawirosetiko, J. S. (2019). Collective sex environments without the sex? Insights from the BDSM community. *Archives of Sexual Behavior*, *48*(1), 63–67. https://doi.org/10.1007/s10508-018-1252-1

Sandnabba, N. K., Santtila, P., Alison, L., & Nordling, N. (2002). Demographics, sexual behaviour, family background, and abuse experience of practitioners of sadomasochistic sex: A review of recent research. *Sexual and Relationship Therapy*, *17*(1), 39–55. https://doi.org/10.1080/14681990220108018

Sandnabba, N. K., Santtila, P., & Nordling, N. (1999). Sexual behavior and social adaptation among sadomasochistically-oriented males. *Journal of Sex Research*, *36*(3), 273–282. https://doi.org/10.1080/00224499909551997

Santtila, P., Sandnabba, N. K., Alison, L., & Nordling, N. (2002). Investigating the underlying structure in sadomasochistically oriented behavior. *Archives of Sexual Behavior*, *31*(2), 185–196. https://doi.org/10.1023/A:1014791220495

Sendler, D., & Lew-Starowicz, M. (2019). Gay BDSM: A cross-cultural comparison of psychiatric wellness of Polish and American professional gay sadomasochist [Meeting abstract]. *European Psychiatry*, *56*, S291.

Sharma, J., & Ghupta, K. (2011). Eroticism, pain and consent: Some reflections from the BDSM community in India. *Culture Health & Sexuality*, *13*, S146–S147.

Sheff, E. (2021). Kinky sex gone wrong: Legal prosecutions concerning consent, age play, and death via BDSM. *Archives of Sexual Behavior*, *50*, 761–771. https://doi.org/10.1007/s10508-020-01866-w

Sheff, E., & Hammers, C. (2011). The privilege of perversities: Race, class, and education among polyamorists and kinksters. *Sexuality and Psychology*, *2*(3), 198–223.

Sheppard, E. (2018). Using pain, living with pain. *Feminist Review*, *120*(1), 54–69. https://doi.org/10.1057/s41305-018-0142-7

Sihvonen, T., & Tuomas Harviainen, J. (2020). "My games are . . . unconventional": Intersections of game and BDSM studies. *Sexualities*, Article 1363460720964092. https://doi.org/10.1177/1363460720964092

Simula, B. (2012). Does bisexuality "undo" gender? Gender, sexuality, and bisexual behavior among BDSM participants. *Journal of Bisexuality, 12*(4), 484–506. https://doi.org/10.1080/15299716.2012.729430

Simula, B. (2013). Queer utopias in painful spaces: BDSM participants resisting heteronormativity and gender regulation. In A. Jones (Ed.), *A critical inquiry into queer utopias* (pp. 71–100). Palgrave Macmillan.

Simula, B. (2014). "Give me a dominant of any gender over any kind of non-dominant": Sexual orientation beyond gender. In T. Weinberg & S. Newmahr (Eds.), *Selves, symbols, and sexualities: An interactionist anthology* (pp. 163–178). Sage Press.

Simula, B. (2019a). A "different economy of bodies and pleasures"?: Differentiating and evaluating sex and sexual BDSM experiences. *Journal of Homosexuality, 66*(2), 209–237. https://doi.org/10.1080/00918369.2017.1398017

Simula, B. (2019b). Power, pain, and pleasure: A review of the literature on the experiences of BDSM participants. *Sociology Compass, 13*(3), Article e12668. https://doi.org/10.1111/soc4.12668

Simula, B., & Sumerau, J. E. (2017). The use of gender in the interpretation of BDSM. *Sexualities, 22*(3), 452–477. https://doi.org/10.1177/1363460717737488

Sloan, L. J. (2015). Ace of (BDSM) clubs: Building asexual relationships through BDSM practice. *Sexualities, 18*(5–6), 548–563. https://doi.org/10.1177/1363460714550907

Smith, J. G., & Luykx, A. (2017). Race play in BDSM porn: The eroticization of oppression. *Porn Studies, 4*(4), 433–446. https://doi.org/10.1080/23268743.2016.1252158

Spengler, A. (1977). Manifest sadomasochism of males: Results of an empirical study. *Archives of Sexual Behavior, 6*, 441–456.

Sprott, R. A. (2020). Reimagining "kink": Transformation, growth, and healing through BDSM. *Journal of Humanistic Psychology*, Advance online publication. https://doi.org/10.1177/0022167819900036

Sprott, R. A., & Hadcock, B. B. (2018). Bisexuality, pansexuality, queer identity, and kink identity. *Sexual and Relationship Therapy, 33*(1–2), 214–232. https://doi.org/10.1080/14681994.2017.1347616

Sprott, R. A., Vivid, J., Vilkin, E., Swallow, L., Lev, E. M., Orejudos, J., & Schnittman, D. (2020). A queer boundary: How sex and BDSM interact for people who identify as kinky. *Sexualities, 24*(5–6), Article 1363460720944594. https://doi.org/10.1177/1363460720944594

Sprott, R. A., & Williams, D. J. (2019). Is BDSM a sexual orientation or serious leisure? *Current Sexual Health Reports, 11*(2), 75–79. https://doi.org/10.1007/s11930-019-00195-x

Steinmetz, C., & Maginn, P. J. (2015). The landscape of BDSM venues: A view from down under. In P. J. Maginn & C. Steinmetz (Eds.), *(Sub)Urban sexscapes: Geographies and regulation of the sex industry* (Vol. 135, pp. 117–137). Routledge.

Tellier, S. (2017). Advancing the discourse: Disability and BDSM. *Sexuality and Disability, 35*, 485–493. https://doi.org/10.1007/s11195-017-9504-x

Thomas, J. N. (2020). BDSM as trauma play: An autoethnographic investigation. *Sexualities, 23*(5–6), 917–933. https://doi.org/10.1177/1363460719861800

Tomazos, K., O'Gorman, K., & MacLaren, A. C. (2017). From leisure to tourism: How BDSM demonstrates the transition of deviant pursuits to mainstream products. *Tourism Management, 60*, 30–41. https://doi.org/10.1016/j.tourman.2016.10.018

Turley, E. L., King, N., & Monro, S. (2018). "You want to be swept up in it all": Illuminating the erotic in BDSM. *Psychology & Sexuality*, 9(2), 148–160. https://doi.org/10.1080/19419899.2018.1448297

Weiss, M. (2011). *Techniques of pleasure: BDSM and the circuits of sexuality*. Duke University Press.

Wignall, L. (2017). The sexual use of a social networking site: The case of pup Twitter. *Sociological Research Online*, 22(3), 21–37. https://doi.org/10.1177/1360780417724066

Wignall, L. (2020). Beyond safe, sane, and consensual: Navigating risk and consent online for kinky gay and bisexual men. *Journal of Positive Sexuality*, 6(2), 66–74.

Wignall, L. (2022). *Kinky in the digital age: Gay men's subcultures and social identities*. Oxford University Press.

Wignall, L., & McCormack, M. (2017). An exploratory study of a new kink activity: "Pup play." *Archives of Sexual Behavior*, 46, 801–811. https://doi.org/10.1007/s10508-015-0636-8

Williams, D. (2006). Different (painful!) strokes for different folks: A general overview of sexual sadomasochism (SM) and its diversity. *Sexual Addiction & Compulsivity*, 13(4), 333–346. https://doi.org/10.1080/10720160601011240

Williams, D., Prior, E. E., Alvarado, T., Thomas, J. N., & Christensen, M. C. (2016). Is bondage and discipline, dominance and submission, and sadomasochism recreational leisure? A descriptive exploratory investigation. *The Journal of Sexual Medicine*, 13(7), 1091–1094. https://doi.org/10.1016/j.jsxm.2016.05.001

Williams, D. J., Thomas, J., & Prior, E. (2014). From "SSC" to "RACK" to the "4Cs": Introducing a new framework for negotiating BDSM participation. *Electronic Journal of Human Sexuality*, 17. http://www.ejhs.org/volume17/BDSM.html

Wilson, A. (2005). German dominatrices' choices of working names as reflections of self-constructed social identity. *Sexuality and Culture*, 9(2), 31–41. https://doi.org/10.1007/s12119-005-1006-9

Winter-Gray, T., & Hayfield, N. (2019). "Can I be a kinky ace?" How asexual people negotiate their experiences of kinks and fetishes. *Psychology & Sexuality*, 12(3), 163–179. https://doi.org/10.1080/19419899.2019.1679866

Wismeijer, A., & van Assen, M. A. L. M. (2013). Psychological characteristics of BDSM practitioners. *The Journal of Sexual Medicine*, 10(8), 1943–1952. https://doi.org/10.1111/jsm.12192

Woltersdorff, V. (2011). The pleasures of compliance: Domination and compromise within BDSM practice. In M. do Mar Castro Varela, N. Dhawan, & A. Engel (Eds.), *Hegemony and heteronormativity: Revisiting "the political" in queer politics* (pp. 169–188). Ashgate.

Wright, S. (2018). De-pathologization of consensual BDSM. *The Journal of Sexual Medicine*, 15(5), 622–624. https://doi.org/10.1016/j.jsxm.2018.02.018

Wuyts, E., De Neef, N., Coppens, V., Fransen, E., Schellens, E., Van Der Pol, M., & Morrens, M. (2020). Between pleasure and pain: A pilot study on the biological mechanisms associated with BDSM interactions in dominants and submissives. *The Journal of Sexual Medicine*, 17(4), 784–792. https://doi.org/10.1016/j.jsxm.2020.01.001

Zambelli, L. (2017). Subcultures, narratives and identification: An empirical study of BDSM (bondage, domination and submission, discipline, sadism and masochism) practices in Italy. *Sexuality and Culture*, 21(2), 471–492. https://doi.org/10.1007/s12119-016-9400-z

Zamboni, B. D. (2018). Experiences of distress by participants in the adult baby/diaper lover community. *Sexual and Relationship Therapy*, *33*(4), 470–486. https://doi.org/10.1080/14681994.2018.1434312

Zamboni, B. D. (2019). A qualitative exploration of adult baby/diaper lover behavior from an online community sample. *Journal of Sex Research*, *56*(2), 191–202. https://doi.org/10.1080/00224499.2017.1373728

Zamboni, B. D., & Madero, G. (2018). Exploring asexuality within an adult baby/diaper lover community. *Psychology & Sexuality*, *9*(2), 174–187. https://doi.org/10.1080/19419899.2018.1459804

1

Research in BDSM

40 Years Along

Thomas S. Weinberg

Introduction

More than 40 years ago the first sociological analysis of BDSM appeared in
the social science literature (Spengler, 1977; Weinberg, 1978, 2020). Since
that time, work in that area has expanded, documented by a literature review and analysis every decade (Weinberg, 1987, 1994, 2006). Since the last
review, there has been an exponential increase in work in BDSM, not only in
sociology but also in related fields such as social psychology, psychology, anthropology, and evolutionary biology.

This chapter reviews and analyzes contributions to the literature on BDSM,
focusing on the work done since the last review, to assess what we now know
about this behavior and what we still must understand. It is not meant to be
comprehensive but is intended to illustrate the breadth of work in the area.
Given the vast number of recent contributions to the field and limited space,
I have had to be selective, choosing research in areas and populations that
had not been previously covered and work that I felt significantly advanced
previous knowledge. The review is broken down topically, noting methodological and theoretical advancements in our knowledge. One important topic
not addressed here, BDSM as leisure, is covered elsewhere in this volume.

The Etiology of Dominance and Submission

Dominance and submission are embedded in the human experience, reflected both in cultures and in individual behavior. They are also a core aspect
of BDSM. Why should this be so? Why and how are they related to sex and
sexuality? These questions have piqued the interest of evolutionary biologists.

Thomas S. Weinberg, *Research in BDSM* In: *The Power of BDSM*. Edited by: Brandy L. Simula, Robin Bauer, and
Liam Wignall, Oxford University Press. © Oxford University Press 2023. DOI: 10.1093/oso/9780197658598.003.0002

In a quantitative study of 688 US participants recruited online, Harris et al. (2016) found that "women were significantly more likely to prefer the trait of dominance in a partner compared to men" (p. 392). Carrascosa (2019) critically reviewed the extant empirical literature on the topic, using both traditional (sexual selection–based and hormone-centric explanations) and modern evolutionary theories such as rational choice to explain researchers' findings. Carrascosa noted that research indicates that there is a relationship between preferences for higher-ranking partners and reproductive success as measured by the number and sex of offspring and close relatives and individual attractiveness. Carrascosa linked preference for dominant partners found in the literature and BDSM thusly: "Therefore, sexual arousal due to overemphasized hierarchy like in a dom/sub relationship may originate in a successful reproductive strategy" (p. 12).

Evolutionary biologist Eva Jozifkova has explored the socio-biological bases for BDSM in a series of papers using a variety of methodologies (Jozifkova, 2013, 2018; Jozifkova et al., 2012, 2014; Jozifkova & Flegr, 2006; Jozifkova & Kolackova, 2017; Jozifkova & Konvicka, 2009). In the first paper (Jozifkova & Flegr, 2006) an internet trap method was used—in which subjects are presented with various options they can select by clicking on a specific "gate" to enter a site—to examine the kinds of choices subjects made regarding gender and dominance/submission. Jozifkova provided "gates" with silhouettes of male–female, male–male, and female–female figures varying in dominant and submissive poses. Jozifkova found that 51% of the sample of 398 men and 41.6% of the 466 women entered the gates that had symbols illustrating an unequal sexual partnership. In a later questionnaire study, Jozifkova (2018) found that similar proportions of a sample of 673 respondents reported being sexually aroused by a dominant or submissive partner.

In other research on dominance and its influence on reproduction, Jozifkova (2013) and Jozifkova and Kolackova (2017) found that both sexually dominant men and submissive women saw themselves as more attractive, and they also reported higher socioeconomic status than non-dominant men and non-submissive women. These variables were interpreted as related to and enhancing mating opportunities and therefore "reproductive success" (Jozifkova & Kolackova, 2017, p. 384), as partly measured by the greater number of offspring produced by dominant men.

While the research on the evolutionary bases of dominance and submission in human social and sexual life is intriguing, it is not a complete explanation for the etiology of BDSM. Unlike other species, human behavior is highly dependent on meaning, which is embedded in culture. Recognizing this, De Neef and colleagues (2019) developed a biopsychosocial model for the convergence of BDSM interests through a meta-analysis of the extant empirical research. The biological factors in their model include gender identity, pain system, reward system, sex hormone levels, and stress system. Psychological factors incorporated in the model are education, personality traits, impulsivity, and attachment style; and sociological factors consist of parenting style, traumatic experiences, and cultural factors. De Neef et al. also present "moderating factors," including partner choices, experiences of BDSM-related play, and accessibility of the BDSM community in their model.

The research on the biological bases of dominance and submission in mate choice is interesting, but there is still a large chasm to bridge in inferring its connection with BDSM, given that this behavior is heavily symbolic, complex, multileveled, nuanced, and not necessarily about sexuality and certainly not about reproduction. Any potential link between the two is probably indirect. More research, like that of De Neef et al. (2019), which examines the interplay of a variety of variables is needed.

Personality Characteristics of BDSMers

Early writers on sadism and masochism (Freud, 1938; Krafft-Ebing, 1886/1965) believed that practitioners were mentally ill or even "sexually perverted" and that their behavior was pathological. Modern scholars have provided evidence that this is not true and that BDSM participants do not significantly differ from non-BDSMers in psychological characteristics. In an online questionnaire survey of 902 BDSMers and 434 controls, using several personality scales, Wismeijer and van Assen (2013) found that, compared to the control group, BDSMers were less neurotic, more outgoing, and more open to new experiences and had a higher subjective sense of well-being.

Hebert and Weaver (2014) compared 80 self-described dominants and 190 submissives recruited from internet BDSM forums. Their survey packet contained several personality scales as well as demographic questions. They found that dominants scored significantly higher on desire for control than submissives, yet both were in the normal range when compared to non-BDSM samples. Both dominants' and submissives' scores on extroversion fell within the normal range, as did their self-esteem and life satisfaction scores.

The researchers concluded that, "The findings that BDSM practitioners do not differ from normative data on a wide variety of personality characteristics suggest that BDSM practitioners are perhaps not so different from people who do not practice BDSM" (p. 114).

Botta et al. (2019) studied the relationship between BDSM role and gender and sexual function and satisfaction in a sample of Italian BDSMers. The 141 men and 125 women were recruited using snowball techniques, which rely on subjects recommending or recruiting other participants. Data were collected through an anonymous questionnaire. Botta and colleagues found that in a comparison with a sample of 200 non-BDSMers, dominant and switch groups expressed fewer concerns about sexual dysfunction than submissive groups and the non-BDSM sample. Additionally, dominants expressed greater sexual satisfaction.

Powls and Davies (2012) reviewed the empirical literature on BDSM with the objective of gaining an "understanding of SM within the context of non-forensic clinical practice" (p. 224). They identified three prevalent traditional psychiatric and psychodynamic theories about BDSM based upon clinical samples: the development of BDSM interests resulting from childhood abuse, an early awareness of BDSM interests, and BDSM as abnormal or deviant sexuality. The authors concluded that none of these beliefs are supported by the empirical evidence. They noted that the vast majority of BDSM practitioners are socially well adjusted, that few of them reported having experienced childhood sexual abuse, and that most became aware of their interests later in life.

Richters and colleagues (2008) conducted a representative telephone survey of 19,307 Australians, asking about their sexual behaviors. They found that those respondents who had engaged in BDSM in the previous year did not report being coerced into this behavior, nor did they indicate unhappiness or anxiety. Male BDSM respondents evidenced less psychological distress than non-BDSM subjects. The authors concluded that BDSM is not pathological or the result of previous abuse but rather a form of sexual activity and a subculture engaged in by a minority of the population.

The findings of contemporary research are consistent. They provide a scientific and objective picture of BDSMers as psychologically normal, strongly discounting the speculations of early writers whose knowledge of this behavior was limited to case studies of their patients. Additional research in this area might focus on sociological variables like the social relationships and adjustments of BDSMers as compared to non-BDSM participants.

Gender and BDSM Role

The earliest sociological writers on BDSM believed that women, other than professional dominatrices, were not part of this scene. Spengler (1977), for example, who studied members of a German BDSM club, did not believe that they existed; and others accepted this view (Weinberg, 1978, 2020). By the late 1980s, however, researchers knew that this was not true, and they began examining the role of women in BDSM (Baumeister, 1988; Levitt et al., 1994; Moser & Levitt, 1987). In the 1990s, BDSM became part of a feminist debate (Hoople, 1996; Hopkins, 1994). Since then, the study of BDSM as it is related to gender has become much more sophisticated (see Rehor, 2015).

In a series of papers, Simula explored how BDSM participants perceive gender, role, and sexual orientation as relevant to interaction (Better & Simula, 2015; Simula, 2012, 2015, 2019a; Simula & Sumerau, 2017), gathering data from 32 semi-structured, in-depth interviews and thousands of pages of discussion board material as well as from informal discussions with BDSMers, coupled with participant observation. There were two main patterns in how participants select partners for BDSM interaction. In the first pattern, gender and BDSM role are equally important in partner choice. However, in the second and most frequent pattern, BDSM role (dominant or submissive) trumped gender and sexual orientation. Simula (2012) also examined the role of gender in BDSM bisexuality, finding that some individuals were able to engage in BDSM with partners of different genders by separating the ideas of "sex" (sexual intercourse and orgasm) and "sexual" (arousal and erotic feelings).

Simula and Sumerau (2017) found that BDSM participants socially construct and maintain their sense of gender in two ways: by downplaying gender and by emphasizing gender. In the first case, people's roles in interaction, their relationships, their individuality, and the scenes enacted were seen as more relevant than their gender. For the second group of respondents, interaction was reinterpreted to confirm gender so that a male's submission was recast as a sign of (masculine) strength (e. g., by demonstrating his ability to withstand pain).

Martinez (2017) was interested in role fluidity (switching) among BDSM participants, especially as it was related to their sexual and gender identities. Martinez's research used both questionnaires administered to 202 volunteers and semi-structured interviews with 25 other respondents. While many respondents acknowledged some degree of BDSM role fluidity, this was most frequently reported by those who self-identified as queer/pansexual. Respondents self-identifying strictly either as submissive, slave, bottom, or masochist or as dominant, master, top, or sadist, all of whom were heterosexual, were strongly attached to their roles and more reluctant to engage in role fluidity. Factors identified as affecting switching included attitude, strength and skill of the respondent and prospective partners, opportunity, and the play context.

Bauer (2008) gathered data from in-person semi-structured interviews with 50 self-identified "dykes, trans people and queers" from the United States and western Europe to examine how they explore gender. BDSM spaces allow them to safely try on and negotiate identities, especially gender identities, and their intersections with age, sexual identity, and class through role play. Bauer (2018) focused on the types of role play in which members of the les-bi-trans-queer BDSM community engage, identifying three types of role play: age play (e.g., daddi, mommi, boi, grrrl), intergenerational play, and kinship play. Each of these types of role play provides benefits to participants, including healing, emotional and physical safety (for those in the becoming-child role), and the opportunity to try on various gender roles and explore various masculinities and femininities.

Until recently, little research was done on women and BDSM, and that quantitative work was based on small samples (Rehor, 2015). We did know that women became aware of their interests as young adults, that they were satisfied with their orientation, that they preferred the submissive role (Levitt et al., 1994), and that they were more inclined to bisexuality than men and more experimental (Moser & Levitt, 1987). The work reviewed here expands on earlier research and provides evidence that gender is not fixed or absolute; it is created, negotiated, and transformed as part of an interactional process. Genders are complex, fluid, and situationally defined. They can be tried on, modified, discarded, and reactivated.

Negotiating Consent and Power Exchange

Negotiating consent is an important concern in BDSM. Dunkley and Brotto (2020) noted that "Negotiation represents an integral precursor to any

BDSM scene or power-exchange" (p. 661) and that the nature and degree of negotiation vary depending on the relationship between individuals and the proposed scene. Setting limits is taken seriously in the BDSM community; violations result in "considerable social repercussions" (p. 662).

In an ethnography of a BDSM community (a technique in which the researcher becomes a participant-observer), Newmahr (2006) addressed the issue of power, seeing it as "a *dynamic* of an interaction, an *idea* rather than a thing or resource, and certainly not a possession wielded by one party over another" (p. 41, italics in original). Newmahr's paper examines three realms of power in the BDSM community:

> the structure of SM play in general—the model according to which newcomers are taught to engage in SM play, and which is, in fact, the norm. The second is the communication and action during play, between the participants, and third are the experiences and understandings of power— and powerlessness—among SM participants. (pp. 41–42)

The "bottom" retains discretion and can exercise it by withdrawing consent and ending the scene, through, for example, the use of safe words. When roles are adopted, "pain is often a central aspect of the scene" (Newmahr, 2010b, p. 394), used as a way "of constructing authentic experiences of power imbalances" (p. 396).

Barker (2013) compared the depiction of consent in BDSM in the popular novel series *Fifty Shades of Grey* with how consent is really negotiated in actual settings. Rather than responsibility for consent residing completely within individuals, as reflected in the novel, Barker showed that consent is potentially impacted by social power dynamics; it is influenced by the participants' social roles and identities such as social status, gender, age, and experience. Barker examined blog postings, some of which illustrate a shift in the locus of responsibility for consent from individuals to a collective responsibility of the BDSM community.

Williams and colleagues (2014) have rethought the ideas presented in the acronyms SSC (safe, sane, and consensual) and RACK (risk-aware consensual kink), proposing a new formulation: 4Cs, which stands for caring, communication, consent, and caution. Williams et al. feel that the addition of caring, which is an ethical consideration; the importance of communication in making explicit individuals' needs; and caution, which considers the variation in individuals' willingness to engage in risk-taking activities, has distinct advantages over SSC and RACK as this motto is easy to remember and provides an important negotiating structure with some flexibility. In addition, it counters the notion held by non-BDSMers that this behavior is coercive and abusive.

Bauer (2020) discussed the issue of consent as it is understood and practiced in the "les-bi-trans-queer" BDSM community, finding that although "basic BDSM technologies of consent are shared across heterosexually dominated and les-bi-trans-queer BDSM contexts" (p. 12), there were important differences between them. In the community that Bauer studied, consent is seen as an active process involving not only the participants but often others like their absent primary partners. Negotiating consent beforehand is not seen as sufficient as scenes are dynamic, so consent is continuous. Verbal communication is often unreliable, so participants must learn to read each other's responses. Members are cognizant of how various power dynamics affect the process of consent. Unlike the situation in the heteronormative BDSM community, the responsibility for withdrawing consent is not placed totally on the bottom; the top and others present also are responsible. Finally, the community creates a culture of consent by educating newcomers and providing and enforcing guidelines.

Faccio et al. (2020) focused on erotic power exchange (EPE), making a distinction between EPE and sexuality. They saw an important difference between "eroticity," which is more abstract, involving imagery and symbolism, and sexuality, which is concrete and more focused. They observed several differences between BDSM and non-BDSM experiences. For example, they noted that satisfaction in BDSM encounters does not necessarily rely upon orgasms. Additionally, they identified some positive outcomes from BDSM activity that may be nonsexual, as in cathartic or therapeutic outcomes. They concluded that, "it would be more appropriate to refer to the EPE experience as an erotic experience rather than a strictly sexual one" (p. 1647).

In sum, the most recent work on consent and power exchange advances our knowledge by viewing negotiation as an ongoing accomplishment, structured by social roles and identities and framed within a larger social context, rather than being a one-time fixed agreement between participants. Consent forms the core of BDSM; it is present in every scenario. Understanding consent and how it is negotiated helps us to understand the complexities of BDSM relationships and practices. What is needed is more work on the role of consent in different BDSM communities and how it works in private situations.

BDSM Subcultures

Subcultures serve a number of functions for their members. They provide access to whatever their members need. They serve to explain, define, justify, rationalize, and neutralize identities and behavior. They create guidelines for acceptable behavior. They often provide protection for their members. Most importantly, subcultures provide a sense of affiliation, support, and belonging. These last functions are especially critical for members of "deviant" groups.

Rather than being an integrated community, BDSM is a collection of many different subcultures. There are, for example, a variety of heterosexual organizations and clubs, the world of the gay leathermen, a variety of women's groups often based on sexual orientation and gender identities (e.g., Bauer, 2008, 2018; Meeker et al., 2021), and special interest groups (Wignall & McCormack, 2017). One of the more interesting subcultural groups is the "pup play" subculture of some gay and bisexual men, in which participants take on the role of puppies or dogs, often using collars, harnesses, leashes, dog masks, and tails. While the experience is seen as sexual by some men, others see their participation in terms of relaxation, receiving petting and cuddling and a way to relax (Wignall & McCormack, 2017).

Sagarin et al. (2019) made the case for using the same type of analysis when studying BDSM collective environments that are used to research other collective sex environments. They pointed out, however, that BDSM settings do not fit the definition of collective sex environments in that participants rarely have sex in these situations and that their motivations extend beyond their choice of partners.

Holmes and colleagues (2017) studied a sample of 10 gay Canadian men involved in the BDSM subculture. The researchers were interested in learning about the "motivations and meanings behind individual desires" (p. 93) and "the pursuit of sexual pleasure . . . at play in BDSM practices" (p. 95). Four major themes were identified in their data: selecting partners, performing BDSM practices, enjoying transgressions, and mitigating risks. In selecting potential partners, respondents considered their appearance, experience, role preference, how they were met, and the type of possible relationship they might form. Performing BDSM practices involved the spaces (public or private) in which interaction occurred, the gear used, a variety of acts, and "indifferen[ce] to receiving genital stimulation and/or reaching orgasm" (p. 107). Enjoying transgressions included physical and psychological pleasure, "a firm resistance to social stratification, and a push to 'normalize' kink" (p. 107). Respondents mitigated risk using several methods of harm reduction such as learning how to perform certain acts properly, careful preparation before the act, using gloves and condoms to reduce the risk of HIV and sexually transmitted disease transmission, emphasis on continuing communication with a partner including prior discussion of limits and the use of safe words, and belonging to a BDSM community.

Two researchers focused on Black participants in the BDSM community. Martinez (2020) addressed the "overwhelming whiteness of BDSM," through interviews with 25 respondents and discussions with 32 participants in an online forum. Using critical discourse analysis, which examines how speech practices are related to power, Martinez found that white respondents explained the low participation in BDSM clubs and settings by people of color in terms of their lack of access to resources, while racialized respondents explained their lack of participation in terms of their experiences of both implicit and explicit racial bias. Martinez theorized that the discursive practices of white BDSMers serve to make their white privilege invisible.

Utilizing textual analysis, websites of Black dominatrices, archival research, email correspondence, and YouTube interviews, Cruz (2015) examined how "Black women facilitate a complex and contradictory negotiation of pain, pleasure and power in their performance in the fetish realm of BDSM" (p. 410). The author noted that, "Despite the growth in BDSM scholarship, Black women's experience with the practice remains undertheorized" (p. 418). Cruz considered the place of race play in BDSM from the points of view of Black female practitioners, noting that some of them do not necessarily see all Black/white BDSM interactions as race play, which is itself a complex interaction requiring skill and training.

The situation of professional dominants was also examined by Pinsky and Levey (2015), who studied the work of 13 professional dominatrices from America and Europe through in-depth interviews, blogs, and published memoirs. The authors emphasized the complexities of the work of "prodommes," which involves emotional labor, seen by their respondents as the most demanding part of their work. "Perhaps most important for our understanding of the emotional labour of the dominatrix," they write, "is the seemingly contradictory, multifaceted performance of emotions that she must execute in a single session" (p. 445).

The research on BDSM subcultures is extensive, illustrating that although they are tremendously varied, subcultures all serve the same functions for their members of accessibility, normalization, protection, and affiliation. There are some BDSM worlds that still need to be studied, such as those of minority participants. Martinez notes the absence of Black participants in BDSM spaces, and Cruz's work was confined to Black professional female dominants, so there is still much to learn. We know little about the BDSMers who do not participate in these worlds or how they differ from subcultural participants.

Affiliation, Support, and Belonging

Webster and Ivanov (2019) studied "munches," described as "events in which no BDSM activities occur but have the intention of enabling members of the community to socialize and introduce new members or curious people to the community" (p. 671). These events, which occur internationally, serve an integrative and socialization function for BDSMers. They found that "the nonplay event is considered an important event for the lifestyle" (p. 674), especially for those first entering the kink/BDSM world, providing them with a sense of belonging to a community.

Graham and colleagues (2016) were interested in how BDSM participants view the role, meaning, and function of BDSM communities in their lives. Their study participants were 48 self-identified members of organized BDSM communities. The analysis identified three themes that developed from discussions: social features, personal expression, and functional resources. Several categories were identified for each theme. Social features included friendships, social networks, meeting lovers, being oneself, and acceptance. Personal expression included expressing one's sexuality, having fun, personal and spiritual growth, and self-acceptance. Functional resources included educational opportunities, information, support, and providing physical safety.

One important function of BDSM communities is to help members deal with stigma. Stiles and Clark (2011) examined how BDSM participants managed a potentially discreditable identity, given the stigma placed on this behavior as abusive and a manifestation of mental illness. Their sample consisted of 42 women and 31 men who self-identified as being in the BDSM lifestyle. Respondents described several levels of concealment of their participation in BDSM. In absolute concealment, which accounted for 38% of the sample, respondents did not reveal themselves to anyone. The 25% of the sample practicing thorough concealment told some, but not all, of their close friends. Scrupulous concealment, reported by 11%, involved disclosing one's behavior only to selected family members. The 18% of respondents engaging in partial concealment revealed themselves to some friends and some family members, while those practicing fractional concealment, representing just 6% of the sample, only conceal their BDSM from one or two people. Only one person in the sample was completely open to everyone. Eight percent of the respondents were intentionally or accidentally exposed by another person. Respondents reported several concealment strategies, including passing, hiding BDSM accoutrements in plain sight, compartmentalizing their public and private behavior, hiding BDSM artifacts, and using cover stories to account for potentially stigmatizing revelations.

Langdridge (2006) addressed stigma using the concept of sexual citizenship as it pertains to BDSM and members of that community. The author noted how the legal system prevents the acceptance of this behavior and/or identity as legitimate. Additionally, the medical/psychiatric profession pathologizes BDSM. Sexual citizenship is "defined by participation in the social and political life of the political community. This involves visibility as an essential component of citizenship, something very lacking with SM" (p. 376). To transform BDSM and make it acceptable requires "reducing the emphasis on sex and violence, the twin sins for citizenship" (p. 380). Langdridge notes that resistance to acceptance of BDSM and its practitioners is being challenged by members of BDSM communities in many ways. However, destigmatizing BDSM is a daunting task, as the research of Faccio and colleagues (2014) illustrates. They found that a quarter of their sample defined their own sexual practices in terms of a continuum of normality versus abnormality.

The affiliation function of "deviant" communities is probably the most important as it provides individuals with emotional support, acceptance, and a feeling of normalcy. Groups can do something that individuals cannot: successfully reject the rejecters and redefine the situation for their members by providing alternative explanations, thus reducing feelings of differentness and stigma. BDSM communities become in-groups, developing their own culture and language to distinguish them from outsiders. The papers reviewed here nicely illustrate the power of groups in providing these functions. Future research should focus on the specific ways in which these communities facilitate their members' self-acceptance.

BDSM Communities and Social Control

All groups, whether conforming or deviant, provide norms and values—guidelines for behavior, definitions of deviance, and engagement in social control. Holt (2016), an ethnographer, discussed how BDSM communities maintain boundaries and how violators are dealt with informally. Boundaries, as noted above, are defined, established, and maintained through pre-scene negotiations; and communication is ongoing.

BDSMers maintain boundaries and protect themselves and others, according to Holt, by "[p]articipating in the community and attending public events" (p. 925). When instances of boundary violations occur, social control is activated within the group. Members are hesitant to involve police for a variety of reasons, including the difficulty of tracking down offenders whose identities have been deliberately concealed. Holt described two ways in which social control is accomplished: "through vigilante justice and through institutionally sanctioned measures" (p. 926). Holt quoted male respondents who described situations in which they physically intervened, sometimes violently, during a scene in which someone was being harmed. Institutionally sanctioned measures include being blacklisted (i.e., ostracized) and banned from participation in the community.

In addition to monitoring interaction within spaces utilized by BDSM participants, BDSM communities serve to protect their members from conflict with police and arrest. Holt provided an instance in which group members were told what to do in case the police showed up. If they were not completely naked and not engaged in sex, they were not violating the law. They were to stay calm and let a lawyer who was present deal with the situation.

Luminais (2015) explained the ambivalence toward police in the BDSM community: "On the one hand, the police are admired and even lionized. On the other, they are feared as agents of oppression" (p. 32). Conscious of laws and how they can be selectively enforced, BDSM groups proactively self-police to avoid trouble. This is done is by limiting attendance at events to those over the age of 18. When alcohol is served at parties, only those over 21 are admitted. Identification is checked, and sex is banned at parties.

Haviv (2016) used semi-structured interviews to gather a snowball sample of individuals contacted through a website for Israeli BDSMers, focusing on how they view the police and their reasons for not reporting assaults that occur within BDSM play. These include fear of being blamed for what happened, fear of being exposed and its possible consequences, shame, and the difficulty of explaining what had happened and providing proof. As reported by participants in Luminais' (2015) and Holt's (2016) samples, Haviv's respondents developed several ways to try to address assaults within their community, including blacklisting violators, using gossip, and outing and banning.

The recent work on social control in BDSM communities illustrates how it is carefully structured by their members, who develop strategies to avoid both internal and external conflicts. Unacceptable behavior is clearly defined and sanctioned in a number of ways (Holt, 2016). As reviewed above (see "Negotiating Consent and Power Exchange"), social control is seen as the responsibility of everyone viewing a scene (Barker, 2013; Bauer, 2020). It would be interesting to see how definitions of deviance and social control vary by specific BDSM subcultures like the gay leathermen's community and various women's communities.

The Development of a BDSM Self-Identity

Participation in BDSM and having BDSM fantasies are not unusual. Holvoet and colleagues (2017) found that almost half of their representative sample of the general Belgian population indicated that they had engaged in a BDSM-related activity, and another fifth of the sample reported having had BDSM fantasies. One-quarter of the respondents acknowledged interest in BDSM. Moreover, 12.5% reported involvement in BDSM regularly. In another report by the same research group (De Neef et al., 2019) the writers identified what they called "the BDSM spectrum," acknowledging degrees of involvement in BDSM and a variety of self-definitions.

Identification with BDSM varies widely among participants. For example, Newmahr (2010a) relates a distinction made by one of the participants in the community studied, who differentiated between "people who *love* SM, and people who *do* SM" (p. 329), making the distinction between those for whom BDSM is an end in itself and those who are primarily interested in it as a prelude to sex. Some researchers found that their respondents conceptualized their BDSM identities as a flow, rather than being fixed. For example, Carlström (2018a) interviewed 29 BDSM practitioners, who commonly conceptualized their identities as a flow of desire, a "becoming" rather than a static state of "being." Similarly, when Sprott and Hadcock (2018) examined the intersection between kink/BDSM and sexual orientation, they noted that, for their respondents, "there was a distinct theme emerging of people identifying with fluidity, rather than just noting changes or shifts in sexual orientation or gender identity over time" (pp. 219–220). Weiss (2006) also noted that "the modernist model of identity does not capture the fluidity, proliferation or community-directed aspects of BDSM" (p. 230). Instead, BDSM "is an identity based on doing" (p. 233).

Yost and Hunter (2012) were interested in how BDSM practitioners conceptualized their initial interest in BDSM. Their sample consisted of 144 women and 128 men. Respondents filled out online questionnaires, with space for them to write comments. An analysis of the data produced two types of narratives that participants used to explain their initial BDSM interests: essentialist (intrinsic) explanations, in which they stated that BDSM was what they were, that these interests had been with them since early childhood, or that there was a biological reason for their feelings (43% of the sample), and constructionist explanations, which were seen as the result of socialization, by a romantic partner or friend or through exposure to media (35.3% of the sample). An additional 21.3% of respondents simply described what they found attractive about BDSM without describing their initial interest.

For some practitioners, the development of a BDSM identity is problematic. Meeker et al. (2021), for example, examined the intersection of feminist and submissive identities in an attempt to understand how women negotiate what appear to be antithetical positions. They found in their interviews with 23 feminist and submissive women that some women accomplished this by identity compartmentalization (e.g., hiding their BDSM interests from non-BDSM feminists), by being around like-minded people, or by reinterpreting submissiveness as compatible with feminism because it incorporates choice.

As Meeker et al. (2021) indicate, one problem that BDSMers face in the development of their identities is information control. Bezreh et al. (2012) asked 20 respondents about their development of identity, focusing on the process of coming out to others. One of the fears expressed by respondents was being labeled and stigmatized. Some of them chose not to reveal themselves. Other respondents "assessed the safety of disclosure based on overall evaluation of a person; being seen as judgmental or narrow was sometimes disqualifying" (p. 48).

The problematic aspect of developing a BDSM identity is illustrated by Hughes and Hammack's (2019) study of 265 international, kink-identified respondents in which they investigated how kinky people construct and maintain an identity by navigating through competing social definitions of kink. The researchers identified four classes of narratives by which this was accomplished. The first category identified was "unelaborated affirmation," in which respondents expressed positive but nondetailed feelings about their kink identities. The second class was "elaborated affirmation," characterized by detailed, varied, and nuanced positive views of their kinky identity. The third category of stories was "compartmentalization," in which respondents reported being selective as to whom they revealed their kink. The last group of stories involved "isolation." These respondents were less likely than the others to have developed positive feelings about their kink. They reported social and geographic isolation from kinky communities and described feelings of depression and suicidal ideation.

The research on BDSM in general, and identities in particular, points out several things. First, practitioners display a variety of BDSM identities, sexual orientations, and gender identities. Second, their development of identity is facilitated by participation in BDSM subcultures. Third, many of them see their gender identities, sexual orientations, and BDSM roles as fluid. What is now needed is work focused on how these identities develop, whether individuals pass through clearly defined stages, how they deal with feelings of cognitive dissonance, and the role of others and the media in recognizing their interests.

Conclusion

This brief review of some of the more recent work in BDSM illustrates how far we have come in developing an understanding of what is a multifaceted, complex phenomenon. So, what have we learned from the explosion of empirical and theoretical work since the last review in 2006? On a macro level, the seminal work of Jozifkova has provided evidence that helps to explain BDSM in terms of a biological imperative for mate selection, based on dominance and submission (Jozifkova, 2013, 2018; Jozifkova & Flegr, 2006; Jozifkova & Konvicka, 2009; Jozifkova et al., 2012, 2014; Jozifkova & Kolackova, 2017). Additionally, De Neef and colleagues (2019) developed a model of differential involvement in BDSM, by integrating biological, psychological, and sociological variables. This work provides a bridge between macro and micro levels of explanation. Ethnographic work (Carlström, 2018a, 2018b;

Carlstrom & Andersson, 2019; Holt, 2016; Luminais, 2015; Newmahr, 2011a; Sagarin et al., 2019; Webster & Ivanov, 2019) and interview data (Haviv, 2016; Simula, 2015, 2019b) have deepened our understanding of the role of the BDSM subculture in supporting, socializing, and protecting its members. On a micro level, we have gained an understanding of the complexities of consent, control, and power exchange as they evolve during a BDSM scene and the varied meaning of pain for participants as it relates to power exchange (Dunkley & Brotto, 2020; Newmahr, 2006, 2011b). Interview data has given us insight into the varieties of commitment to BDSM and the process of becoming a BDSMer (Bezreh et al., 2012; Carlström, 2018a; Yost & Hunter, 2012). Simula (2012, 2015) and Simula and Sumerau (2017) examined the varied ways in which participants view gender, sex, sexual orientation, and BDSM roles. In so doing, the ways in which some BDSMers separate sex and sexuality have been clarified.

There is still much to learn. A number of writers acknowledge gaps in their data collection. One of these is that while we are beginning to understand a good deal about those individuals who are involved in public or semi-public BDSM scenes, usually recruited from organizations, websites, chatrooms, etc., we know little about those people who are not part of any group because they have not been studied. How they differ from individuals who are part of a BDSM community is an important question. Another area of research is the participation of ethnic/racial minorities in BDSM.

An important development in the study of BDSM is that we now are accumulating a body of research from other countries. Research is being done on samples in Belgium, the Czech Republic, Germany, Israel, Italy, the Netherlands, Portugal, South Africa, Australia, Sweden, and the United Kingdom, joining that done in the United States, Canada, and Finland. However, these are all developed nations. We know little about BDSM in Global South countries or even if it exists in those places.

References

Barker, M. (2013). Gender and BDSM revisited. Reflections on a decade of researching kink communities. *Psychology of Women Section Review*, *15*(2), 20–28.

Bauer, R. (2008). Transgressive and transformative gendered sexual practices and white privileges: The case of the dyke/trans BDSM communities. *Women's Studies Quarterly*, *36*(3), 233–253. https://doi.org/10.1353/wsq.0.0100

Bauer, R. (2018). Bois and grrrls meet their daddies and mommies on gendered playgrounds: Gendered age play in the les-bi-trans-queer BDSM communities. *Sexualities*, *21*(1–2), 139–155. https://doi.org/10.1177/1363460716676987

Bauer, R. (2020). Queering consent: Negotiating critical consent in les-bi-trans-queer BDSM contexts. *Sexualities*, *24*(5–6). https://doi.org/10.1177/1363460720973902

Baumeister, R. F. (1988). Gender differences in masochistic scripts. *Journal of Sex Research*, *25*, 478–499.

Better, A., & Simula, B. L. (2015). How and for whom does gender matter? Rethinking the concept of sexual orientation. *Sexualities*, *18*(5–6), 665–680.

Bezreh, T., Weinberg, T. S., & Edgar, T. (2012). BDSM disclosure and stigma management: Identifying opportunities for sex education. *American Journal of Sexuality Education*, *7*(1), 37–61. https://doi.org/10.1080/15546128.2012.650984

Botta, D., Filippo, M. N., Tripodi, F., Silvaggi, M., & Simonelli, C. (2019). Are role and gender related to sexual function and satisfaction in men and women practicing BDSM? *Journal of Sexual Medicine*, *16*(3), 463–473. https://doi.org/10.1016/j.jsxm.2019.01.001

Carlström, C. (2018a). BDSM: Becoming and the flows of desire. *Culture Health & Sexuality*, *21*(4), 404–415. https://doi.org/10.1080/13691058.2018.1485969

Carlström, C. (2018b). BDSM—The antithesis of good Swedish sex? *Sexualities*, *22*(7–8), 1164–1181. https://doi.org/10.1177/1363460718769648

Carlström, C., & Andersson, C. (2019). The queer spaces of BDSM and non-monogamy. *Journal of Positive Sexuality*, *5*(1), 14–19.

Carrascosa, C. (2019). *Fifty shades of ape: Exploring the evolutionary explanations behind BDSM* [Unpublished thesis for Bachelor's of Arts and Sciences]. University of Amsterdam. https://doi.org/10.13140/RG.2.2.35231.61609

Cruz, A. (2015). Beyond black and blue: BDSM, internet pornography, and black female sexuality. *Feminist Studies*, *41*(2), 409–436.

De Neef, N., Coppens, V., Huys, W., & Morrens, M. (2019). Bondage–discipline, dominance–submission and sadomasochism (BDSM) from an integrative biopsychosocial perspective: A systematic review. *Journal of Sexual Medicine*, *7*(2), 129–144. https://doi.org/10.1016/j.esxm.2019.02.002

Dunkley, C. R., & Brotto, L. A. (2020). The role of consent in the context of BDSM. *Sexual Abuse*, *32*(6), 657–678. https://doi.org/10.1177/1079063219842847

Faccio, E., Casini, C., & Cipolletta, S. (2014). Forbidden games: The construction of sexuality and sexual pleasure by BDSM "players." *Culture, Health & Sexuality: An International Journal for Research, Intervention and Care*, *16*(7), 752–764. https://doi.org/10.1080/13691058.2014.909531

Faccio, E., Sarigu, D., & Iudici, A. (2020). What is it like to be a BDSM player? The role of sexuality and eroticization of power in the BDSM experience. *Sexuality & Culture*, *24*, 1641–1652. https://doi.org/10.1007/s12119-020-09703-x

Freud, S. (1938). *The basic writings of Sigmund Freud* (A. A. Brill, Trans. & Ed.). Modern Library.

Graham, B. C., Butler, S. E., McGraw, R., Cannes, S. M., & Smith, J. (2016). Member perspectives on the role of BDSM communities. *Journal of Sex Research*, *53*(8), 895–909.

Harris, E. A., Thai, M., & Barlow, F. K. (2016). Fifty shades flipped: Effects of reading erotica depicting a sexually dominant woman compared to a sexually dominant man. *The Journal of Sex Research*, *54*(3), 386–397. https://doi.org/10.1080/00224499.2015.1131227

Haviv, N. (2016). Reporting sexual assaults to the police: The Israeli BDSM community. *Sexuality Research and Social Policy, 13*, 276–287. https://doi.org/10.1007/s13178-016-0222-4

Hebert, A., & Weaver, A. (2014). An examination of personality characteristics associated with BDSM orientations. *The Canadian Journal of Sexuality, 23*(2), 106–115.

Holmes, D., Murray, S. J., Knack, N., Mercier, M., & Fedoroff, J. P. (2017). BDSM, sexual subcultures, and the ethics of public health discourse. In D. Holmes, S. J. Murray, & T. Foth (Eds.), *Radical sex between men: Assembling desiring-machines* (pp. 93–116). Routledge. https://doi.org/10.4324/9781315399546

Holt, K. (2016). Blacklisted: Boundaries, violations, and retaliatory behavior in the BDSM community. *Deviant Behavior, 32*(8), 917–930. http://dx.doi.org/10.1080/01639625.2016.1156982

Holvoet, L., Huys, W., Coppens, V., Seeuws, J., Goethals, K., & Morrens, M. (2017). Fifty shades of Belgian gray: The prevalence of BDSM-related fantasies and activities in the general population. *Journal of Sexual Medicine, 14*(9), 1152–1159. https://doi.org/10.1016/j.jsxm.2017.07.003

Hoople, T. (1996). Conflicting visions: SM, feminism, and the law. A problem of representation. *Canadian Journal of Law and Society, 11*(1), 177–220.

Hopkins, P. D. (1994). Rethinking sadomasochism: Feminism, interpretation, and simulation. *Hypatia, 9*, 116–141.

Hughes, S. D., & Hammack, P. L. (2019). Affirmation, compartmentalization, and isolation: Narratives of identity sentiment among kinky people. *Psychology & Sexuality, 10*(2), 149–168. https://doi.org/10.1080/19419899.2019.1575896

Jozifkova, E. (2013). Consensual sadomasochistic sex (BDSM): The roots, the risks, and the distinctions between BDSM and violence. *Current Psychiatry Reports, 15*, Article 392. https://doi.org/10.1007/s11920-013-0392-1

Jozifkova, E. (2018). Sexual arousal by dominance and submissiveness in the general population: How many, how strongly, and why? *Deviant Behavior, 39*(9), 1229–1236. https://doi.org/10.1080/01639625.2017.1410607

Jozifkova, E., Bartos, L., & Flegr, J. (2012). Evolutional background of dominance/submissivity in sex and bondage: The two strategies? *Neuroendocrinology Letters, 33*(6), 636–642.

Jozifkova, E., & Flegr, J. (2006). Dominance, submissivity (and homosexuality) in general population. Testing of evolutionary hypothesis of sadomasochism by internet-trap-method. *Neuroendocrinology Letters, 27*(6), 711–718.

Jozifkova, E., & Kolackova, M. (2017). Sexual arousal by dominance and submission in relation to increased reproductive success in the general population. *Neuroendocrinology Letters, 38*(5), 381–387.

Jozifkova, E., & Konvicka, M. (2009). Sexual arousal by higher- and lower-ranking partner: Manifestation of a mating strategy? *Journal of Sexual Medicine, 6*, 3327–3334.

Jozifkova, E., Konvicka, M., & Flegr, J. (2014). Why do some women prefer submissive men? Hierarchically disparate couples reach higher reproductive success in European urban humans. *Neuroendocrinology Letters, 35*(7), 594–601.

Krafft-Ebing, R. von. (1965). *Psychopathia sexualis.* (F. S. Klaf, Trans.). Stein & Day. (Original work published 1886)

Langdridge, D. (2006). Voices from the margins: Sadomasochism and sexual citizenship. *Citizenship Studies, 10*(4), 373–389. https://doi.org/10.1080/13621020600857940

Levitt, E. E., Moser, C., & Jamison, K. V. (1994). The prevalence and some attributes of females in the sadomasochistic subculture: A second report. *Archives of Sexual Behavior, 23*, 465–473.

Luminais, M. (2015). Stating desire: Sexuality, the state, and social control. In T. S. Weinberg & S. Newmahr (Eds.), *Selves, symbols and sexualities* (pp. 31–44). SAGE.

Martinez, K. (2017). BDSM role fluidity: A mixed-methods approach to investigating switches within dominant/submissive binaries. *Journal of Homosexuality, 65*(10), 1299–1324. https://doi.org/10.1080/00918369.2017.1374062

Martinez, K. (2020). Overwhelming whiteness of BDSM: A critical discourse analysis of racialization in BDSM. *Sexualities, 24*(5–6). https://doi.org/10.1177/136346072 0932389

Meeker, C., McGill, C. M., & Rocco, T. S. (2021). Negotiating self: Navigating feminist and submissive identities. *Identity, 21*(3), 238–254. https://doi.org/10.1080/15283 488.2021.1903900

Moser, C., & Levitt, E. E. (1987). An explorative-descriptive study of a sadomasochistically oriented sample. *The Journal of Sex Research, 23*, 322–337.

Newmahr, S. (2006). Experiences of power in SM: A challenge to power theory. *Berkeley Journal of Sociology, 50*, 37–60.

Newmahr, S. (2010a). Rethinking kink: Sadomasochism as serious leisure. *Qualitative Sociology, 33*, 313–331.

Newmahr, S. (2010b). Power struggles: Pain and authenticity in SM play. *Symbolic Interaction, 3*, 389–411.

Newmahr, S. (2011a). *Playing on the edge: Sadomasochism, risk, and intimacy.* Indiana University Press.

Newmahr, S. (2011b). Chaos, order, and collaboration: Toward a feminist conceptualization of edgework. *Journal of Contemporary Ethnography, 40*(6), 682–712.

Pinsky, D., & Levey, T. G. (2015). "A world turned upside down": Emotional labour and the professional dominatrix. *Sexualities, 18*(4), 438–458.

Powls, J., & Davies, J. (2012). A descriptive review of research relating to sadomasochism: Considerations for clinical practice. *Deviant Behavior, 33*(3), 223–234. https://doi.org/10.1080/01639625.2011.573391

Rehor, J. E. (2015). Sensual, erotic, and sexual behaviors of women from the "kink" community. *Archives of Sexual Behavior, 44*, 825–836.

Richters, J., de Visser, R. O., Rissel, C. E., Grulich, A. E., & Smith, A. M. (2008). Demographic and psychosocial features of participants in bondage and discipline, "sadomasochism" or dominance and submission (BDSM): Data from a national survey. *Journal of Sexual Medicine, 5*(7), 1660–1668. https://doi.org/10.1111/j.1743-6109.2008.00795.x

Sagarin, B. J., Lee, E. M., Erickson, J. M., Casey, K. G., & Pawirosetiko, J. S. (2019). Collective sex environments without the sex? Insights from the BDSM community. *Archives of Sexual Behavior, 48*, 63–67. https://doi.org/10.1007/s10508-018-1252-1

Simula, B. L. (2012). Does bisexuality "undo" gender? Gender, sexuality, and bisexual behavior among BDSM participants. *Journal of Bisexuality, 12*, 484–506.

Simula, B. (2015). Give me a dominant of any gender over any kind of non-dominant. In T. S. Weinberg & S. Newmahr (Eds.), *Selves, symbols and sexualities* (pp. 163–177). SAGE.

Simula, B. L. (2019a). A different economy of bodies and pleasures? Differentiating and evaluating sex and sexual BDSM experiences. *Journal of Homosexuality, 66*(2), 209–237. https://doi.org/10.1080/00918369.2017.1398017

Simula, B. L. (2019b). Pleasure, power, and pain: A review of the literature on the experiences of BDSM participants. *Sociology Compass, 13*(3), Article e12668. https//doi.org/10.1111/soc4.12668

Simula, B. L., & Sumerau, J. (2017). The use of gender in the interpretation of BDSM. *Sexualities, 22*(3), 452–477. https://doi.org/10.1177/1363460717737488

Spengler, A. (1977). Manifest sadomasochism of males: Results of an empirical study. *Archives of Sexual Behavior, 6*, 441–446.

Sprott, R. A., & Hadcock, B. B. (2018). Bisexuality, pansexuality, queer identity, and kink identity. *Sexual and Relationship Therapy, 33*(1–2), 214–232. https://doi.org/10.1080/14681994.2017.1347616

Stiles, B. L., & Clark, R. E. (2011). BDSM: A subcultural analysis of sacrifices and delights. *Deviant Behavior, 32*(2), 158–189.

Webster, C., & Ivanov, S. H. (2019). Events are bound to happen, spank you very much: The importance of munch events in the BDSM community. *Event Management, 23*, 669–684.

Weinberg, T. S. (1978). Sadism and masochism: Sociological perspectives. *Bulletin of the American Academy of Psychiatry and the Law, 6*(3), 284–295.

Weinberg, T. S. (1987). Sadomasochism in the United States: A review of recent sociological literature. *The Journal of Sex Research, 2*, 50–69.

Weinberg, T. S. (1994). Research in sadomasochism: A review of sociological and social psychological literature. *Annual Review of Sex Research, 5*, 257–279.

Weinberg, T. S. (2006). Sadomasochism and the social sciences: A review of the sociological and social psychological literature. *Journal of Homosexuality, 50*(2–3), 17–40.

Weinberg, T. S. (2020). The beginning of the sociological study of BDSM: A personal reflection. *Sexualities, 24*(5–6), 825–831. https://doi.org/10.1177/1363460720961288

Weiss, M. (2006). Working at play: BDSM sexuality in the San Francisco Bay area. *Anthropologica, 8*, 229–245.

Wignall, L., & McCormack, M. (2017). An exploratory of a new kink activity: "Pup play." *Archives of Sexual Behavior, 46*, 801–811. https://doi.org/10.1007/s10508-015-0636-8

Williams, D. J., Thomas, J., Prior, E., & Christensen, M. (2014). From "SSC" and "RACK" to the "4Cs": Introducing a new framework for negotiating BDSM participation. *Electronic Journal of Human Sexuality, 17*. http://www.ejhs.org/volume17/BDSM.html

Wismeijer, A. J., & van Assen, M. A. L. M. (2013). Psychological characteristics of BDSM practitioners. *Journal of Sexual Medicine, 10*(8), 1943–1952. https://doi.org/10.1111/jsm.12192

Yost, M. R., & Hunter, L. E. (2012). BDSM practitioners' understandings of their initial attraction to BDSM sexuality: Essentialist and constructionist narratives. *Psychology & Sexuality, 3*(3), 244–259. https://doi.org/10.1080/19419899.2012.700028

2

The Role of the Internet in Research on BDSM

Liam Wignall

The Internet's Impact on Sexuality

The internet has transformed sexual cultures (Döring, 2009), providing a generally accessible platform which can connect people across social, cultural, and geographical divides (James, 2018), particularly for those who speak English. It has allowed sexual minorities pathways to explore their sexual orientation (Gudelunas, 2012) and connect to others with similar sexual interests or preferences (Miller, 2015; Pacho, 2018); it provides ways for individuals to learn about sex and sexuality (McCormack & Wignall, 2017), including access to sexual health resources (Pedrana et al., 2013). New technologies using the internet allow individuals to find people to have sexual encounters with offline (Wignall, 2022) as well as engage in sex in online spaces (Daneback et al., 2005), which was especially welcome during social lockdowns due to COVID-19 (Banerjee & Rao, 2021; Cascalheira et al., 2021). There has been a proliferation of individuals using the internet to engage in sex work (Sanders et al., 2020; Schrimshaw et al., 2017), including fan-based sites like OnlyFans (Ryan, 2019). While the full scope of the internet's impact on sexuality is beyond this chapter (there are books dedicated to the topic, e.g., Manderson, 2012; Nixon & Düsterhöft, 2018; Sanders et al., 2020), the internet has been recognized as having a transformative impact on sex, sexuality, and sexual cultures. However, it is important to note that this is predominantly the case for those who have access to internet resources and some level of computer literacy.

The internet has been especially useful for sexual minorities, allowing for the development of online sexual subcultures and communities (Fox & Ralston, 2016). Earlier examples of these online subcultures used online bulletin boards and online forums to connect with others (Burke, 2000;

Liam Wignall, *The Role of the Internet in Research on BDSM* In: *The Power of BDSM*. Edited by: Brandy L. Simula, Robin Bauer, and Liam Wignall, Oxford University Press. © Oxford University Press 2023.
DOI: 10.1093/oso/9780197658598.003.0003

Campbell, 2014). However, technological advances which focused on connecting people globally led to fundamental changes with the internet and how it was used (Baym, 2015). One such change was the creation of social networking sites (SNSs) like Facebook. SNSs allowed users to construct an online profile within the website's framework, generate connections with other users, and explore the social networks of other users (boyd & Ellison, 2007, p. 211). While Facebook and Twitter are for general audiences, there are also SNSs specifically for sexual minorities, including the Gay Youth Corner (GYC), which is based in the United Kingdom, and the Asexual Visibility and Education Network (AVEN), which is predominantly based in the United States. Despite further technological advances and many of these sites moving away from websites in traditional computer browsers to smartphone applications, their functions have predominantly remained the same—connecting users and facilitating communication (Meier et al., 2016; Mowlabocus, 2016). Indeed, there are now numerous mobile apps classified loosely as SNSs for sexual minorities, including Grindr, Her, Lex, and Taimi, as well as those for people who participate BDSM, such as KinkD, Kinkoo, and Kinkr.

Given the various ways in which sexual SNSs are used, such as to facilitate sexual encounters and engage with sexual subcultures (e.g., Jaspal, 2017; Renninger, 2019), it seems inaccurate to label them as solely *social* networking sites. Instead, as argued elsewhere (Wignall, 2017, 2022), they are more accurately labelled as *socio-sexual* networking sites (SSNSs). This label acknowledges the dual nature of the sites, recognizing the importance of social communication occurring on these sites alongside the opportunities for sexual encounters, as well as their primary demographic being sexual minorities. As such, I will now refer to them as SSNSs.

"Here's to (Fet)Life": BDSM SSNSs

The internet has also had a huge impact for people who engage in BDSM (Simula, 2019), allowing people to explore their BDSM interests through SSNSs and pornography (Wignall, 2019; Wignall & McCormack, 2017), access BDSM-related resources (Graham et al., 2016), join local and international communities (Fay et al., 2016; Wignall, 2017), and find others to engage in BDSM with, both online and offline (Denney & Tewksbury, 2013). While a panoply of SSNSs exist to cater for the diverse interests of people interested in BDSM, one of the most popular BDSM-based SSNSs is FetLife. Due to the centrality of FetLife within academic research (Colosi & Lister, 2019; Wignall, 2022), its popularity among people who engage in BDSM, and how many of the features of FetLife mirror other BDSM SSNSs, this section will go into further detail about the site and how it is used by its members.

FetLife describes itself as "the Social Network for the BDSM, Fetish & Kinky Community . . . Like Facebook, but run by kinksters like you and me." FetLife is a BDSM SSNS that caters to all genders, sexual orientations, and BDSM interests but has a predominantly heterosexual/pansexual userbase (McCabe, 2015). The site's main function has remained the same since its creation in 2008—to provide a platform for people with BDSM interests to interact online with others with shared interests, mirroring how SSNSs are used generally (Mowlabocus, 2016). This is achieved through users interacting with other FetLife users (currently at almost 10 million globally, with the majority based in the United States and the United Kingdom), posting to online discussion threads (approaching 11 million), joining interest groups (nearly 150,000), and posting blogs (almost 4 million).

Like most SSNSs, users create an online profile outlining demographic information and general interests, upload profile pictures and photos into public and private albums, and publicly connect with other profiles. However, owing to its BDSM nature, FetLife also allows users to add BDSM-related information to their profiles, including specific BDSM interests and FetLife groups of which the user is a member and BDSM-style relationships with other FetLife users (such as dominant, submissive, master, pup; see Hebert & Weaver, 2015).

While describing itself as a "social network site," FetLife is unique from other general SSNSs for two reasons. First, it is predominantly a website-based platform. FetLife does not have an app in App Store or on Google Play (where mobile apps are traditionally located), compared to some other BDSM SSNSs (e.g., Recon). However, users can download an app directly from the website, but this depends on the type of device they have. Second, FetLife strongly encourages participation in an online community through forum discussions on a range of topics (BDSM-related, non-BDSM-related, and nonsexual), allowing users to publicly display their engagement in BDSM (e.g., listing BDSM relationships with others) and list fetish interest groups in profiles. In this way, FetLife promotes a sense of online community among its members and boasts an all-encompassing profile of one's BDSM identity (Jaspal, 2017).

There is limited research which has explored FetLife in particular, and BDSM SSNSs more generally. In their master's thesis, McCabe (2015) conducted a discursive analysis of user-generated content on FetLife, demonstrating how "the site's structural and social affordances [give] rise to novel and unconventional forms of sexual expression" (p. 66). McCabe argues that the site has been constructed to create a strong community feeling among its members through promoting interactions and encouraging group discussions. However, most of the user-generated content (including blog posts, examples of BDSM scenes, and pornographic content) often follow conventional pornography tropes which focus on young, white, feminine, attractive, cisgender women. This is especially notable in the content that users are suggested they might like in the "kinky and popular" tab (see also Jones, 2020).

More recently, Colosi and Lister (2019) interviewed FetLife users about their experiences of navigating BDSM identities online and associated stigma particularly in non-BDSM settings. Participants felt that their sexualities were policed on general SNSs, such as Facebook or Tumblr, and that sites like FetLife helped them to express an authentic version of themselves. FetLife also provided a safe space for users to form online communities and learn from other members about BDSM practices and lifestyles. Interestingly, communications online did not always extend to offline interactions in this study, raising questions about how online BDSM communities can operate offline.

FetLife is often referenced in academic literature on BDSM. However, scant research explores the complex interactions which occur on FetLife, instead using it to recruit participants or mentioning it in interview schedules. Similarly, there is little research on other SSNSs. Recently, I (Wignall, 2022) explored two other BDSM SSNSs which are primarily aimed at gay and bisexual men, Recon and ClubCollared. Immersing myself on these SSNSs and conducting interviews with users, I found that these sites served two primary purposes for their users: to allow individuals to feel connected to an online community and maintain a presence within the online BDSM world and to facilitate BDSM hookups offline. Moreover, Recon and ClubCollared allowed individuals who were not immersed in BDSM communities offline to learn about BDSM and interact with others with shared interests—a different narrative from earlier research on BDSM which outlined how people needed to invest resources (predominantly time) to gain knowledge of BDSM subcultures (e.g., Graham et al., 2016; Newmahr, 2011; Rubin, 1991).

I argue that the increased visibility of the "non-community" individual, who engages in BDSM but does not immerse themselves in BDSM communities (both offline and online), is partly due to the increased accessibility of BDSM SSNSs (see also Zambelli, 2017).

BDSM Research Moving Forward

Research is continuing to recognize the important role that BDSM SSNSs have in helping people explore their BDSM interests and connect with others who share similar interests, alongside how SSNSs like FetLife help to foster a sense of community within BDSM subcultures (Hughes & Hammack, 2019). However, as previously stated, BDSM SSNSs are often not the focus of academic research; instead, their importance is acknowledged in how they are used as a recruitment tool for research on BDSM. The difficulty of recruiting individuals to participate in research on BDSM without preexisting links to BDSM communities has been well documented (see Weinberg, 2006; see also Chapter 1 in this volume), and BDSM SSNSs provide an easy and convenient way of recruiting participants. However, there are several problems with how research has traditionally engaged with BDSM SSNSs.

Firstly, despite their importance, there is relatively little academic research on the complex social worlds, online communities, and public/private interactions that occur on BDSM SSNSs. There is growing recognition and scholarship on the complex digital worlds created on SNSs (e.g., Grieve et al., 2013; Murthy, 2018), and this has expanded to consider gay men's online sexual cultures (Mowlabocus, 2016); yet the significance of online community and social identity remains underplayed as BDSM research focuses on offline BDSM communities. This may be partly due to the physical and interpersonal nature of BDSM activities and the misunderstanding that BDSM only happens in person. Perhaps one of the impacts of COVID-19 will be to draw more attention to the use of online spaces for diverse forms of sexual exploration, including BDSM.

Secondly, research should explore the interactions that occur within online communities and how these translate to offline interactions (including more formal BDSM events but also personal interactions). My research (Wignall, 2017) on Pup Twitter, for example, showed that people interested in pup play developed their social BDSM identities online, through creating

Twitter accounts for their pup identity and crafting them to reflect the personality of this pup identity (e.g., profile images featuring pup hoods, "bios" which described aspects of their pup identity). However, the presence of Pup Twitter and an online community transformed how pup play was practiced in community venues, with the online and offline influencing each other; people would often ask for a Twitter handle when at offline events, pictures were taken purposefully to upload online, and pups having never met before knew of each other through online networks. Relatedly, it is notable how much excellent research on BDSM communities does not consider online spaces as part of BDSM communities (see Wignall, 2022, for this critique). It would be beneficial for research on BDSM communities to include the internet more routinely and SSNSs as topics for interview schedules or as topics to consider in observations and ethnographies.

Thirdly, despite a range of BDSM SSNSs being available, researchers often only recruit through FetLife. This may partly be explained by researchers using preexisting networks to recruit participants or by the difficulty in gaining access to other BDSM SSNSs (e.g., Hughes & Hammack, 2022). However, the consequence of predominantly using one BDSM SSNS is that, rather than research exploring all individuals who engage in BDSM, research into BDSM provides insights into FetLife users. Given that FetLife is predominantly used by heterosexual/pansexual individuals, there is a significant lack of insight into the experiences of individuals who participate in BDSM who identify as LGBTQ+. Furthermore, BDSM SSNSs which specifically cater to a particular BDSM interest or a specific geographical region are often understudied, despite evidence that they can differ from some of the bigger BDSM SSNSs (e.g., see Chapter 5 in this volume). Research needs to engage with a range of BDSM SSNSs when recruiting participants.

Finally, research needs to move beyond recruiting people who are immersed in communities. This can be partly addressed through recruiting people who engage in BDSM and sign up to BDSM SSNSs but are less active members. Related to the previous point, given the focus on community within BDSM promoted by FetLife, research may only be recruiting people who are immersed in BDSM communities, rather than the range of people who engage in BDSM (Zambelli, 2017). My (Wignall, 2022) research on the non-community participant highlights this group, and my recruitment process that facilitated this process used Recon and ClubCollared.

Research could move beyond recruiting people who practice kink on BDSM SSNSs, instead potentially exploring more general (non-BDSM-focused)

SSNSs (e.g., Wignall, 2017). There are numerous SSNSs which provide ways of expressing an interest in BDSM, such as the "leather" tribe on Grindr (see Conner, 2019), BDSM tags on GayRomeo (García-Iglesias, 2020), or through pictures displayed on more traditional SNSs (see Chapter 4 in this volume). Exploring how BDSM interests are negotiated and discussed in these online spaces would also be a fruitful area of research.

However, there are ethical considerations when recruiting participants through BDSM SSNSs and engaging in these online spaces, as with research in online spaces more generally (e.g., Eynon et al., 2009; Winter & Lavis, 2020). Researchers may need permission from the sites to collect certain forms of data, particularly if they are not already members of these online spaces, or indeed the BDSM communities the sites serve. Most BDSM SSNSs require people to create accounts to join, raising questions about the public nature of these profiles and ethics of collecting data from participants—this has been recognized by some users of BDSM SSNSs who, despite not adding any legal rights, state something like the following on their profile:

> WARNING: Any institution or person using this site or any of its associated sites for study, projects, or personal agenda do not have my permission to use any of my profile or pictures in any form or forum, both current or future. You do not have my permission to copy, save, or print my pictures for your own personal use, including, but not limited to, saving them on your computer, posting them on any other website, or this one and passing them off as your own. If you have or do, it will be considered a violation of my privacy and will be subject to all legal remedies.

While BDSM SSNSs may offer a novel way to recruit people who participate in BDSM and provide opportunities to explore how BDSM is practiced in online spaces, there must be careful consideration before conducting research in these online spaces.

To conclude, the transformative effect of the internet on almost all aspects of social life has started to be understood in sexology and critical sexuality studies. Yet, BDSM studies has not been at the vanguard of this scholarship, tending to engage with the internet reluctantly or as an incidental aspect of BDSM practices and communities. In this brief chapter, I hope to have drawn attention to key ways that scholars of BDSM can consider the role of the internet more fully and develop a critical account of the internet's impact on the lives of people who engage in BDSM.

References

Banerjee, D., & Rao, T. S. (2021). "#Intimacy" at times of COVID-19: The renewed impetus behind cybersex. *Journal of Psychosexual Health*, *3*(1), 13–17. https://doi.org/10.1177%2F26318318211004397

Baym, N. K. (2015). *Personal connections in the digital age*. John Wiley & Sons.

boyd, D. M., & Ellison, N. B. (2007). Social network sites: Definition, history, and scholarship. *Journal of Computer-Mediated Communication*, *13*(1), 210–230. https://doi.org/10.1111/j.1083-6101.2007.00393.x

Burke, S. K. (2000). In search of lesbian community in an electronic world. *CyberPsychology & Behavior*, *3*(4), 591–604. https://doi.org/10.1089/109493100420197

Campbell, J. E. (2014). *Getting it on online: Cyberspace, gay male sexuality, and embodied identity*. Routledge.

Cascalheira, C. J., McCormack, M., Portch, E., & Wignall, L. (2021). Changes in sexual fantasy and solitary sexual practice during social lockdown among young adults in the UK. *Sexual Medicine*, *9*(3), Article 100342. https://doi.org/10.1016/j.esxm.2021.100342

Colosi, R., & Lister, B. (2019). Kinking it up: An exploration of the role of online social networking site FetLife in the stigma management of kink practices. In *British Criminology Conference* (Vol. 19). British Society of Criminology.

Conner, C. T. (2019). The gay gayze: Expressions of inequality on Grindr. *The Sociological Quarterly*, *60*(3), 397–419. https://doi.org/10.1080/00380253.2018.1533394

Daneback, K., Cooper, A., & Månsson, S. A. (2005). An internet study of cybersex participants. *Archives of Sexual Behavior*, *34*(3), 321–328. https://doi.org/10.1007/s10508-005-3120-z

Denney, A. S., & Tewksbury, R. (2013). Characteristics of successful personal ads in a BDSM on-line community. *Deviant Behavior*, *34*(2), 153–168.

Döring, N. M. (2009). The internet's impact on sexuality: A critical review of 15 years of research. *Computers in Human Behavior*, *25*(5), 1089–1101. https://doi.org/10.1016/j.chb.2009.04.003

Eynon, R., Schroeder, R., & Fry, J. (2009). New techniques in online research: Challenges for research ethics. *Twenty-First Century Society*, *4*(2), 187–199. https://doi.org/10.1080/17450140903000308

Fay, D., Haddadi, H., Seto, M. C., Wang, H., & Kling, C. (2016). An exploration of fetish social networks and communities. In *International conference and school on network science* (pp. 195–204). Springer.

Fox, J., & Ralston, R. (2016). Queer identity online: Informal learning and teaching experiences of LGBTQ individuals on social media. *Computers in Human Behavior*, *65*, 635–642. https://doi.org/10.1016/j.chb.2016.06.009

García-Iglesias, J. (2020). Wanting HIV is "such a hot choice": Exploring bugchasers' fluid identities and online engagements. *Deviant Behavior*, *41*(10), 1232–1243. https://doi.org/10.1080/01639625.2019.1606617

Graham, B. C., Butler, S. E., McGraw, R., Cannes, S. M., & Smith, J. (2016). Member perspectives on the role of BDSM communities. *The Journal of Sex Research*, *53*(8), 895–909. https://doi.org/10.1080/00224499.2015.1067758

Grieve, R., Indian, M., Witteveen, K., Tolan, G. A., & Marrington, J. (2013). Face-to-face or Facebook: Can social connectedness be derived online? *Computers in Human Behavior*, *29*(3), 604–609. https://doi.org/10.1016/j.chb.2012.11.017

Gudelunas, D. (2012). There's an app for that: The uses and gratifications of online social networks for gay men. *Sexuality & Culture, 16*(4), 347–365. https://doi.org/10.1007/s12119-012-9127-4

Herbert, A., & Weaver, A. (2015). Perks, problems, and people who play: A qualitative exploration of dominant and submissive BDSM roles. *The Canadian Journal of Human Sexuality, 24*(1), 49–62.

Hughes, S. D., & Hammack, P. L. (2019). Affirmation, compartmentalization, and isolation: Narratives of identity sentiment among kinky people. *Psychology & Sexuality, 10*(2), 149–168.

Hughes, S. D., & Hammack, P. L. (2022). Narratives of the origins of kinky sexual desire held by users of a kink-oriented social networking website. *The Journal of Sex Research, 59*(3), 360–371. https://doi.org/10.1080/00224499.2020.1840495

James, J. (2018). Love at our fingertips: Exploring the design implications of mobile dating technologies. In P. G. Nixon & I. K. Düsterhöft (Eds.), *Sex in the digital age* (pp. 57–67). Routledge.

Jaspal, R. (2017). Gay men's construction and management of identity on Grindr. *Sexuality & Culture, 21*(1), 187–204. https://doi.org/10.1007/s12119-016-9389-3

Jones, Z. (2020). *Pleasure, community, and marginalization in rope bondage: A qualitative investigation into a BDSM subculture* [Doctoral dissertation, Carleton University]. Curve. https://doi.org/10.22215/etd/2020-14247

Manderson, L. (2012). *Technologies of sexuality, identity and sexual health*. Routledge.

McCabe, C. S. (2015). *"Facebook for kinky people": A discursive analysis of FetLife* [Doctoral dissertation, Simon Fraser University]. Summit. http://summit.sfu.ca/item/15574

McCormack, M., & Wignall, L. (2017). Enjoyment, exploration and education: Understanding the consumption of pornography among young men with nonexclusive sexual orientations. *Sociology, 51*(5), 975–991. https://doi.org/10.1177%2F0038038516629909

Meier, A., Reinecke, L., & Meltzer, C. E. (2016). "Facebocrastination"? Predictors of using Facebook for procrastination and its effects on students' well-being. *Computers in Human Behavior, 64*, 65–76.

Miller, B. (2015). "They're the modern-day gay bar": Exploring the uses and gratifications of social networks for men who have sex with men. *Computers in Human Behavior, 51*(Part A), 476–482. https://doi.org/10.1016/j.chb.2015.05.023

Mowlabocus, S. (2016). *Gaydar culture: Gay men, technology and embodiment in the digital age*. Routledge.

Murthy, D. (2018). *Twitter*. Polity Press.

Newmahr, S. (2011). *Playing on the edge: Sadomasochism, risk, and intimacy*. Indiana University Press.

Nixon, P., & Düsterhöft, I. (2018). *Sex in the digital age*. Routledge.

Pacho, A. (2018). "Cake is better than sex"—AVEN and asexuality. In P. G. Nixon & I. K. Düsterhöft (Eds.), *Sex in the digital age* (pp. 113–123). Routledge.

Pedrana, A., Hellard, M., Gold, J., Ata, N., Chang, S., Howard, S., Asselin, J., Ilic, O., Batrouney, C., & Stoove, M. (2013). Queer as f** k: Reaching and engaging gay men in sexual health promotion through social networking sites. *Journal of Medical Internet Research, 15*(2), Article e25. https://doi.org/10.2196/jmir.2334

Renninger, B. J. (2019). Grindr killed the gay bar, and other attempts to blame social technologies for urban development: A democratic approach to popular technologies and queer sociality. *Journal of Homosexuality, 66*(12), 1736–1755. https://doi.org/10.1080/00918369.2018.1514205

Rubin, G. (1991). The Catacombs: A temple of the butthole. In M. Thompson (Ed.), *Leatherfolk: Radical sex, people, politics, and practice* (pp. 119–141). Alyson Books.

Ryan, P. (2019). Netporn and the amateur turn on OnlyFans. In *Male sex work in the digital age* (pp. 119–136). Palgrave Macmillan.

Sanders, R., Brents, B., & Wakefield, C. (2020). Sex without touch: Consumers of the webcam market. In *Paying for sex in the digital age: US and UK perspectives* (pp. 161–185). Routledge.

Schrimshaw, E. W., Siegel, K., & Meunier, É. (2017). Venues where male sex workers meet partners: The emergence of gay hookup apps and web sites. *American Journal of Public Health, 107*(12), 1866–1867. https://doi.org/10.2105%2FAJPH.2017.304118

Simula, B. L. (2019). Pleasure, power, and pain: A review of the literature on the experiences of BDSM participants. *Sociology Compass, 13*(3), Article e12668. https://doi.org/10.1111/soc4.12668

Weinberg, T. (2006). Sadomasochism and the social sciences: A review of the sociological and social psychological literature. *Journal of Homosexuality, 50*(2–3), 17–40. https://doi.org/10.1300/j082v50n02_02

Wignall, L. (2017). The sexual use of a social networking site: The case of pup twitter. *Sociological Research Online, 22*(3), 21–37. https://doi.org/10.1177%2F1360780417724066

Wignall, L. (2019). Pornography use by kinky gay men—A qualitative approach. *Journal of Positive Sexuality, 15*(1), 7–13. https://doi.org/10.51681/1.512

Wignall, L. (2022). *Kinky in the digital age: Gay men's subcultures and social identities.* Oxford University Press.

Wignall, L., & McCormack, M. (2017). An exploratory study of a new kink activity: "Pup play." *Archives of Sexual Behavior, 46*(3), 801–811. https://doi.org/10.1007/s10508-015-0636-8

Winter, R., & Lavis, A. (2020). Looking, but not listening? Theorizing the practice and ethics of online ethnography. *Journal of Empirical Research on Human Research Ethics, 15*(1–2), 55–62. https://doi.org/10.1177%2F1556264619857529

Zambelli, L. (2017). Subcultures, narratives and identification: An empirical study of BDSM (bondage, domination and submission, discipline, sadism and masochism) practices in Italy. *Sexuality & Culture, 21*(2), 471–492. https://doi.org/10.1007/s12119-016-9400-z

PART II
PLAY AND PRACTICES

3

The World of Rope Bondage

Belonging, Resistance, and the "Infinite Possibilities" of Community

Zoey Jones

Introduction

Rope bondage is a type of BDSM activity that involves playing with a physical, often fetishized material (rope) along with a range of engagements with power, pain, pleasure, or skill development (Martin, 2011; Ordean & Pennington, 2019). It is often classified as a form of "edge play," a type of BDSM activity that carries a high level of physical, psychological, or emotional risk (Lee et al., 2015; Newmahr, 2011). Rope bondage is described by its practitioners as a physical activity, a form of intimacy, a sexual outlet, a style of expression, a type of art, an athletic endeavor, a creative adventure, and countless other things. Within the pansexual BDSM subculture, many rope bondage practitioners operate within their own sub-subculture and community(ies) focused on exploring, understanding, and displaying this practice.

Not all people who practice rope bondage engage with the subculture, but many do; and the scope of this social sphere is enormous. Practitioners gather in person and online to share information, build relationships, practice, play, and create art. These experiences are informed by wider BDSM subculture (see Bauer, 2008; Newmahr, 2011; Simula, 2019; Wignall, 2022; several chapters in this volume) as many rope bondage practitioners begin their journeys in more general BDSM practices and social connections. The ebb and flow of practices, meanings, and relations that make up the rope bondage world transcend geospatial boundaries, while often being quite

Zoey Jones, *The World of Rope Bondage* In: *The Power of BDSM*. Edited by: Brandy L. Simula, Robin Bauer, and Liam Wignall, Oxford University Press. © Oxford University Press 2023. DOI: 10.1093/oso/9780197658598.003.0004 firmly contained within the social boundaries of the subculture. Adam, a white cisgender man in his early 30s (rope top, bottom, self-tier[1] educator, and performer) explained, "there is a separate rope community. It's like a subculture in some ways, in that the punk scene is a subculture of the greater culture of music."

Rope bondage subculture is characterized by traditions, norms, ethics, symbols, language, and activities that are relatively self-contained within its proverbial borders. In this world, rope bondage practitioners in small-town Ontario may have more in common (and correspond more frequently) with a rope bondage practitioner in Austin than a whips enthusiast who lives down the street or a non-kinky coworker they sit beside during their workday. Rope bondage practitioners interact with each other to share passions and develop relationships but also to share the knowledge and skills required to pursue their practice. Rope bondage subculture is structured by many levels, types, and expressions of community that are both subjective and intersubjective; these communities are at times as small as a single friend group and at other times as large as every person networked together in the global rope bondage scene.

Research almost solely conducted by graduate students has begun to establish and explore rope bondage as a specific BDSM practice. For example, Ordean and Pennington (2019, p. 68) describe rope bondage as "not a unified body of techniques but rather a growing collection of styles and approaches," not all of which are identified by their participants as BDSM. They highlight a wide range of purposes and practices within rope bondage, including aesthetics, sex, and performance, as guiding priorities and philosophies. Pennington (2017) studies rope bondage as performance, separating it conceptually from BDSM practice and examining its context within contemporary and historical Japanese tradition. Galati (2017) adopts a similarly corporeal understanding of rope bondage, describing the rope bondage community in the United Kingdom as empowering and inclusive and the practice itself as therapeutic. Sheela (2008, p. 6) alternatively finds that "the BDSM body in Singapore is gendered, classed and racially marked" and particularly explores the positioning of Chinese men at the bottom of this social hierarchy with respect to rope bondage practice and spaces.

This scarce but rich research on rope bondage can be supplemented by knowledge that resides mostly in non-academic instruction manuals, internet blogs, formal and informal gatherings, and word of mouth (see Harrington & RiggerJay, 2015; Kent, 2010; Midori & Morey, 2002; Nawakiri, 2017; Wiseman, 1996). These varied sources indicate that rope bondage in BDSM subculture is mostly associated with two formal forms of learning: Western rope bondage and *shibari* (or *kinbaku*)/Japanese rope bondage. There are myths and norms associated with each, although they have not as yet been thoroughly documented in academic research. Popular wisdom within BDSM communities often claims that *shibari* draws from an ancient Japanese martial art (Martin, 2011), and this influence can be seen in many trappings that surround *shibari* practice such as Japanese characters and words, the use of kimono during performance/play, and a deference in the United States and Canada to rope practitioners who are or learn from Japanese teachers. Ordean and Pennington (2019, p. 66) resist this easy history by drawing attention to how "the ostensible origins of rope bondage in feudal Japan" are used to validate rope bondage practice without basis in recorded evidence. Western rope bondage, on the other hand, holds its origins in the early days of rope bondage pornography in the United States (Sisson, 2007).

While rope as a practice is beginning to be explored, the unique and disparate social world of rope bondage has rarely been the focus of academic inquiry. Therefore, I use data I have gathered via interviews with rope bondage practitioners alongside personal experiences in this practice and world to describe the subculture (see Wilkinson & Kitzinger, 2013). In this chapter I use *subculture* to refer to the overarching culture of rope bondage or BDSM-related norms, relationships, and activities, while *community* refers to a more micro type of social organization constructed and developed by the everyday interactions of people (Bessant, 2018). We can also understand *subculture* to be an umbrella underneath which "communities" operate; the framework of rope bondage subculture influences the interactions that take place within communities (Wignall, 2022).

This chapter will explore the social and personal realities of being a rope bondage practitioner. These experiences provide critical insights that may aid us in understanding the wider dynamics at play in BDSM subculture—from the sense of belonging and joy that motivates people to invest in these spaces to the marginalization and oppression that people relate experiencing within both the rope bondage and the BDSM scenes. This includes contrasting ideas of what community is along with rich descriptions of their social and personal experiences of rope and its related social world.

Method

This chapter is informed by my doctoral research study, a qualitative exploration of the lived experience of rope bondage practitioners (see Jones, 2020, for an in-depth description of methodology). This work is grounded in an insider perspective as well as a critical theoretical understanding of the social world as shaped by power dynamics and oppression. The theoretical orientation of this work consists of two pieces: a critical overarching approach to society, power, and oppression that is influenced by feminist theory (hooks, 1992), critical race theory (Delgado & Stefancic, 2017), and critical disability studies (Goodley, 2013) and a symbolic interactionist approach to the meaning people ascribe to their actions. Symbolic interactionism holds that social reality is constructed and experienced in interactions, and this type of inquiry generally involves a micro-scale investigation of subjective human experiences and meaning-making (Blumer, 1969). Symbolic interactionism lends itself well to the interpretivist paradigm that I adopt in this research, which understands reality and knowledge as socially constructed (Tracy, 2013).

Participants

Participants were recruited from Fetlife (a well-known social networking site for BDSMers) and Twitter in 2018. There were several inclusion criteria: people could volunteer if they (a) were at least 18 years old, (b) currently resided in Canada or the United States, and (c) had been practicing rope bondage for at least 6 months (broadly interpreted). There were two exclusion criteria centered on mitigating a potential risk of insider research: Potential participants were excluded if we had a current or past romantic or sexual relationship or a current or past dominant/submissive relationship where I was the dominant partner.

Given the high number of people who responded to my call for participants, after initial recruitment I incorporated quota sampling in four major categories: race/ethnicity, gender, sexuality, and ability (Kilty, 2014). This sampling method prioritized the selection of at least two people of color, at least two people with a disability, at least two people with a queer and/ or LGBTQIA+ sexuality, and at least two gender-diverse (e.g., transgender, genderfluid, genderqueer, agender, two-spirit) people. Table 3.1 provides demographic information on the participants who were selected.

Procedure

I interviewed local participants ($n = 12$) in person and non-local participants ($n = 11$) via Skype and telephone calls. Semi-structured interviews were used and ranged from 40 minutes to 150 minutes. Questions primarily focused on exploring the experience of "doing rope," discussing rope bondage subculture, and communities and their connections to them.

Analysis

I conducted an iterative analysis (Tracy, 2013) of the results of data collection using several different methods. Each stage of analysis included in-depth discussion with my doctoral supervisor. First, I wrote memos after each interview to capture my initial impressions, and so a quiet kind of analysis began after the first interview. When transcriptions were finished, I developed a descriptive codebook of preliminary-cycle codes that described the literal words of my participants. These codes were simple ones like *origin stories*, *pictures*, and *money*. This process allowed me to separate types of stories and commentaries into large thematic *buckets* instead of coding minutely at the start. Some of these buckets were as large as *ROPE*² (with subcategories for practice, play, styles, materials); *knowledge and information*; *social, inside*, and *social, outside*. One of the most surprising and rewarding categories emerged during data immersion as *pleasure* and morphed into *sensation, feelings, pleasure*, to encompass all of the accounts and thoughts about people's feelings about or during rope play. This code resulted in 144 references, the third largest after *social, inside* (280) and *ROPE* (174).

After primary-cycle coding, I developed a second-level or analytical codebook by repeating the above process with the codes I chose to focus on: discussions of community/subculture, experiences of marginalization by race and disability, and experiences of pleasure. These choices were informed primarily by the prevalence and size of the code in addition to unique academic value (e.g., little research explores racism and ableism within BDSM

Table 3.1 Participant Demographics[a]

	Number of participants
Age (years)	
21–25	5
26–30	7
31–35	4
36–40	3
41–45	3
46–50	1
Gender	
Transgender women	2
Cisgender women	11
Transgender/questioning men	1
Cisgender men	5
Nonbinary/genderqueer	3
Agender	1
Sexuality	
Heterosexual/straight	6
Bisexual	5
Pansexual	5
Demisexual[b]	3
Asexual	1
Homoflexible	1
Queer, otherwise not specified	4
Race	
White	16
Multiracial	1
Black	3
Asian	3
Disability	
Identified a disability	11
Did not identify a disability	12

[a]Local and non-local participants are all included in this table. Aside from some slight age trends (more younger participants interviewed locally), demographics had similar ranges across these two groups, and for this chapter they were treated as one data set.

[b]Three participants identified as demisexual in addition to another sexuality.

or rope bondage subcultures). This cycle of thematic coding was informed by the participants' accounts and the project's theoretical orientation and examined themes like *challenges, discrimination*; *joy, happiness*; *resistance*; and *racism*.

The full analysis did not show differences between people's accounts based on location aside from region-specific details (e.g., physical availability of events from one city to the next), and the themes reported in this chapter—*pleasure, exclusion, community*—were drawn across the full set of both local and non-local participants.

Ethics

This study followed institutional and methodological standards of ethics, alongside the ethics of the kink scene. In some ways, the latter standard is higher than those held by ethics review boards as kink etiquette and approaches to consent often focus on micro-interactions between individuals (Bauer, 2020). For example, people in progressive kink communities and spaces are increasingly working on respecting and using appropriate pronouns, gaining explicit consent before even mild physical contact, being transparent about motivations and intentions, and prioritizing enthusiastic informed consent which should be ongoing and revocable at any time. I have held these principles close throughout this study, and they informed the ethics protocol and application. To maintain anonymity, each participant was offered the opportunity to choose their pseudonym; roughly half of participants chose this, and the others were assigned a random name.

Insider Research and Reflexivity

Navigating my insider status was complex. As an insider who used my networks for recruitment, I leveraged my personal connections and reputation to gain the trust of (and access to) people normally wary of researchers. I felt that my intentions were good and the process transparent, and I received only positive feedback on my recruitment, design, and final published dissertation. I was (and am) accountable to my community for my actions as a researcher and the results that I publish. This influenced my actions primarily through a dedication to transparency and knowledge translation as I ensure that community members, particularly participants, have access to resulting publications, are regularly informed of how this data is being used, and are invited to share feedback with me without consequence.

Constructing, Experiencing, and Resisting Rope Bondage Subculture and Community

Tying and Being Tied: Defining and Understanding Rope Bondage

At its most literal, rope bondage is the practice of tying a person with rope, tying oneself in rope, and/or being a person tied by another in rope. These people can be of any gender, ethnicity, race, body shape and size, dis/ability, class, sexual orientation, and more and may tie in any power configuration one can imagine. Every aspect of rope bondage can (and often does) have meaning for rope bondage practitioners.

Rope can be made of many flexible natural and synthetic materials, but the types most commonly used in bondage are natural fiber rope made of jute, hemp, or cotton (see Nawakiri, 2017) and synthetic rope, which is usually made of nylon, polyester, or artificial hemp. The tactile experience of rope is one of the elements around which people's passions can be organized. When I asked Adam what rope bondage means to him, he said, "So much of rope bondage for me is in the texture, the feeling, the smell, and . . . just the total sensory experience of the rope itself." These qualities differ wildly depending on how a piece of rope is constructed and conditioned. Hemp may smell like grass or like a barnyard; jute may smell like beeswax; nylon may be thrilling in its softness; paracord may be deliciously painful in its thinness. Tara, a bisexual, white, cisgender woman in her late 20s (rope top, bottom, and self-tier), explained how the physical qualities of rope and its manufacture can impact a person's physical, emotional, and sensory experience:

> From the first point where you hear the jute come out and it's a little bit creaky, and then the jute dust when you open the first coil, and the dust goes like a little explosion in the air. A lot of the times they're treated with beeswax or jojoba oil or something, so it's always really smooth and usually really shiny, and often this deep gold, like a lion's mane kind of color. . . . From the first touch of the rope on my skin, it's like when you're listening to a beautiful piece of music and you get the goosebumps and all

your hairs stand up on end, and your whole body from your head to your toes has shivers. That's how I get as soon as rope touches me with the intention to start a scene.

Past the physical details of the material, rope bondage as a critically visceral and potentially disruptive experience resists definition. Practitioners describe rope bondage as "infinite expression," as "all-consuming of my intention," and as "paradoxically freeing." Participants reported that rope bondage is an expressive human experience, a sadomasochistic pursuit, a high art, an athletic endeavor, a personal grounding technique, a connective practice, a tool for intimate communication, a sexual experience, and more.

When considering sexuality and rope bondage, participants expressed complicated perspectives on the pleasure of rope bondage. It is not simply that rope bondage is or is not sexual but that the complexity of feelings, sensations, pleasures, and emotions that people experience do not neatly fit into a single descriptive box like *sex*.

Grappling with Rope Bondage "Community"

Participants in this study reported that social networks, community, and/ or subculture were critical aspects of their experiences with rope. For a small few these narratives were strictly positive or neutral, but for most they were a tense series of stories and feelings that left them with mixed feelings. Their stories of rope were often bound up in and integrally linked to their experiences of the social; similarly, their belonging in some of these social worlds was conditionally connected to their ongoing rope bondage practice. When people stopped doing rope (or being able to do rope, as in the case of a temporary or permanent disability), they told me their stories of "leaving" community or "taking a break"; when people felt themselves alienated from or pushed out of social spaces, they frequently recounted feeling disconnected from and disillusioned about their private and personal rope play.

Bird, a pansexual, demisexual, white, cisgender woman in her early 30s (rope top, bottom, and "some self-tying"), is one practitioner whose accounts reflected a common (but not universal) understanding of "community" that applies both to what you do and where you go and to the people that you feel affinity with:

There's two very distinct communities in my head that are mine. There is a local one, and I think that comes from the side of me that organizes events and is trying to make a difference here. So I think [about] the rope people in [city] and how to do things that might help [city] people. But . . . my rope community is as much about beliefs as it is about location. So I have this second one that's less of the organizer brain and more of the "this is where I feel like I belong." And those are the ones that share similar values . . . like bottoming has become valued more, or people who think that consent is not simple and it should be explicit and it's for everything. . . . And so for me it's almost like that's my second community, is people who are . . . not same-minded, but like-minded. And are into rope bondage, obviously.

For Bird, some people overlapped between these communities, but there was a functional difference between the community that she organizes in— her local community, open to anyone interested in and physically able to attend—and her community of affinity and belonging, which included local as well as national and international connections.

Like Bird, many rope bondage practitioners felt it was important to de-lineate between communities that they consciously contributed to which aligned with their values and beliefs and communities that they belonged to by virtue of shared practice and/or physical space. Personal communities were relayed as critical to a participant's sense of self, with some of the most meaningful relationships in their life in these communities, while other manifestations of community were described in apathetic or value-neutral tones. For example, Evelyn, an East Asian cisgender woman rope switch (a label adopted by some people who both tie and enjoy being tied) described community as follows: "I mean, you go to a party and odds are you'll rec-ognize a bunch of people, and those people will also recognize a bunch of people."

Some rope bondage practitioners invest a great deal of energy into the cre-ation and support of their communities. Angel, a pansexual, white, trans-gender woman in her mid-40s (rope bottom), was setting up her own event; within the context of her interview at this point, *community* seemed to mean the collection of events and people in her local area, which require energy and investment from its members to thrive. However, when asked what she meant by "rope community," she answered,

Well, I mean there's the general rope community to include everyone in the world obviously. You know, I think rope is, excuse the pun, it's very binding. . . . you've got your local communities that, you know, we visit people who you get to practice with, you get to know.

Yet, some participants recognized that (a) community[3] exists and conceptualized themselves as not belonging to it. Chen, an East Asian gender-questioning man in his early 20s (rope bottom), sometimes attended events, but he felt uncomfortable:

> I've been to [around 10–15] events, but after that not a lot because . . . well, to be honest, I don't feel people really go there to learn. They more go there to try out new stuff, and also for people without partners. Especially me being male biologically, it's not that easy to find a good partner as well. And also it feels like there's kind of a barrier. It may be cultural, I don't know, for me to feel good to talk to people . . . to talk to a total stranger in that kind of setting. I don't feel very comfortable, and I wasn't able to find a good partner. So I just don't bother going there anymore.

He had neither a close friendship-based type of rope bondage community nor a geographical one despite attempts to attend local events and make friends. Chen's experience is reflective of Pohtinen's work (2017, p. 29) on Finnish kink communities, which argues that "a lonely individual who is not actively invited to participate may indeed feel estranged and not very safe" in community. Pohtinen (2017) argues that physical presence at events is not enough to be welcomed into kink community and that the experience of a "not-so-warm welcome" can be alienating and agonizing, as it was for Chen.

These complex themes of contrasting communities, energy investment, and alienation wove through many of the participants' accounts of community and contribute to building an overarching understanding of rope bondage subculture. Althea, a bisexual, white, cisgender woman in her early 30s (rope bottom), explained that her community was complicated and shaped by recent interpersonal turmoil:

> [The rope bondage community] looks very divided. And it looks very confused, and that makes me really sad. And sometimes the rope community looks helpful, especially when the parts that are divided can come together. . . . I've come back from [events] feeling, feeling a high because of within that rope community, like sure we're being tied up with each other and we're all giggling, but people are braiding my hair. . . . in these

communities when it feels good in the rope community is when I can really embrace parts of myself.

There are two different approaches to community in these accounts that are remarkably clear reflections of Bessant's (2018) *intentional communities*, built on communion, shared values, and beliefs, and *communities of practice*, which arise from a shared foundation of collective experience, knowledge, and information transference. Rope bondage practitioners reported both types of community, which sometimes overlapped, and often had qualitatively different impacts on their lives. Some rope bondage practitioners who did not feel they could attend local events due to their own values and beliefs—for example, if education was taught by a known consent violator or if a venue was owned by an overtly racist person—explained how they had lost access to important information that they needed to pursue advanced parts of the practice semi-safely, like suspension and sadomasochistic ties.

"Colonial Ideas" versus "Sexy Fun": Alienation and Exclusion in Rope Bondage Spaces

Participants who shared stories of being pushed out of or alienated from their local communities of practice were disproportionately people of color and disabled kinksters. These practitioners shared feelings ranging from abandonment, despair, frustration, sadness, and anger to a disconnection from their craft and even themselves. Some attempted to address the problems they witnessed, such as writing and developing safer space policies for an event, working to improve local consent practices through education, and conducting anti-racist activist work within the scene. Often, though, practitioners chose to partially or fully avoid "community" virtual and/or physical spaces as they did not want to continue suffering ongoing microaggressions, occupying a space that did not feel safe, or implicitly supporting hosts, educators, and venue owners who did not reflect their values. In many cases people reported moving from one end of this engagement spectrum to the other as their capacity and enthusiasm for community work waxed and waned.

Adrien, a queer, demisexual, Black, non-binary/genderqueer person in their early 30s (rope bottom and self-tier), shared their accounts of attempting to organize or find intentional and inclusive community spaces both locally and internationally, which was an uphill battle:

> I'm finding myself incredibly frustrated with folks I see in community organizing who are constantly trying to . . . appeal to people who don't care about things like making sure that the space isn't racist. [Laughs] Like, who don't care about things like making sure that the space is accessible to people economically, who don't care about building a space for other people, they want to build a space for their own egos. . . . If someone isn't interested in building a safer space, meaning sort of in the activity sense of a space that is as safe as possible for the people in it, so that it's not racist, it's not being homomisic,[4] that oppressive and colonial ideals are not being upheld within that space, if they don't *care* about making sure that that's not *happening* and making sure that that space is being deconstructed in a way that makes it safe for everyone, then I don't personally really care about having that person in my space. If their need to have sexy fun is more important than making sure that people who are in the space feel welcome and safe? Then we have different goals, and I'm not organizing for those people in that case.

The kind of engagement with community that Adrien describes is representative of a small number of organizer-type participants who work to create separate spaces that affirm their values and resist some of the problems (like racism) that pervade the mainstream kink scene (Cruz, 2016; Feast, 2020).

Each of the seven racialized participants described an overwhelmingly white local scene where they were hyper-visible when they chose to attend. When I asked Kristen, a demisexual, Black, cis woman in her early 40s (rope bottom and self-tier), about other Black people in her community, she said,

> They exist. A lot of them . . . you won't see a lot of [them]. Every time I go out, if I go to a rope thing, it's guaranteed I will be one of two. Because there's another one that comes up from the south. If I go to a dungeon, there's a good chance I'm going to be the only one. . . . Like I'll go to some of the [major metropolitan area] ones. And I've been to like the [more rural] ones, and . . . yeah, I was the only person in the room. The only African American in the room. And I know there are more in the community.

Relatedly, Ewok, a straight, Black, cis man in his mid-20s (rope top), said, "I would say I'm not seeing a *single* rope top that [is] not white. I'm not just saying like African American, I'm saying was not white." Adrien theorized about this phenomenon when they explained that "it's not that kinky people of color don't exist, it's that there are so few of us, and when you don't see people like you in spaces, you don't feel safe going into spaces."

They painted a picture of an exhausting and white-dominated scene that drains and alienates people of color, leading their visible presences to be brief, signaling to other racialized folks that those spaces are not safe. Adrien felt that the lack of safety may be overt, as in the case of "racist assholes"; but they also identified a passive type of danger from complacent white people who claim to want diverse and safe spaces but "don't want to put the work in to change it" from the (unsafe) current environment.

Disabled rope bondage practitioners' accounts of community were similarly laden with stories of exclusion and discrimination from rope bondage communities and/or spaces. In some cases, a participant was both racialized and disabled, like Adrien. Of the 23 participants interviewed for this project, 11 of them identified as having some type of disability, with some using mobility devices such as canes and a large proportion experiencing chronic pain.

When participants spoke of personal barriers to their full and enjoyable participation in rope bondage, they sometimes commented on challenges with their own disabilities but more commonly cited social discrimination, inadequate educational opportunities, and inaccessible locations as the true barriers. For example, Robin, a queer, white, non-binary person in their late 20s ("self-rigger, bottom, top, in that order"), explained that she came to self-tying as a way to play with rope despite a difficulty finding partners:

> Being a disabled bottom, it's really hard to find partners. So, I just kind of paid attention to the few times I was suspended, or I'd pay attention to classes where I was bottoming. I'd watch other people suspend. And once you've done enough floor work, like moving to self-suspending is not super difficult as long as you're paying attention to what all the riggers are saying.

Robin had not been to a "rope event" in 2 years or more because when she did go, she found they taught a "very specific way of tying for a very specific body" that did not suit her:

A lot of that doesn't work for me. Like even the standard hip harness. I can't put weight on my waist because I have a paralyzed digestive system that makes me feel really sick. But I can put a lot of weight on my hips because my bones really don't care about anything anymore. So, like, a lot of the common ways to teach tying don't work for me. Or they expect you to weigh less than I do.

In some ways, Robin's experiences with chronic illness and disability gave them strengths as a rope bottom that they otherwise may not have had, from being able to manage a lot of weight on their bones to pain processing skills. Robin worked with rope and their body, picking up further tools and skills where they could, and self-taught to find out what worked for them. Their trial and error process (which they described as "well, that hurts, that didn't work. Or oh, that really helps!") led them to a style of tying that meets their needs and desires and works for their body absent the opportunities of their abled peers. Still, they explain that they are often infantilized and desexualized as a disabled person, a phenomenon that is replicated outside of rope bondage spaces as well (Kattari, 2015; Reynolds, 2007).

"The Rope Community Is Love": Belonging, Pleasure, and Resistance

The pleasures of rope bondage are a driving factor of why people continue to engage with rope bondage community and subculture even when there is potential for harm, alienation, and oppression. These pleasures motivate some people to belong to, and fight to improve, this world even while experiencing adversity. For many participants, rope—and even rope bondage community—provides something valuable and compelling that they cannot find elsewhere. The meaning and purpose of rope, as both a practice and a social world, were regularly described in terms almost indescribable. For example, Olivia, a Black, bisexual, cis woman in her early 40s (self-tier and rope bottom), said,

Rope in particular, because I experience it not just as bondage, it's just infinite possibilities. It's art, it's communication, it's all sorts of things. It's a lens and a focus. It's just a wonderful medium for expression that I found for myself. And that applies to all of my roles—as a top, as a bottom, as a switch, as a self-suspender. It's just infinite in a way that so few things are.

As Althea outlined, "rope has facilitated therapy, in times where I've needed to *belong* somewhere, may it be as part of the community with rope, or just physically tied down." When practitioners did leave the community and/or the practice due to the bad parts, as in the case of Adrien and others, losing the good left them with feelings of loss, alienation, nostalgia, and sometimes anger.

Celeste, a white, queer, cis woman in her early 20s (rope bottom), explained what it means to say that her life is centered on rope bondage:

> It's like all of my life. I mean, it's my job, it's my passion, it's my way of having sex with someone, for the most part. Not to say that I have necessarily a lot of sex in rope. . . . But rope is my primary way of having sexual contact with other people. . . . it's my job. It's my community. It's my primary source of friends and social interaction. Rope bondage is everything to me.

Celeste was one of the few participants who was a professional rope bondage player, teacher, and performer but their sentiment was reflected by more than half of participants: rope bondage is everything. It stands for something deeply private and personal as well as something social and external. The connection between private play and public engagement frequently overlapped like this, suggesting that one cannot be considered without the other.

For some rope bondage practitioners, accessing these feelings and spaces is relatively easy, particularly if they do not experience the alienation and oppression reported by others. For the more marginalized practitioners, finding relationships and spaces safe enough to practice rope and find their joy took work. They reported creating their own events, teaching their friends and partners, engaging in herculean efforts to try to fix problematic spaces, and more. For example, Stephanie, a bisexual, white, cis woman in her late 20s (rope top, bottom, and self-tier), explained battling the financial barriers to rope education:

> It started out with a lot of book learning and then just hands-on practicing. And then I started learning more options for getting in-person education. And they were super, super financially inaccessible because I'm a single parent who was on social assistance. So I started organizing my own events.

G, a white, agender, asexual person in their late 30s (rope switch), shared their experience looking for a safe enough place that they could practice rope and connect with people in a way that honored their gender and sexuality:

> I tried to get into the rope scene in [city] but the 3 big riggers here were not open to me because of my bigger body, because of my gender, because I didn't want to have sexual play with one of the persons. So I saw a posting about [event] in [another city] and drove 2 hours, and it was one of the best experiences I ever had just right off the bat. And I've never missed an [event name] since. Now I'm hosting some of the [event name]s.

Olivia explained how and why she consciously occupies space as an instructor:

> Race, definitely, I think has an impact [on my experience]. My body size, because I'm not a standard rope model size by, you know, the American average. . . . I get a tremendous amount of support and positivity from people who are happy to see people who look like them. Actually it's one of the things that pushed me to be an instructor. Because there just aren't a lot of people who look like me with the presenter badge.

She later explained how this dynamic motivates her photography and modeling as well: "part of the thing that has motivated me to document and photograph my journey is just to be like, 'hey, I would like to see more fat, 40-year-old Black women out in rope. So I'm going to take some pictures.'"

This work, and the dedication to fulfilling their desires, can be understood as a process of resistance (Hannem, 2012) as these participants refused to allow axes of oppression that play out in rope subculture—like racism, cis normativity, ableism, and fat phobia—to prevent their engagement in and with rope bondage. Being in these social spheres of like-minded friends, lovers, acquaintances, teachers, and even strangers was often framed as a person's reprieve from a less accepting wider world, a place where they were able to be themselves.

Post-interview, I asked each participant if there is anything they wish people outside of the community knew about rope bondage. Althea answered,

I wish that they knew the love that it feels in your heart, that makes rope *so* important. I feel like they just look at these pictures and I understand why there's that disconnect, but they don't know that. Sure I'm being tied in this really strange position, but before it happened, I was asked how my day was. And I was fed. And I was taken care of. And I was loved.

This quote perfectly exemplifies why participants were so consistent in connecting their experiences of community with their pleasure and joy in rope.

Discussion

Considering the intricacies of rope bondage subculture and community allows us to take a lesson from kinksters and engage with the complexity of a thing that causes both pleasure and pain. Being bound to rope bondage communities can be, like rope play itself, pleasurable, painful, expressive, connective, and transformative; it can be a site of abuse and a site of empowerment. Rope is simultaneously a tool, a passion, and a fulcrum around which a subculture and its communities turn.

The intricacies of rope bondage communities shed light on the overarching social structure of rope bondage subculture. The subculture is the environment within which these communities and individuals operate and communicate with one another, borrowing techniques, words, norms, etiquettes, values, and even people across and between one another. This subcultural environment encompasses a social sphere where communities do not act or exist in isolation. From the accounts of these practitioners—people connected to the pansexual BDSM subculture who connect at least partly online—that subculture is characterized by complicated interplays of pleasure, power, oppression, joy, and resistance as people connect and communicate over rope. Some rope bondage practitioners, particularly people marginalized by race and disability, report experiences of oppression and power differentials within this subculture that reflect and, sometimes, even exceed the oppressions they face outside of BDSM. These perspectives intertwine when rope bondage practitioners grapple with their love and disillusionment with rope bondage and the potential utopia that some glimpse during their rope bondage careers.

Notes

1. A *self-tier* is someone who ties themselves in rope. Spelling varies between *tier* and *tyer*, with some using a hyphen and some not.
2. I wrote this code in all capitals initially because it felt ridiculous and too obvious to code for *rope* during a rope bondage study. Later I found that having such a code was critical during data analysis.
3. Even the grammar ranged between and through interviews, from *community* as an abstract concept (e.g., "it is hard to find community") to *a/the community* as a noun or object (e.g., "I joined the community").
4. *-misic* or *-misia* (suffix): Evolving language to replace *-phobia* as a suffix when speaking of bigotry to center hatred rather than fear. For example, *transmisic* instead of *transphobic* and *homomisia* instead of *homophobia*.

References

Bauer, R. (2008). Transgressive and transformative gendered sexual practices and white privileges: The case of the dyke/trans BDSM communities. *Women's Studies Quarterly*, *36*(3/4), 233–253. https://www.jstor.org/stable/27649798

Bauer, R. (2020). Queering consent: Negotiating critical consent in les-bi-trans-queer BDSM contexts. *Sexualities*, *24*(5–6), 1–17. https://doi.org/10.1177/136346072 0973902

Bessant, K. C. (2018). *The relational fabric of community*. Palgrave Macmillan.

Blumer, H. (1969). *Symbolic interactionism: Perspective and method*. Prentice-Hall.

Cruz, A. (2016). *The color of kink: Black women, BDSM, and pornography*. New York University Press.

Delgado, R., & Stefancic, J. (2017). *Critical race theory: An introduction* (3rd ed.). New York University Press.

Feast, F. (2020). *Users on a site for kink people say the racism has become unsustainable*. Buzzfeed News. https://www.buzzfeednews.com/article/fancyfeast/fetlife-racism-kink-alt-right-anti-semitism

Galati, M. (2017). *The therapeutic impact of rope bondage: A case study in the UK* [Unpublished master's thesis]. University College London.

Goodley, D. (2013). Dis/entangling critical disability studies. *Disability & Society*, *28*(5), 631–644. https://doi.org/10.1080/09687599.2012.717884

Hannem, S. (2012). Theorizing stigma and the politics of resistance. In S. Hannem & C. Bruckert (Eds.), *Stigma revisited: Implications of the mark* (pp. 10–28). University of Ottawa Press.

Harrington, L., & RiggerJay. (2015). *Shibari you can use: Japanese rope bondage and erotic macramé* (2nd ed.). Mystic Productions Press.

hooks, b. (1992). *Black looks: Race and representation* (1st ed.). South End Press.

Jones, Z. (2020). *Pleasure, community, and marginalization in rope bondage* [Unpublished doctoral dissertation]. Carleton University.

Kattari, S. K. (2015). "Getting it": Identity and sexual communication for sexual and gender minorities with physical disabilities. *Sexuality and Culture, 19*(4), 882–899. https://doi.org/10.1007/s12119-015-9298-x

Kent, D. (2010). *Complete shibari: Land* (Vol. 1). Mental Gears Publishing.

Kilty, J. M. (2014). The evolution of feminist research in the criminological enterprise: The Canadian experience. In J. M. Kilty, M. Felices-Luna & S. C. Fabian (Eds.), *Demarginalizing voices: Commitment, emotion, and action in qualitative research* (pp. 125–146). UBC Press.

Lee, E. M., Klement, K. R., & Sagarin, B. J. (2015). Double hanging during consensual sexual asphyxia: A response to Roma, Pazzelli, Pompili, Girardi, and Ferracuti (2013). *Archives of Sexual Behavior, 44,* 1751–1753. https://doi.org/10.1007/s10508-015-0575-4

Martin, R. J. (2011). *Powerful exchanges: Ritual and subjectivity in Berlin's BDSM scene* [Unpublished doctoral dissertation]. Princeton University.

Midori, & Morey, C. (2002). *The seductive art of Japanese bondage.* Greenery Press.

Nawakiri, S. (2017). *Essence of shibari: Kinbaku and Japanese rope bondage* (1st ed.). Mystic Productions Press.

Newmahr, S. (2011). *Playing on the edge: Sadomasochism, risk, and intimacy.* Indiana University Press.

Ordean, I.-C., & Pennington, H. (2019). Rope bondage and affective embodiments: A rhizomatic analysis. *Revista Corpo-grafías: Estudios críticos de y desde los cuerpos, 6*(6), 64–77. http://hdl.handle.net/11349/18331

Pennington, H. (2017). Kinbaku: The liminal and the liminoid in ritual performance. *Performance of the Real, 1*(1), 42–51. https://www.otago.ac.nz/performance-of-the-real/otago666946.pdf

Pohtinen, J. (2017). Creating a feeling of belonging: Solidarity in Finnish kink communities. *SQS, 10*(1–2), 21–34. https://doi.org/10.23980/sqs.63645

Reynolds, D. (2007). Disability and BDSM: Bob Flanagan and the case for sexual rights. *Sexuality Research & Social Policy, 4*(1), Article 40. https://doi.org/10.1525/srsp.2007.4.1.40

Sheela, C. S. (2008). *The state of discipline: Chinese masculinity and BDSM in Singapore* [Unpublished master's thesis]. National University of Singapore.

Simula, B. L. (2019). Pleasure, power, and pain: A review of the literature on the experiences of BDSM participants. *Sociology Compass, 13*(3), Article e12668. https://doi.org/10.1111/soc4.12668

Sisson, K. (2007). The cultural formation of S/M: History and analysis. In D. Langridge, M.-J. Barker, & C. Richards (Eds.), *Safe, sane and consensual: Contemporary perspectives on sadomasochism* (pp. 16–40). Palgrave Macmillan.

Tracy, S. J. (2013). *Qualitative research methods: Collecting evidence, crafting analysis, communicating impact.* Wiley-Blackwell.

Wignall, L. (2022). *Kinky in the digital age: Gay men's subcultures and social identities.* Oxford University Press.

Wilkinson, S., & Kitzinger, C. (2013). Representing our own experience: Issues in "insider" research. *Psychology of Women Quarterly, 37*(2), 251–255. https://doi.org/10.1177%2F0361684313483111

Wiseman, J. (1996). *SM 101: A realistic introduction.* Greenery Press.

4

Play, Performativity, and the Production of a Pup Identity in the United States

Robert M. Matchett and Dana Berkowitz

Introduction

Pup play is a socio-sexual kink in which a human actor's role play incorporates the affective, behavioral, and cognitive performances of young dogs (pups); pup play is associated with the actor accessing a distinct "pup identity,"[1] which sometimes is embodied through the application of specialized gear (Lawson & Langdridge, 2020; Wignall & McCormack, 2017). Emerging out of the BDSM and leatherman communities (Lawson & Langdridge, 2020), pup play accentuates play and the forging of a pup identity. Leathermen ascribed to a strict regimen of protocols, including a hierarchical structure in which actors engaging in leather scenes took on and performed various roles, including sirs, doms, daddies, masters, subs, boys, and slaves (Bauer, 2019; Moskowitz et al., 2011; St. Clair, 2015). Most of these performative roles fit into binary categories of dominants or subordinates (Martinez, 2018; St. Clair, 2015). When protocols were violated, punishments were used to train the subordinates. One punishment was being reduced to the role of a dog-slave, with the role stripping the boys of their humanity by requiring them to be on all fours and to eat and drink from a dog bowl and forbidding them from communicating verbally (Daniels, 2006; Lawson & Langdridge, 2020; St. Clair, 2015). Importantly, while the dog-slave role was a punishment, some participated in this activity for the humiliating and dehumanizing components absent of punishment (Wignall, 2022).

While some incorporate humiliation and dehumanization into their versions of pup play, others stray from the subcommunity's historical conceptualizations. The "new puppy movement" signifies a shift in ideology

Robert M. Matchett and Dana Berkowitz, *Play, Performativity, and the Production of a Pup Identity in the United States*
In: *The Power of BDSM.* Edited by: Brandy L. Simula, Robin Bauer, and Liam Wignall, Oxford University Press.
© Oxford University Press 2023. DOI: 10.1093/oso/9780197658598.003.0005

from the "Old Guard"[2] perspectives and centers the core focus around play (St. Clair, 2015). As a result, if present at all, rules became more flexible, and pups employ this role by choice. This erasure of rules (regardless of how strict) also fits in with newer kink narratives that emphasize play (Wignall, 2022).

Play is such an essential element that it is built into all facets of the pup subculture. As Langdridge and Lawson (2019) point out, play's importance is highlighted by the choice to embody pups rather than dogs, due to their playful nature (p. 2209). Play is a core element of our developmental process that originates in childhood and lasts through adulthood; it is pleasurable, intrinsically motivated, freely chosen, actively engaged, imaginative, non-literal, and transcendent (White, 2013). As we age, play becomes more evolved and complex; we can take on various roles and build elaborate imaginary universes (White, 2013). We do not usually associate adults with playfulness, and play is seen as childish and immature. However, some researchers have challenged this perspective and explored how play can be a regular and normal function of adulthood (Aune & Wong, 2002; Brown & Stenros, 2018; Paasonen, 2018). One way adults engage in play is sexual play. The enmeshing of sex and play centers sexuality in pleasure, and elements of play, including toys, gear, and role-playing, have long been used as elixirs to treat a dimming relationship (Paasonen, 2018). Grey (2011) discusses several ways that play benefits individuals including reducing stress, improving cognition, regulating emotions, making friends, and experiencing joy.

One central element of engaging in sexual play that is well known within BDSM subcultures is the notion of a *headspace*, described as a state of mind that allows participants to engage with a role they are taking on; variations can include *subspace*, *top space*, and *pup headspace* (Simula, 2017). This has been described in research on pup play (Wignall, 2022; Wignall & McCormack, 2017), where an individual becomes so focused on the play that they begin to forget about the world around them. Connecting with pup headspace can be challenging; while some pups can simply enter headspace through the application of gear, others must engage with a more arduous process. Pup headspace manifests in multiple variations and can bring out an uninhibited pup identity that is somewhat distinct from an individual's human identity. The experience of becoming a pup allows individuals to engage in self-discovery through a nonhuman role (Langdridge & Lawson, 2019).

Theorizing Pup Play

Sexuality scholars studying pup identities could benefit from sociological theories that explore how individuals create, navigate, and perform their identities. Sociologist Erving Goffman famously said, "All the world is not, of course, a stage, but the crucial ways in which it isn't are not easy to specify" (1959, p. 72). Perhaps the struggle in specifying why the world is not a stage is that the human experience is centered in interactions, which follow social rules, causing the acting to happen subconsciously. While Goffman's work provides insight into how individuals perform aspects of their daily lives, it is a limited framework through which to understand the pup experience in the sense that Goffmanian performers do not know that they are acting (Schechner, 1988).

More relevant to our study is Schechner (1988), a performance scholar who expanded on Goffman's work to examine the experiences of individuals who intentionally shift between roles. Schechner's (1988) theoretical constructs can be applied to pup play as pups engage in a transformative and transportive process as they shift between their persona and pup identity. Much like the professional actors Schechner studied, individuals come into pup play already socialized; they must engage in identity work and deconstruct themselves into bits, which are "the smallest repeatable strips of action" (Schechner, 1988, p. 321). Once their identity is deconstructed into bits, the individual can reconstruct themselves into their pup identity. This deconstructive–reconstructive process is a profoundly reflexive practice. For pups, this means that they must send their human self to the backstage role as an observer and bring their pup identity to the front stage as the actor. This intensive process requires individuals to deconstruct and reconstruct themselves multiple times as they intentionally shift between roles. Thus, adopting the pup role and providing a genuine performance necessitates a great deal of identity work.

Arlie Hochschild's work on emotional labor is also a useful lens through which to view pup identity work (1983). Hochschild documented how flight attendants managed their affective performances to ensure that clients had an enjoyable travel experience. Hochschild coined the term *emotion labor* to capture this type of impression management, which involves manipulating one's feelings to transmit a certain impression. Hochschild documented that the flight attendants engaged in different layers of acting to achieve these workplace performances—surface acting and deep acting. Whereas in surface acting, the subject manipulates their expressions to display a particular emotion that they do not feel, in deep acting, the subject produces the internal emotions of the performance. While Hochschild's work initially explored the emotion work of flight attendants, these concepts have been applied to convenience store cashiers, fast food workers, hair stylists, ride operators at Disneyland, lawyers, and detectives (Steinberg & Figart, 1999). Hochschild's concepts of emotion work, surface acting, and deep acting are useful tools to conceptualize how pups move through different dimensions of pup headspace. For instance, whereas new pups may only be able to engage in surface acting due to the difficulty of accessing the pup headspace, seasoned pups can access the pup headspace through deep acting. Finally, some pups may transcend deep acting and access a state of genuine acting where they can maintain the pup headspace for long periods of time. Taken together, Goffman's, Schechner's, and Hochschild's works provide us with the conceptual scaffolding through which to understand how subjects maneuver their identities when engaging in pup play.

Method

The first author collected data from spring 2020 to summer 2020. During data collection, the United States was under a stay-at-home order due to the COVID-19 pandemic. As a result, all recruitment efforts took place online. Following previous research (Wignall, 2017), we turned to social media platforms with large pup communities such as Instagram, Twitter, and Facebook. Additionally, the Center for Positive Sexuality, a non-profit organization that addresses social issues through sex-positive research and education, endorsed the project and released a call for participants on its website and social media.

Participants

Thirty pups participated in the interviews. The ages of the participants ranged from 18 to 48 (mean = 28). In terms of race, 26 individuals self-identified as white, one identified as Asian, two identified as Black, and one identified as mixed-race. The sample included one individual who identified as queer and agender, one pansexual woman, one lesbian woman, one bisexual transwoman, two bisexual men, and 23 gay men. One participant was from the Northeast, four participants were from Midwestern states, seven participants were from the Western states, seven participants were from Southwestern states, and 11 participants were from the Southeast. With regard to educational background, three participants had high school diplomas, one attended vocational school, eight had completed some college, seven had bachelor's degrees, five had master's degrees, and one had a doctoral degree. Lastly, in terms of employment, five were full-time students, 19 were employed, and six were unemployed.

Procedure

Interviews were conducted using a semi-structured approach. The first author conducted all interviews on Skype, on Zoom, or over the telephone. Several pups interviewed online wore their gear as an extra measure to preserve anonymity. Further, pseudonyms were assigned to the participants to protect their identities. The interview guide began with demographic questions and progressed through key themes. To understand how respondents conceptualized pup play, they were asked questions such as the following: Pretend for a moment you are talking with someone who has no understanding of what pup play is or how it works. How would you explain the concept to them? Next, to gauge the respondents' history with pup play, they were asked questions such as the following: How did you first learn about pup play? Then, to process how individuals become pups, respondents were asked questions such as the following: What steps do you take to solidify your pup identity? Lastly, the interviews concluded by asking respondents if there was anything else that they thought we should know about the subculture. While the interview guide was extensive and covered a range of topics, the present chapter focuses on themes related to play, performativity, and the creation of pup identities.

Following a constructivist grounded theory approach, we engaged in close coding of the data early on (Charmaz, 2014). During initial coding, we identified themes; and once we had a set of tentative codes, we were able to process larger amounts of data. We moved beyond initial coding into focused coding to advance our codes' theoretical direction (Charmaz, 2014). Focused coding allowed us to fully engage with our initial codes and make comparisons within and between codes. It is in this way that the data analysis was an iterative process that emphasized theoretical construction.

Becoming and Being a Pup

Our findings are organized into three main sections. First, we detail the processes by which individuals are introduced to pup play. Next, we explore how pups use the internet and social media to forge and maintain relationships and community. We then shift our analysis to a discussion of how participants construct their pup identity and how this is both an embodied and a psycho-social process.

Getting Started

In line with previous research (Wignall & McCormack, 2017), pups in our sample were introduced to pup play by an individual who was already integrated into the pup community. When asked about getting involved with pup play, Venom, a white, 28-year-old, gay pup from the Southwest, reflected as follows:

> I was in [Southwestern state], and I was going to meet up with this guy who was already a pup. We had met a couple of times, and he was like, I want to show you something. I had heard about pups before but had never gave it much serious thought. He let me borrow one of his hoods, which is a full wrap-around mask, and one of his tails, and it was just like a switch flipped, you know?

Other pups echoed Venom's experience of having someone introduce them into the subculture. Some pups, like Dodgr, a white, 21-year-old, gay pup from the Southeast, suggested seeking out other pups as a starting point. "I would say first, really finding a pup, just finding somebody who already does it, or who already has an interest in it, and then getting more involved with it." Additionally, connecting with other pups served as a source of inspiration for potential pups. CB, a white, 22-year-old, gay pup from the West, said, "It's kind of difficult to describe how to be a pup, so if you are able to see other people get into the headspace, it makes the journey just a little bit easier."

These narratives highlight the importance of networking in the process of becoming a pup in the ways said networks provided valuable socialization through the transmission of shared knowledge.

Even though many described the pup community as an accepting place where anyone can be a pup, our findings reveal that subtle forms of racial inequality permeated the subculture. For example, Scooter, a 36-year-old, Black, gay pup from the Southeast, discussed how the pup subculture is mainly comprised of white men and that pups of color were a "very small community." Baxter, a white, 23-year-old, trans female pup from the Midwest, also expressed about her pup community:

> There's like a large black population on the south side, and white affluent people on the north side and the north side is where all of the gay neighborhood stuff is. That doesn't change with pups either. I live on the south side; my boyfriend is black. They don't really do any outreach down here. I talked to the board members[3] constantly about the need to bring something to the south side, and I keep getting pushback. They're saying they don't want to ostracize the people who are already on the north side because their primary audience is on the north side.

Four of the 30 pups interviewed identified as pups of color. While our data is limited, it does suggest that pup play is experienced differently for racial minority pups, mirroring findings documented in the broader BDSM community (Cruz, 2016; Martinez, 2021).

Constructing Pup Communities Through Social Media

Technological advances, especially the internet, have dramatically changed how we construct our identities, cultivate our bodies, and develop communities (Anderson & McCabe, 2012). Scholars studying sexual minority subcultures have found that the internet has transformed how individuals in these subcultures connect (Döring, 2009; Hillier & Harrison, 2007; McKenna & Bargh, 1998; Wignall, 2017). Along these lines, we found that social media and messaging apps were central to how pups developed and maintained community. Hermes, a white, 33-year-old, gay pup from the Southwest, who was new to the world of pup play at the time of the interview, discussed how he used social media to connect with other pups:

A majority of my interactions have been on Instagram. Just seeking out other pup profiles, and then you know if I really like the content of their post or that they like what I'm posting, we will start messaging, and talking, and making friendships or connections. It's wonderful in that social media allows us to interact with anybody in the world . . . . So, it's nice to have an outlet with such a vast and diverse connection.

Twenty-eight of the 30 pups in our sample reported that they used some form of technology to connect with other pups. Nightwing, a 35-year-old, white, gay pup, and his husband Scooter were an interracial married couple from the Southeast. Like other participants, Scooter and Nightwing also used social media to connect with a pup community when they first got into pup play. Scooter shared the following:

A lot of it [connecting with the pup community] has been social media . . . Nightwing had met some people on Reddit who are also from [state in the Southeast], and they said, "Oh, join this Telegram thing." So, he joined and started talking to them, and then I joined afterwards. . . . People find out you're a pup, and then other pups find out you're a pup, and they all kind of start gravitating towards you and adding you.

In a separate interview, Nightwing brought up the same story, reflecting on how he used Reddit to engage with other pups who directed him toward other social media platforms to connect with other pups in the community.

While most pups referenced Facebook, Twitter, Instagram, and Telegram, several others mentioned additional social networking platforms and messaging apps, including Reddit, Scruff, FetLife, Recon, and Grindr. Crash, a white, 27-year-old, gay pup from the Southeast, stated the following:

I am very open on sites like Recon, Scruff, or FetLife, where pups are pretty heavily into things. I have a Twitter account where I do some more stuff and share my stuff, and Telegram has been a real game-changer for finding pups, furries, whatever. It's so easy to go, "Oh, there's not a pup group, I'll go and make a Pup Telegram channel" and I'll put it on the Telegram list, and maybe people will join or not.

Each social networking site and messaging app served a unique purpose for pups. For instance, while pups tended to post visual content in all these digital spaces, Tumblr and Twitter have been known to contain more explicit content (Wignall, 2017). Resulting from the 2018 porn ban on Tumblr, Twitter remains one of the only social media platforms where pups can post sexually explicit content. Dodgr even described Twitter as a "spank bank."[4]

Multiple participants explained how even though there is sexually suggestive material on Instagram, it is significantly more censored than other apps. Even though pups chatted on almost all these apps, Twitter, Facebook, and Telegram were the primary forms of social media pups used to engage in communication and community building. Telegram is a messaging app that allows users to message each other and create group chats and appeals to pups because of its focus on privacy. Lastly, gay dating apps such as Grindr and Scruff and apps designed for kinky communities, such as FetLife and Recon, were also used to connect pups. While participants had personal accounts on these social media platforms, they also maintained pup accounts to display and perform their pup identities. These digital performances aided not only in the construction of a community but also in the creation and presentation of pup identities.

Constructing a Pup Identity

Many pups in our sample crafted their pup identities and gear with meaningful components from their personal and professional identities. For example, Nightwing had a deep interest in comics and built in elements of DC Comics into his pup identity. For instance, some of his Instagram content depicts him wearing a Nightwing bodysuit or a Harley Quinn–inspired T-shirt that reads "Daddy's Little Pup" with her signature bat. His husband Scooter, an avid motorcyclist, would often integrate motorcycle gear and instruments into his pup identity. For example, he added an adhesive red mohawk accessory, like the one used on biker helmets, to his pup hood. Scooter also incorporated musical instruments into his pup identity since he was a musician.

Hermes shared how he modeled his pup identity after the Egyptian god Anubis, with his pup hood having a large muzzle and ears which were elongated and came to a point like a Doberman's. His hood was constructed of black leather with gold accents. About his hood, he explained,

Growing up as a kid, I always kind of loved Egyptian mythology. I was fascinated with the role of Anubis as the protector of souls, and a lot of people misconstrued him as the god of death. He is the god of, if you will, the transition from the living world to the afterlife and the protector of the souls in between. That really tied into who I was in my professional life as a nurse, you know, working in the [intensive care unit].

Hound, a white, 27-year-old, gay pup from the Southeast, was another pup who chose to customize his hood in a way that incorporated his professional identity:

I worked with an artist . . . to make the design. I said I want blue, black, and a little bit of white, and then I sent him some circuit patterns, the nose is a processer, and these ears are code that I have written in the past. This is RSA encryption in JavaScript I work in information security, so it means something for me there, and then this is an encrypted backup code for a project that I did for my first job.

Like other BDSM practices, pup play is characteristic of a "consumer sexuality" whereby capitalism, sexual identities, and sexual desire are intimately connected (Weiss, 2012). As pup play grows in popularity, so does the market value for gear. Like BDSM gear, the availability of pup gear has extended beyond specialized retailers to large digital distributors and other online platforms (Weiss, 2012). The wide availability of pup gear means that there are more toys, clothing, and technology that pups can add to their collection.

One key piece of gear that is important to pup play is the hood. While most of the gear can be deemed superfluous, the hood has a powerful transformative property because it gives the subject pup-like features, such as whiskers and a muzzle. Purchasing and customizing hoods was a common way that pups molded their pup identities. As with most BDSM gear, pup hoods can be pricey. Even though one online retailer offers a standard neoprene puppy hood in 10 colors for $27.98, some pups who purchased their hood from this retailer expressed dissatisfaction with the quality. Dodgr stated,

I hate talking about the [online retailer] hoods because I have such a strong opinion on why they suck, and I always tell people, "just get a credit card and buy a Mr. S hood and pay it off as you can" . It's really worth it because now they've started releasing really nice custom ones.

Mr. S Leather, a specialty store that has top-quality bondage, leather, rubber, and neoprene clothing, sells several versions of pup hoods, crafted from neoprene, leather, or rubber. The standard neoprene puppy hood design had a retail value of $109.99, with custom hoods starting at $179.95. Upgrading to a standard leather puppy hood ran pups $349.95, with custom puppy hoods starting at $379.95. While the pup hood is an important accessory, collars, dog tags, bandanas, leashes, harnesses, jockstraps, tails, mitts, and other toys are common accoutrements of the pup wardrobe.

Amassing all this gear quickly adds up, and not all pups had the financial means to spend hundreds of dollars on their hoods and accessories. As such, some, like Max, a white, 34-year-old, gay pup from the Southeast, downplayed the importance of gear to his pup identity:

> Ninety-nine percent of the time, I'm literally just in my hood wearing jeans and a T-shirt, and that's it. On occasion, I will stick my tail[5] in if I'm, you know, feeling froggy, you know, and a jockstrap maybe, but that's kind of it. . . . There are some pups that have incredible stuff, and I'm like, I'm not that rich, so I can't afford this crap.

Max's narrative is illustrative of one of the many ways that participation in the pup subculture is shaped by Western consumerism and deeply influenced by social class. In addition to the cost of gear customization, some pups pay membership dues to pup organizations, and specialized pup events have fees paired with traveling dining and leisure expenses. The financial constraints felt within the pup community are not unique as this has also been reported by members of other kinky subcultures (Weiss, 2012; Wignall, 2022).

Perhaps this is why some pups, such as Dodgr, emphasized the importance of the desire to be a pup instead of focusing on the gear:

> It's not necessarily a gear thing. Most pups think, oh, I have to have a hood to be a pup, or I have to have a collar, or a leash, and all these harnesses and underwear. No! You don't have to have any of the gear to get started. You just have to have that mindset.

Dodgr's statement reveals how decorating one's body in gear is only part of the transformation into pup headspace, a topic to which we now turn.

Mind, Body, and Soul: Entering Headspace

Headspace is an alternative state of mind that an individual can achieve when role-playing. Various forms of headspace exist within the wider BDSM community, such as *dom space*, *sub space*, and *pup headspace* (Simula, 2017). When in a pup headspace, an individual adopts the affective, behavioral, and cognitive performances of puppies. While pups do access a different frame of mind in pup headspace, it is important to note that they do not abandon their sense of reason and can still understand consent and the difference between right and wrong (Wignall & McCormack, 2017). Entering headspace can be challenging for some pups, requiring deep concentration, scripted behaviors, and the application of gear. The pups in our sample described two techniques that aided them in achieving a pup headspace: (1) scripted behaviors or rituals and (2) the application of gear.

Some participants spoke about how pup play's scripted behaviors, such as getting on all fours, becoming non-verbal, and being petted by their handler—an individual who takes on the role of the human companion who takes care of the pup once they are in pup headspace—transported them into the pup headspace. Flower, a white, 32-year-old gay pup from the West Coast, was one of the few participants who interviewed without his pup gear on, though he was not shy about showcasing the gear he owned. Flower discussed how individuals transform from human to pup:

> Some pups use putting on gear almost like a way to get into puppy space. So, some handlers will like to help them get dressed and like, you know, pet them or call them a good boy while they are helping them. Others kind of use it as a meditation, like taking deep breaths and kind of finding that place of calm relaxation while they are putting on their gear.

As Flower explained, the process of getting into pup headspace resembles something different for each pup. New pups may not be able to connect with headspace as deeply without having other people give them verbal cues, having people help them get dressed, and using relaxation techniques such as meditation. Seasoned pups can access this state of mind more easily by simply applying the hood. However, some pups preferred putting on the hood last, at the end of the ritualistic dressing experience, because of its transformative power. For instance, Pablo, a white, 38-year-old, gay pup from the Southeast, reflected as follows:

> Initially, it was as simple as putting on the hood, but because it is not ideal to fall directly into a deep headspace, it has become kind of a routine or ritual. I start by putting on shorts and a shirt, I have a belt with a tail, and then I put my mitts on one at a time slowly. As I'm putting things on, I can feel myself slipping slowly into a deeper headspace.

While scripted behaviors and rituals were one way for pups to enter into the pup headspace, another technique that pups used was applying gear. While we discuss these methods of entering headspace separately, there is overlap in the sense that putting on gear can be ritualized.

Whereas collars, leashes, and harnesses are optional, a hood, regardless of how elaborate, is an important tool used to facilitate pup headspace and the pup transformation process. While a pup headspace can be achieved without gear, the hood's visceral sensations have powerful effects on the individuals who are wearing them. Pup hoods are often made of neoprene or leather and have ears and a muzzle, which gives off a canine appearance and impacts on how people interact with the pup. Pablo shared why he believed hoods were essential to moving into pup headspace:

> Some of it is that there's a little bit of a confining pressure, and so you kind of focus on that. It also narrows your field of vision and it kind of cuts off your hearing. It reduces your sensations to some degree. I don't know if there's just something primal about us that that triggers, but it just instantly snaps me into a state of mind, and it can take me a long time to come out of it even if I just wear it for a couple of minutes. It can take me some time to readjust afterwards.

The way the hood compresses the subject's head alters their vision and distorts their hearing, all serving to transform the subject, transporting them into pup headspace. Having experienced this process for the first time, some pups struggled to find the words to describe who they had become. Reflecting on his first experience in a hood, Venom said,

I compare it to how in the Spiderman Universe, where Venom takes over Spiderman, and he kind of assumes a new identity. It felt just like that. I didn't recognize the thing that I had transformed into, but I knew that it was completely different, and I could make that thing whatever I wanted it to be.

As each piece of gear is applied to the body, human features are masked, and abilities are constrained, helping pups move deeper into the pup headspace. For instance, while not all the pups in our sample wore mitts, limiting dexterity was one way some used props to push themselves deeper into the pup headspace. Thus, even though it is not required, gear serves a critical function in the pup transformation process.

The process of entering headspace and engaging with one's pup identity was significantly more involved than engaging in scripted behaviors and decorating bodies in gear; it required a great deal of work to transform themselves into the playful, energetic, happy, confident, and sexy character of the pup. Parker, a white, 25-year-old, gay man, who's pup persona was built around Marvel's Spiderman, said,

I would say it makes you feel playful. Not that I'm not happy, but it just makes you really happy and playful, like goof around and not worry about things that are like serious all the time. You can just jump around and pretend to be a dog. You can just roll on the floor and give each other belly rubs, give each other snacks, and just fool around.

Parker's narrative illustrates what Hochschild (1983) refers to as deep acting, a form of emotion work in which actors manage both their external impressions and their internal feelings to align with the organizational or, in this case, the subcultural expectations. Rolling around on the floor, giving each other belly rubs, becoming non-verbal and barking are examples of deep acting activities that pups engaged in. Distinct from surface acting, where pups fake the required emotions and are arguably alienated from their sensibilities, deep acting involves producing the emotions necessary for the performance. As they engage in deep acting, pups turn off the human thoughts that limit their ability to perform, a process that requires a deal of emotion work.

Some pups could transcend the deep acting described by Parker and enter what Ashforth and Humphry (1993) refer to as "genuine acting." Genuine acting is when pups achieve the feelings when taking on a role (Ashforth & Humphrey, 1993). Pups attained this state of genuine acting when they entered headspace completely without having to put in the work. In short, the actor and character became completely integrated. Genuine acting was seemingly effortless, and some described it as "flow" or "trance." Trance was a state of mind where "the feelings associated with the transformation become so powerful that it overcomes the knowing and observing half of the performer" (Schechner, 1988, p. 316). For example, Flower elaborated, "I can only really identify it as flow like that aspect of being so in the zone like time passes by super-fast because you are having so much fun or you are so in it." Similarly, Pablo described the ways that headspace transformed him into his pup character and transported him to an alternate reality:

> Since you're in headspace, you're not thinking. You'll do things you don't normally consider doing because you're reactionary. I broke my teeth, my front teeth, the first time that I was in headspace in a public place and didn't realize it until after.

Since headspace can be achieved at various levels, it was important for pups to take safety precautions before entering pup headspace. Flower detailed the importance of having other pups or handlers there with him to make sure he was safe and stayed hydrated throughout the scene. For other pups, these safety precautions included wearing knee pads, elbow pads, or mitts and making the environment "pup-proof" before engaging in play.

A consequence of becoming fully immersed into pup headspace through genuine acting was that subjects found it difficult to get out of pup headspace and transport back into the human world. Much like individuals who enter sub space, pups who were in the genuine acting phase of their performance became so deeply immersed in their roles that the world around them faded; they were in a deep state of concentration where even perceptions of time were interpreted differently. Pups also discussed the importance of aftercare when coming out of pup headspace. Much like Schechner's (1988) concept of cooling off where performers leave the performance and engage in reflection, aftercare is the period when pups exit pup headspace. They take off their gear, engage in relaxing activities like cuddling, and debrief about their experiences. Not all pups needed to engage in this cool-off period, which only came up when pups were either deep in pup headspace or building other kinks and sexual activities into their pup performances. Aftercare is not unique to the pup community. It is an important and common activity across various kink communities and usually focuses on participants who are bottoms or submissives (Newmahr, 2011; Pitagora, 2013). Consent, trust, and open communication before and after engaging in a scene were crucial because entering pup headspace rendered pups vulnerable in some situations. The more often that pups could enter pup headspace across time, the easier it was to disconnect from the human observer during the performance.

Conclusions

In this chapter, we explored the processes by which those involved in the pup subculture construct and negotiate their pup identities and create and maintain pup communities increasingly through social media and messaging apps. Pups used social networking to learn about the subculture, acquire inspiration for their pup identities, and forge digital communities across the globe. In addition, drawing on theories of performativity and identity work, we demonstrated how pups engage in a multidimensional identity-building process to access headspace and cultivate their pup identity. Our theoretical approach to understanding pups can inform how scholars understand other kink subcultures.

Our findings should be viewed in light of our limitations. Our sample was comprised of predominantly gay, white, cisgender men. Pup culture, much like the wider BDSM community, is overwhelmingly white (Martinez, 2021). As such, future research should use an intersectional lens to explore the experiences of heterosexual pups, pups of color, women pups, and transgender pups. Moreover, most of the studies that have been conducted on pup culture are exploratory in nature and based on data from qualitative convenience samples. Our study, which is the first sociological analysis of pups in the United States, suffers from this methodological shortcoming. Future research would benefit from more diverse sampling and research methodologies. For example, quantitative studies are necessary to provide data about the number of individuals who comprise the subculture and the demographic characteristics of these participants. Cross-cultural research on pup communities is also warranted, as are longitudinal studies exploring the social–sexual careers of pups. In addition, scholarship would benefit from more ethnographic work on pup communities. Lastly, while not discussed in our chapter, pup packs are a unique and important part of the pup community as they operate as a pup's "chosen family" (Wignall et al., 2022). Future research should explore pup packs as well as the dynamics that exist within them. Although it is a relatively new sexual subculture, a sociological lens on pup play can tell us a great deal about the ways that those in sexually stigmatized subcultures navigate desire, identity, and community.

Notes

1. Here, we use *pup identity* to describe the role identity individuals assume when engaging in pup play. *Role identities* are the meanings people use to define who they are when occupying roles in the social structure (Stryker, 2002).
2. Here, we are using *Old Guard* in the same way that Rubin (1998) discusses the Old Guard, exploring some of the more traditional aspects of the SM/leather scene.
3. The executive board of an organization in its local area that was created for pups and handlers.
4. A term used to describe a collection of explicit pictures that people, particularly men, masturbate to.
5. This is an insertable butt plug that gives the appearance of a tail.

References

Anderson, L., & McCabe, D. B. (2012). A constructed world. *Journal of Public Policy & Marketing, 31*(2), 240–253. https://doi.org/10.1509/jppm.08.043

Ashforth, B. E., & Humphrey, R. H. (1993). Emotional labor in service roles: The influence of identity. *Academy of Management Review, 18*(1), 88–115. https://doi.org/10.5465/amr.1993.3997508

Aune, K. S., & Wong, N. C. H. (2002). Antecedents and consequences of adult play in romantic relationships. *Personal Relationships, 9*(3), 279–286. https://doi.org/10.1111/1475-6811.00019

Bauer, R. (2019). BDSM relationships. In B. Simula, J. Sumerau, & A. Miller (Eds.), *Expanding the rainbow: Exploring the relationships of bi+, polyamorous, kinky, ace, intersex, and trans people* (pp. 135–147). Brill.

Brown, A. M. L., & Stenros, J. (2018). Adult play: The dirty secret of grown-ups. *Games and Culture, 13*(3), 215–219. https://doi.org/10.1177/1555412017690860

Charmaz, K. (2014). *Constructing grounded theory* (2nd ed.). SAGE Publications.

Cruz, A. (2016). *The color of kink: Black women, BDSM, and pornography*. New York University Press.

Daniels, M. (2006). *Woof! Perspectives into the erotic care & training of the human dog*. Nazca Plains.

Döring, N. M. (2009). The internet's impact on sexuality: A critical review of 15 years of research. *Computers in Human Behavior, 25*(5), 1089–1101. https://doi.org/10.1016/j.chb.2009.04.003

Goffman, E. (1959). *The presentation of self in everyday life*. Doubleday.

Grey, P. (2011). The decline of play and the rise of psychopathology in children and adolescents. *American Journal of Play*, 3(4), 443–463.

Hillier, L., & Harrison, L. (2007). Building realities less limited than their own: Young people practising same-sex attraction on the internet. *Sexualities*, 10(1), 82–100. https://doi.org/10.1177/1363460707072956

Hochschild, A. R. (1983). *The managed heart: Commercialization of human feeling*. University of California Press.

Krasnor, L., & Pepler, D. (1980). The study of children's play: Some suggested future directions. *New Directions for Child and Adolescent Development*, 1980(9), 85–95.

Langdridge, D., & Lawson, J. (2019). The psychology of puppy play: A phenomenological investigation. *Archives of Sexual Behavior*, 48(7), 2201–2215. https://doi.org/10.1007/s10508-019-01476-1

Lawson, J., & Langdridge, D. (2020). History, culture and practice of puppy play. *Sexualities*, 23(4), 574–591. https://doi.org/10.1177/1363460719839914

Martinez, K. (2018). BDSM role fluidity: A mixed-methods approach to investigating switches within dominant/submissive binaries. *Journal of Homosexuality*, 65(10), 1299–1324. https://doi.org/10.1080/00918369.2017.1374062

Martinez, K. (2021). Overwhelming whiteness of BDSM: A critical discourse analysis of racialization in BDSM. *Sexualities*, 24(5–6). https://doi.org/10.1177/1363460720932389

McKenna, K. Y. A., & Bargh, J. A. (1998). Coming out in the age of the internet: Identity "demarginalization" through virtual group participation. *Journal of Personality and Social Psychology*, 75(3), 681–694. https://doi.org/10.1037/0022-3514.75.3.681

Moskowitz, D. A., Seal, D. W., Rintamaki, L., & Rieger, G. (2011). HIV in the leather community: Rates and risk-related behaviors. *AIDS and Behavior*, 15(3), 557–564. https://doi.org/10.1007%2Fs10461-009-9636-9

Newmahr, S. (2011). *Playing on the edge: Sadomasochism, risk, and intimacy*. Indiana University Press.

Paasonen, S. (2018). Many splendored things: Sexuality, playfulness and play. *Sexualities*, 21(4), 537–551. https://doi.org/10.1177/1363460717731928

Pitagora, D. (2013). Consent v coercion: BDSM interactions highlight a fine but immutable line. *The New School Psychology Bulletin*, 10(1), 27–36. https://doi.org/10.1037/e543732013-004

Rubin, G. (1998). Old guard, new guard. *Cuir Underground*, 4(2). http://www.black-rose.com/cuiru/archive/4-2/oldguard.html

Schechner, R. (1988). *Performance theory*. Routledge.

Simula, B. L. (2017). A "different economy of bodies and pleasures"? Differentiating and evaluating sex and sexual BDSM experiences. *Journal of Homosexuality*, 66(2), 209–237. https://doi.org/10.1080/00918369.2017.1398017

St. Clair, J. (2015). *Bark!* Nazca Plains.

Steinberg, R. J., & Figart, D. M. (1999). Emotional labor since: The managed heart. *The Annals of the American Academy of Political and Social Science*, 561(1), 8–26. https://doi.org/10.1177/000271629956100101

Stryker, S. (2002). *Symbolic interactionism: A social structural version*. Blackburn Press.

Weiss, M. D. (2012). *Techniques of pleasure: BDSM and the circuits of sexuality*. Duke University Press.

White, R. E. (2013). *The power of play: A research summary on play and learning.* Minnesota Children's Museum.

Wignall, L. (2017). The sexual use of a social networking site: The case of Pup Twitter. *Sociological Research Online, 22*(3), 21–37. https://doi.org/10.1177/1360780417724066

Wignall, L. (2022). *Kinky in the digital age: Gay men's subcultures and social identities.* Oxford University Press.

Wignall, L., & McCormack, M. (2017). An exploratory study of a new kink activity: "Pup play." *Archives of Sexual Behavior, 46*(3), 801–811. https://doi.org/10.1007/s10508-015-0636-8

Wignall, L., McCormack, M., Cook, T., & Jaspal, R. (2022). Findings from a community survey of individuals who engage in pup play. *Archives of Sexual Behavior, 51,* 3637–3646. https://doi.org/10.1007/s10508-021-02225-z

5

Perverting Innocence in Age Play?

Using Little Space to Explore Vulnerability, Innocence, and Discipline in Adultist Society

Robin Bauer

Introduction

Children's sexuality is under intense scrutiny and regulation in today's Western societies, if its existence is not downright denied. For the purpose of this chapter, *age play* is defined as an erotic, sexual, or asexual practice in which one or more adults role-play as babies, children, or adolescents. While the scripts of some of these age play scenes may resemble pedophilia, incest, or sexual abuse, age play is not to be confused with pedophilia, given that only adults are involved who play-act as minors. Age play is also distinct from incest or child abuse because these practices (e.g., a spanking as punishment) are consensual.

Some types of age play are considered edge play within the BDSM community as edge play is about engaging with and transgressing boundaries during BDSM encounters, including playing on cultural taboos like incest, sexual violence, or the abuse of power, which can all be part of age play dynamics (Bauer, 2014, 2018; Weiss, 2011). When adults enter the head/affective space of a baby, child, or adolescent in an intimate, erotic, or sexual role-playing context (*little space*), they engage in a practice that may be associated with incest and pedophilia and that therefore raises concern or leads to stigmatization. Therefore, age players often try to distance themselves from real-life pedophilia or incest (Bauer, 2018; Lewis, 2011), for instance, by spelling their roles *boi* instead of *boy* or *grrrl* instead of *girl* and by emphasizing that they desire the adult bodies behind the role. On the other hand, the taboo-breaking nature of such practices may result in an especially intense emotional, intimate, and/or sexual experience.

Robin Bauer, *Perverting Innocence in Age Play?* In: *The Power of BDSM.* Edited by: Brandy L. Simula, Robin Bauer, and Liam Wignall, Oxford University Press. © Oxford University Press 2023. DOI: 10.1093/oso/9780197658598.003.0006

Other types of age play resemble what appear to be among the "sweetest" types of role-playing in BDSM communities and their fringes, such as wearing children's clothes and/or diapers, sucking on pacifiers, cuddling with stuffed animals, playing children's games and with children's toys, eating children's food, and being nurtured by a loving caregiver, often without any sexual acts involved. Yet even these activities can be considered edge play in that they transgress the boundaries of what is deemed acceptable behavior for adults.

This chapter is based on two qualitative studies and seeks to address the following questions: How is age play constructed in different community contexts? How is childhood innocence constructed (and deconstructed) in age play? This chapter analyzes age play as situated in cultural contexts that consider particular notions of adulthood as a norm that devalues other modes of existence such as being or acting like children (i.e., adultist societies) to better understand what is at stake and to engage with the effects such practices have.

Adult Littles, Diaper Lovers, and Other Childish Delights—Adult Age Playgrounds

The terminology among age players to categorize their own practices has become increasingly differentiated. In the online forum I studied for this chapter, members were never able to reach a consensus on definitions; and moreover, any debate turned into a meta-discussion about the (non)sense of categories themselves. In this chapter, I will use the gender-neutral *caregivers* and *adult littles* as well as *age play* as umbrella terms. For the purpose of this chapter, I define *age play* as all activities (solitary or in collaboration with others) where at least one chronologically adult participant takes on a role and/or enters a state of being that resembles and/or is experienced as infancy, childhood, or adolescence (*little space*). Since age players are all adults who are aware of the fact that all participants are adults, it is fundamentally different from pedophilia (Bauer, 2018, pp. 144–145). Therefore, I use the term *adult littles* to clarify that these are adults who role-play or live out a partial identity/aspect of their self (e.g., self-defining as boy/boi, girl/grrrl, brat, adult baby, etc.). *Caregiver* denotes an adult who performs the role of the responsible adult (e.g., self-defining as big, daddy/daddi, mommy/mommi, etc.).

Some age players are very specific about the age they are entering as their adult littles, while others cannot pinpoint an exact age, or the age fluctuates depending on circumstance. Moreover, some create their own complex layers of age regarding their adult littles, as one forum user in my study[1] explained in a thread discussing why so many littles wear diapers at a little age where chronological children would not typically use diapers anymore: "My little is an eight-year-old who wishes to be three or four again being allowed to wear diapers." It therefore cannot be assumed that wearing a diaper or using a pacifier means that the adult little is an adult baby; rather, forum members created their own versions of ages that are not necessarily consistent with children's normative age stages, as one user put it: "The appeal [of age play] lies in being able to pick and choose the best from all ages and not being so limited." Many explained that they enjoyed the emotions diapers and pacifiers gave them, but they otherwise preferred an age range that provides them with a more active and self-determined being in the world and specific "fun" activities such as playing with Lego. Using *adult little* as an umbrella term therefore also has the advantage of including both, *adult babies* and *adult children* and those who do not fit easily into these categories. The term *diaper lover* is used by those whose emotional, sensual, or sexual focus lies on wearing diapers (some call it a fetish), in combination with or independently of role-playing as littles. Individuals in my studies did not describe themselves as diaper lovers (although there exists some overlap between the age play and diaper lover communities), and it is therefore not engaged with in greater detail.

While there is a growing body of academic writing on BDSM, there is little non-pathologizing research on age play. In a body of work on adult babies and diaper lovers from a clinical and mostly pathologizing perspective, authors either discuss clinical cases or conduct quantitative analyses of online samples (for an overview, see Lasala et al., 2020). Non-clinical and qualitative research usually includes age play as part of a larger BDSM study (e.g., Bauer, 2007, 2014, 2018; Brame et al., 1993; Tiidenberg & Paasonen, 2018; Weiss, 2011). Tiidenberg and Paasonen have framed age play as play "practiced for its own sake" (2018, p. 2), questioning the normative limiting of play that is "just for play" (as opposed to adult playing which serves purposes beyond the activity itself) to childhood (p. 9). In my own work (Bauer, 2007, 2014, 2018) I have focused on the meaning of age play for les-bi-trans-queer BDSM practitioners, for instance, becoming children of a different gender.

Age Play in an Adultist Context

Childhood studies is an interdisciplinary research perspective that analyzes how childhood is a social construction that is subject to historical change, varies geographically, is class-specific, and is differentiated by gender and how such constructions of childhood affect the lives of children (Kehily, 2009). In modern Western nuclear middle-class families, children have become increasingly economically redundant but are accorded great emotional value (Gittins, 2009, p. 43), while in other geopolitical contexts, children are, for instance, part of the workforce to sustain their families. From this particular Western perspective, childhood can be "lost" by what are considered age-inappropriate experiences (Kehily, 2009, p. 3). This middle-class ideal of childhood was eventually universalized as normative for all classes (Gittins, 2009, p. 45).

The analytical term *adultism* describes a social power structure that privileges adulthood and adults over childhood and children; adult points of view dominate in society (Wall, 2019, p. 4). Adulthood is naturalized as an "unmarked age" (p. 5), that functions as a taken-for-granted standard against which childhood is measured. Wall (2019) holds that, contrary to adultist beliefs, children possess agency and are "constructors of meaning in their own right" (p. 7). Adultism stands out among other forms of oppression since everyone has experienced it first-hand in their own childhood. When adults play as children, they therefore enter the position of an "other" to their current status, while also re-connecting to something familiar from their own biography.

The child has been constructed as an "unrealized adult" from an adultist perspective (Jenks, 2009; Walkerdine, 2009): Children are not judged on their own account but are measured against an idealized version of adulthood. Adulthood is conceptualized not only in terms of a body that has stopped growing (grown-up) but also as a state of supposedly fully realized maturity and rationality. Children are supposed to reach this endpoint by going through normative developmental stages (Jenks, 2009, p. 95). One of the most influential developmental psychologists, Piaget (1977), judges children's play as trivial; but to children, play is essential in meaning-making and acquiring competencies (Jenks, 2009, p. 98). In adultism, adult perspectives are considered to be authoritative rather than starting with the meanings children assign their own practices. Moreover, anyone who (supposedly) is not able or takes longer to reach the final stages of development is excluded from adulthood and therefore considered an inadequate human being.

Therefore *sanism*, the ideology of equating being fully human with possessing certain kinds of cognitive and rational capacities, lies at the heart of adultism (and many other forms of oppression). Most obviously, animals, children, and the so-called mentally disabled are excluded from rationality. Furthermore, sanism has been used to construct all kinds of groups as inferior by claiming they are not capable of rational thought and deed (LeFrancois & Coppock, 2014) and constructing them as overtly emotional, irrational, irresponsible, etc. (cf. Piper, n.d., p. 31, on women as historically constructed as child-like; cf. Keating, 2016, on constructing Black men as irrational and therefore aggressive).

Adultism has an effect not only on the subordinated group (children), or other subordinated groups, but also on the privileged group (adults). Walkerdine (2009) points out that any instability in adults is seen as child-like and developmentally regressive rather than simply human (p. 117). So to become fully accepted as adults, individuals have to learn not to show their insecurities or emotions (especially not in public) and not to display what are negatively labeled "childish" interests and behaviors, such as certain kinds of playing, being silly, being naive, etc. Some age players build on these notions to make sense of their own non-conforming emotions and needs.

In the adult–child binary that is created through sanist–adultist ideologies, children are constructed as "the other" to how adults construct themselves, for instance, as irrational and incapable of deciding for themselves. Here, I will briefly sketch the construction of children as innocent as it is pertinent to my data. One understanding of children as innocent can be traced back to Rousseau's (1889) romanticist view of children as symbolizing and literally embodying a return to (unspoiled) nature. According to Rousseau, the child needs time to develop at its own pace while being sheltered from the malignant influence of society. Given that children are always already part of society, this ideal seems impossible to achieve in reality. Sexual ignorance has become one crucial element in conceptualizing the innocence of children, in opposition to the sexually knowledgeable adult (Piper, n.d., p. 9). At the same time, children's assumed sexual innocence builds the ground for eroticizing children as the ultimate cultural transgression. This can be observed in age play as well, where experiencing arousal is especially transgressive and therefore a "hot button issue" (Weiss, 2011, p. 214) when juxtaposed with the normative image of the innocent child (Tiidenberg & Paasonen, 2018, p. 384). The construction of children as sexually innocent makes it impossible to conceive of children as possessing sexual agency. If they are sexually knowledgeable (a minimum prerequisite to possessing sexual agency), they lose their unspoiled status of innocence and are deemed "corrupted" (Piper, n.d., p. 14; Robinson, 2012, p. 264). Thus, the notion of children as innocent constructs them as asexual beings. At the same time though, *hetero*sexualization of children's everyday life is encouraged (e.g., through mock weddings, kiss and chase, or role-playing as mommies/daddies), while moral panics erupt once children transgress heteronormative expectations (Robinson, 2012, p. 268).

Historically, childhood innocence and vulnerability have only been applied to white children acting in accordance with heteronormative expectations, while Black children have been constructed as resilient, immoral, and devilish in general (Rand, 2019, p. 257). The construction of sexual purity of girls was also class-specific: Middle-/upper-class girls were considered pure in the 19th-century United Kingdom, while lower-class girls were seen as sexually active and available to older wealthy men (Kehily & Montgomery, 2009, p. 75). So innocence is a major element in the construction of children and often equated with sexual ignorance, but non-white or lower-class/poor children are not necessarily provided the protection that innocence grants some children.

In Christian theology, children have also been attributed innocence. For instance, the child stood for perceiving the world as new and beautiful (Davis, 2011, p. 384). So a child's pre-rational state was interpreted as so immediate and pure that it could teach adults how to better relate to the world (p. 385). Davis calls this notion "radical innocence" (pp. 389–390) and claims this perspective can open up spaces for other ways of being adult—spaces that age players often crave and seek out in their practices.

Method

This chapter is based on two qualitative empirical studies. The first is an interview study of les-bi-trans-queer BDSM practices (Bauer, 2014), referred to as the "interview study." Between 2003 and 2008 I conducted

49 semi-structured face-to-face interviews with self-defined lesbian, bi-/pansexual and queer cis women, femmes, butches, transwomen, transmen, and genderqueers whose ages were spread out evenly between 20 and 60 in the United States and Western Europe who practiced BDSM. Participants were not asked about age play in particular but discussed age play practices and identities when answering questions about identities, power, or personal growth/healing. The sample was mainly recruited through networks and snowball sampling from various trans-inclusive women's BDSM communities. While this les-bi-trans-queer community was highly diverse when it comes to gender, body types, age, sexuality, and relationship practices, it was mostly populated by white and often highly educated individuals. This is reflected in my sample as well. Interviews were transcribed verbatim, anonymized, and edited for grammar; and research participants were given the opportunity to authorize the transcripts. The study was conducted within the framework of grounded theory (Strauss & Corbin, 1990), which seeks to generate theories from empirical data. Interviews were analyzed through a close line-by-line reading of each interview, resulting in codes that were then compared across interviews and further grouped into overarching categories.

The second study is a content analysis of a German open message board for age players, which I refer to as the "forum study." 270 thematic threads assembled under a category encouraging posts on everything related to "age play and being little" were analyzed and coded into various subcategories. These threads included a total of 2747 posts between the start of this online forum in 2016 and February 2021, which were analyzed through the same coding techniques as in the interview study. Posts varied in length, but issues were often elaborated on in some detail, with contributors describing their own experiences or perspectives. All threads and posts that were subject to analysis were public, with no registration necessary to access them. In terms of research ethics (Rodham & Gavin, 2006), these messages were therefore considered public acts that need no further consent to be gathered as data, while the portal and the contributors were anonymized and the posts translated into English (and deliberately not offered in the German original) to avoid identification of individuals. Most contributions were posted by the same circle of active members, who mostly described heterosexual encounters, fantasies, and relationships, including a minority of individuals with gay preferences and practices as well as members whose activities as littles were cross-gender (mostly cis men playing and/or identifying as little girls, which confirms Brame et al.'s [1993, p. 138] earlier observation that many cis men play as baby girls). Controversial discussions centered around whether age play is sexual or not and part of BDSM or not. Many members characterized their age play activities as asexual, which confirms the findings of studies from other geographical contexts that many motivations given for adult baby/diaper lover play are not sexual in nature (Hawkinson & Zamboni, 2014). Some forum members expressed an interest in playing with other adult littles independently of gender. Studies have pointed to the possibility that adult littles use their age play practices as coping mechanisms for incontinence related to disability or traumatic childhood experiences (Brame et al., 1993; Lasala et al., 2020; Speaker, 1980, p. 72). Some members in the forum study also disclosed physical or mental disabilities such as being diagnosed with Asperger's syndrome. When brought up, such posts insinuated that their age play interests were somehow connected to their (dis)abilities. No contributors to the forum described themselves as Black, Indigenous, or people of color; but sociodemographic data in general could not be accessed through this format. Class and race were not discussed in any thread, which is typical for hegemonic German culture where whiteness often functions as an invisible standard. Therefore, in regard to both samples, the space to explore age provided by these different communities may not be equally accessible to all individuals or may play out differently for other individuals/communities.

Given that perspectives on caregiving were hardly present in the forum study, I focus on the adult little perspective for better comparison between these groups.

Social (Re)Constructions of Childhood Innocence in Age Play

Various ways of constructing childhood in age play practices emerged in the analysis of the data. For this chapter, I will restrict the analysis to how childhood innocence is constructed and deconstructed during age play practices, starting with little space as a space for vulnerability as this is the framework for children's innocence. I will also take a look at one counter-discourse to innocence, that of the bad child in need of discipline.

Space for Vulnerability

In the forum study, adult littles often used the concept of "*little space*" in a similar way as "*sub space*" is referred to in the overall BDSM community. One post described in more detail how intensely this space can be experienced as a

> pretty complete regression. There are a few potential triggers, and when one of these appears, my perception shrinks to a radius of maybe four meters around me, everything outside simply ceases to exist, and everything inside is extremely intense and interesting and is experienced in a partly very sensual way. I also have a closer relationship to persons who enter this circle in such a stage. . . . During these stages of regression, which can last about one or two hours, I am mostly busy playing—with stuffed animals, with toy blocks, toy trains, and other toys.

Adult littles stressed how deeply they are entering an alternate state of consciousness. The term *trigger* refers to the process of being "triggered" into little space, not triggered by past trauma, although in some cases this may overlap: One adult little in the forum study described triggers for their anxiety disorder which simultaneously triggered them into little space. In general, adult littles described becoming highly vulnerable in little space. As in this quote, they sometimes used the term *regression* to express a state of being that makes them feel like a little child with all senses. Because children are constructed as unrealized adults, it is tolerated that they show emotions in general, and vulnerability and dependence in particular, while this is not or is less tolerated in adults. Adult littles in both studies felt a desire to express vulnerability in a safe(r) space, and they found that in age play, as queer femme Teresa from the interview study explained: "It's kind of what a little girl persona feels like to me. Being valued for my vulnerability, being valued for how much strength it takes in this world to be vulnerable, to not shut down." The role of an adult little gave age players permission to embrace and show various kinds of vulnerabilities and, as in Teresa's perspective, reconceptualize vulnerability as strength, especially in sanist–adultist society.

Children are constructed as cute and innocent, which is a two-edged sword given that they are therefore considered to be worthy of protection, their weaknesses are more easily forgiven, and they are generally constructed as lovable, which creates an idealistic age play space for adult littles to feel safe in.[2] On the other hand, because of their construction as cute and innocent, children are not taken seriously; and the delight adults take in children's cuteness plays a part in obscuring the fact that children are actually denied agency in adultist society. Teresa had to play the sweet, innocent little girl in her chronological childhood to appease her abusive father, while playing as little girl for butch or trans daddies made her feel differently:

> And it's good to have someone powerful and masculine tell me I'm cute, tell me I'm sweet, sit me on their lap, pat my head, that kind of stuff. And feel really loved and nurtured and having mostly that with not super fucked-up people. That is healing, continually. They also respect my autonomy, that I don't have to take any of their shit.

While her role in the abusive nuclear family depended on the figure of the innocent girl-child being denied her agency, in queer age play contexts, properties like sweetness and cuteness were nonetheless associated with autonomy, therefore not robbing her of her knowledge and agency through the construct of innocence but reconstructing the girl-child as someone whose boundaries are respected and who is also valued for her strength.

Constructing Children as (Sexually) Innocent

The construction of children as innocent through constructing them as sexually ignorant or asexual can also be witnessed in age play. Tiidenberg and Paasonen also observed this in what they refer to as the symbolic, cultural figure of the child, which is based on stereotypes of childhood rather than one's real experiences (2018, pp. 383–384). Some posts in the forum study considered naivety as a trademark of children that they valued highly. In the interview study, several participants described the innocence of children as a limit to making their age play sexual (in a normative, genitally focused sense), as queer transman BJ explicitly stated: "There's just something about children, they're pure, they're innocent. I'm not saying that sex cannot be pure and innocent and sweet and good, I'm just saying, that is just a line even in age play I cannot broach." So, while BJ states that sex can also be sweet and innocent, it seems to be a different kind of innocence that children are attributed: an innocence that is constructed as asexual.

In the interview study, les-bi-trans-queer BDSM practitioners were engaging in sexual age play, even those who stressed that there were nonsexual
elements to their adult littles or that they could not go beyond a certain imaginary age (like BJ). In contrast, in the forum study, many adult littles stressed
that their age play was completely asexual. This was commonly substantiated
with the resemblance to real-life childhood, taking the construction of childhood as asexual for granted. Moreover, sexual activities as adult littles were
never discussed explicitly in this online community, even though some
adult littles stated that their play is erotically charged or sexual and even
though other activities were described in great detail. References to real-
life children's "age-appropriate" and consensual sexual explorations such as
"playing doctor" were notably absent, with just a few posts mentioning the
existence of children's sexuality as a general fact, and even that was contested.
Children were often constructed as asexual in statements like this: "When
being little I sense and feel like a small child would, so anything sexual is not
suitable for me at all." Quotes like these create the impression that these age
players are ignorant of or in denial of children's sexuality, reproducing hegemonic adultist views of children as lacking sexual desire and agency. Some
age players admitted to developing erotic feelings or arousal, for instance,
while being diapered or being close to their caregivers, but reluctantly so and
claiming it had nothing to do with eroticizing their little role. Possibly, the
specter of pedophilia was behind the disavowal and/or secrecy or the need to
justify sexual pleasure in age play:

> It's about the joint play, about the joint living out of something one carries
> deep inside and desires in a bonding way. To me that creates a wish or desire
> for intimacy and sexuality, and whether you are still in the little role or not
> does not really matter, since I desire an adult person.

So the desire for sexual activity was explained via an experience of intimacy with one's adult partner, while any eroticization of the caregiver–adult
little dynamic was disavowed. Some adult littles also distinguished between sensual and sexual activities to distance themselves from sexual desire: "To me, there are also diverse forms of sensual, but precisely not sexual
satisfaction—among those to me for instance cuddling, sucking or relieving
yourself in your diapers, thus things that feel good and trigger contentment."
Interestingly, sucking and playing with the relaxation of the anal muscle resemble textbook examples of the oral and anal stages of children's sexual

development according to Freud (1968, pp. 73–107), one of the most influential scholars of sexuality. Age players seemed to follow common popular
beliefs that children are asexual and that their pleasurable exploration of
their bodies is anything but sexual. In following this logic, they also inadvertently re-established a narrow heteronormative understanding of sexuality as
genital intercourse rather than embracing the non-normative pleasures that
simulating children's sexuality might have to offer to expand the realm of the
sexual. Positing sexuality as a distinguishing feature between adults and children furthermore reproduces the child–adult binary.

Interestingly though, this discourse of asexual innocence was disrupted
by one individual who pointed out repeatedly that she discovered sexuality
early in her own childhood: "Even if it is embarrassing: I have discovered
my sexuality as a child so early on that I cannot even remember a time before. Therefore, this aspect belongs to being little for me." That she starts with
a disclaimer ("embarrassing") demonstrates how dominant the discourse
about children, and by extension adult littles, as asexual was in this online
community. Nonetheless, she had the courage to acknowledge that children
are sexual and that it is therefore a valid element to age play. Another individual also tried to intervene by stating, "Let's be honest: Even real children
can get erections, it's simply a sensitive area down there." So only a minority
in the forum study tried to counter the common narrative of children's asexuality, while sexuality and sexual identity played a more explicit role in the
interview study. Participants were playing with the taboo-breaking nature of
sexualizing children and minors, sometimes even in public. Queer femme
Zoe described a scene in which she took a trans lover who was 29 chronologically but, due to his stage in transitioning to a man, "looks like he's twelve
now" to a hairdresser's shop as part of a scene:

> I'm having him get this little marine haircut and he says to [the hair-
> dresser]: "Yeah, I'm thinking about going to military school." . . . And she
> looks at him and says: "How come you're not in school?" And he looks at
> me kind of sly and says: "I'm being home schooled."

Zoe's lover was perceived as a schoolboy in this occurrence, and both seemed
to take pleasure in being able to break a taboo in public, posing as a couple
involving presumably a teenage boy and a woman in her 40s (who he had once
called his "soccer mom"). And it was the adult little (boy) who did not correct
the age misperception of the hairdresser (which would have immediately

distanced them from associations with pedophilia or child abuse) but rather made a double-edged comment that positioned him as a schoolboy (associated with innocence) while simultaneously hinting at inappropriate sexual relations with Zoe and thereby demonstrating that he possesses sexual desires and is a sexual subject. The playing at "realness" in this situation that presented itself by chance possibly made the taboo-breaking nature of their sexual BDSM relationship more intense (and simultaneously provided comic relief as gay men witnessing this scene were in on the joke and started "snickering"). Transgressing such taboos or social boundaries is a common strategy in BDSM to generate intense pleasures (Bauer, 2014; Weiss, 2011), and in this regard the dominant discourse in the online community seemed to differ from that in les-bi-trans-queer BDSM communities in trying to "sanitize" age play into a more respectable, asexual activity.

Participants in the interview study also resisted the heterosexualization of childhood in their age play practices. Queer femme Emma described her adult little style: "Combat boots with skirts and things like that, that kind of style. And that to me is a dyke style, it's a grrrl style." Emma was using the spelling *grrrl* to distance herself from pedophilia (Bauer, 2018, pp. 144–145) and to associate herself with the riot grrrl movement, which used this "growling" respelling to reclaim the term *girl* from its common use to belittle women. So to Emma it was important that her adult little was presenting as a dyke or riot grrrl, making sexual nonconformity among children/adolescents visible and thereby granting them desire and sexual agency in the pursuit of that desire.

Innocence and Truth

Innocence in children is often associated with (sexual) ignorance, in other words a lack of knowledge. But childhood innocence is also connected to a presumably unmediated, more "natural" access to truth, as explained above in regard to Christian notions of radical innocence (Davis, 2011). In other words, children possess knowledge that adults may have lost along with their "lost innocence." In this discourse, children know and speak the truth, while adults have been corrupted by society. In this sense, innocence is constructed as moral purity that children naturally and still possess but that is in danger of being lost by growing up. For instance, in the forum study, one adult little considered it valuable that they had "rescued a little bit of children's affect and vulnerability into my adult life." They made this comment in a post about how their adult little self was capable of feeling unfiltered rage about social injustice or animal cruelty. That empathy toward suffering animals or humans and expressing this affect are only deemed appropriate for children shows how much the standard for ethical and political reasoning is constructed as purely rational in sanist–adultist society. So, on the one hand, children have unmediated access to certain truths, for instance, without being corrupted by economic interests; but, on the other hand, their truth is affective and therefore only romanticized but ultimately not as authoritative as rationalist claims to truth. According to age players, as their adult little selves, they were capable of drawing on these in their eyes valuable innocent children's perspectives just like actual children. For instance, they used children's/adult littles' assumed capacity to speak with greater honesty to mediate in relationship conflicts. As transgender butch Jacky from the interview study put it, communication from adult littles "comes more unfiltered." Therefore, Jacky and their partner, who both switched between the roles of adult littles and caregivers in their relationship, used their adult littles for "difficult conversations."

Innocence's Counter-discourse: Constructing Children as Bratty and Disobedient

A counter-discourse to children as sweet and innocent emerged in both studies as well; in the forum study, one adult little proclaimed,

> Sassiness is one of the four cardinal virtues, or not? That is why provocative behavior is a moral duty for each proper child . . . . After all, adults have long unlearned what is really important, and when presented with the alternatives of playing Lego or eating cabbage, then the priorities are self-evident. That there will be protest, for certain as well.

So children's resistance to rules imposed on them by adults and the underlying adultist views were an inspiration for age players to construct their adult littles as bratty or sassy individuals who questioned the caregiver's authority. On the one hand, this can be a way to question sanist–adultist values such as that duties come before pleasure. Again, children's views were constructed as purer (they have unmediated knowledge about the value of life; they are not yet corrupted by productivity-oriented capitalist society) and capable of showing adults an underlying truth about what is important in life. Disobedience was thus still grounded in these notions of innocence as truth. One adult little posted a very explicit dismissal of social values in productivity-oriented capitalist society: "We do not like the system if you will. I'd rather play than work and I have actually never done the latter. And I am beyond 30 by now." After this almost revolutionary rejection of society's demand to become a productive citizen, the post quickly started to explain this with a lack of maturity caused by psychological disorder. Yet this self-pathologization did not stop this adult little from asserting their own values, and they claimed that as adult littles, "we have no desire to adjust to this stupid world."

On the other hand, sassiness was often discussed in conjunction with rules as an integral element of age play:

> I am someone who really likes to provoke! At least in little space I love to test my limits and wait for the reaction of my counterpart. I especially love to have inflexible rules as part of the play and transgress them often in order to be punished.

So the role that rules from adults play in children's lives is presented as a welcome framework to engage in playing with power, discipline, and punishment.

BDSM or not BDSM? Rules and Control as Integral to Children's Experience

In the interview study, participants were recruited as BDSM practitioners and discussed their age play practices as part of their BDSM. In the forum study, the message boards were dedicated to age play, and not everyone participating in this online community identified as a BDSM practitioner. Yet, elements related to the power imbalance between caregivers and adult littles were considered crucial to age play. Rules determined by the caregiver, control and punishment, as well as some play described as bullying and humiliation among adult littles would clearly qualify as dominance/submission from a BDSM perspective. Forum posters stressed that adult littles were often not allowed to make their own decisions such as what to wear or when to eat and that the caregiver had to control the adherence to everyday rules such as whether the adult little had properly brushed their teeth. These practices were seen as replicating authentic adult–child relations and therefore as indispensable in age play, as one forum poster summarized it: "Children cannot decide for themselves yet in many instances and therefore they have to be put under control and surveillance." Here, the construction of children as unrealized adults and lacking in agency is reproduced and used to enhance the age play experience. One adult little in the forum study had to switch off all electronic devices when going to sleep and was video-surveilled by their caregiver. This tempted them to break the rules and play with their mobile devices rather than going to sleep:

> So in order to avoid the light of the display being visible, I pulled the blanket over myself and hoped that it would not be apparent that the mobile phone was not in its proper place. Then I really felt like a child; put back into those times in which one was still secretly reading with a flashlight under the blanket, despite having to go to school early in the morning.

So, first and foremost, rules called for breaking them, which provides an interesting dynamic to play with. Secondly, rules that resemble typical childhood rules and that one recalls from one's own childhood could facilitate entering a little space that felt really authentic. Such rules could transport the adult little back into past childhood memories and affects, intensifying the experience of little space.

Related to the issue of whether age play is about striving for authenticity or about inventing one's own version of childhood, a discussion erupted on the forum about what kinds of rules are appropriate in age play, with one position summarized in this post: "In general I like a lot of things, that one would also do with a biological child, but not necessarily anything that goes further [than what is acceptable to do with biological children]." Appropriate rules for forum age players in this sense were those that stressed that one is little and dependent, effectively providing a feeling of being taken care of and protected. So rules were deemed legitimate if they are implemented to protect the adult little like actual children, for instance, holding an adult's hand when in public or bedtimes, which not only restrict self-determination but communicate that someone cares about your comfort and safety. The authenticity criterion was also evident in the following post:

I therefore only wish for one rule: **Treat me like a child!** THE PARENTS
ALWAYS DETERMINE THE RULES! . . . It's my job to find out what the
dos and don'ts are. I mean when a child is born into the world, then it also
learns all by itself to adhere to certain rules, because the big ones teach them
that. . . . The nice thing about it is that one really totally naïvely and stupidly,
yes directly childishly, approaches things and possibly even makes mistakes
unintentionally. If that does not make you become little again, then I don't
know what else to say. (Emphasis in original post)

Repeatedly, certain dynamics were sought that would enable the adult little
to feel like a real child. This was also evident in forum discussions about appropriate punishments, which often found most approval when resembling
those deemed appropriate punishments for real children aimed at their
proper development, such as "loving admonishment" or, for serious mis-
behavior, a temporary prohibition of TV time or candy (while some adult
littles also enjoyed corporal punishment as a BDSM as opposed to a realistic
variant of age play). One post pointed to the various layers of experience or
realities in age play in regard to the adult little's ambiguous relationship to
punishments:

On the one hand, they demonstrate in a great way, that one is not allowed to
decide what one wants to do. On the other hand, they are also disagreeable
(and they necessarily have to be, in order to be authentic), because they are
usually unpleasant and one wants to rather avoid them. A good punishment
to me, as in the education of biological children, is directly connected to the
deed and should more follow as a "consequence" from the deed rather than
an artificially chosen punishment.

So punishments signaled to the adult consciousness during age play that the
person was actually put into the position of a (real) child via the loss of self-
determination, so punishments were welcome in that sense. But entering
little space, they simultaneously were to be avoided given that they were
connected to unpleasant affects. They could not be enjoyable as this would
render them inauthentic and therefore not fulfill the function of assisting in
entering an authentic little space (as opposed to a supposedly inauthentic
little space, in which spanking creates sexual arousal or other kinds of not
child-like transgressions). This discussion served to distance age play from
BDSM, even though it closely resembles BDSM-typical pleasures. Possibly

this emphasis on authenticity was also strong because, as opposed to many other BDSM-related role-playing scenarios, every adult has autobiographical first-hand experience of what it means to be a child and individual memories of their actual childhood. Yet one does also not simply play oneself because one has passed into adulthood since and is therefore also embodying an experience of otherness in age play.

Adult littles in the forum also stressed how everyday rules and controlling these rules enhanced intimacy in a relationship in comparison to a regular adult relationship: "But when diapers of one's partner are checked and whether the teeth are brushed . . . that is somehow . . . real bonding and symbiosis." Boundaries are crossed in caregiving and control that are usually left intact in adult relationships. These consensual transgressions enhanced intimacy, just like many other boundary-transgressing BDSM practices (Bauer, 2014; Newmahr, 2011). Rules and control also expanded the felt presence of the partner because even in their absence "the partner is always present through their things, through rules and agreements," as one adult little experienced it.

Conclusion

The German online community of age players was comprised in part of individuals who reported in posts that they were also active in BDSM communities, while others distanced themselves from BDSM by drawing on notions of the authenticity of their little space, which relied on social constructions of children as innocent, asexual, and in need of non-erotic types of control and punishment. From a BDSM perspective, this attempt to distinguish age play from BDSM is not necessarily convincing, given that nonsexual motives and authenticity also play a role for many BDSM practitioners. The authenticity claimed is also in part dubious, given that age players tend to pick and choose what elements of chronological children's material life they draw on to enhance their affective, sensual, and sexual experiences in little space. So why do some age play communities feel the need to distance themselves from BDSM communities? Possibly, this is connected to the ongoing stigmatization of BDSM in general and the edgy nature of age play, with its danger of being conflated with pedophilia in the eyes of the public, in particular. In the interview study, those individuals who identified with queer, anti-normative politics, in contrast, saw value and pleasure in transgressive sexual age play practices; but even some of them encountered limits, such as BJ in regard to the imagined age that could be embodied in sexual age play.

The activities adult littles enjoy are considered to be child-like, childish, or unreasonable in adultist society. The strategy of using little space as a safer space to reclaim certain vulnerabilities and behaviors for adults has various effects: Relying on the concept of little space constructs these little selves in opposition to their adult selves and therefore tends to reinscribe adultist norms rather than questioning their foundation like the adult–child binary. At the same time, for some the space age play creates also opens a door to question adultist or social norms like productivity-oriented capitalist society in general. This is often accomplished by relying on popular constructions of children as innocent, therefore carving out spaces to move beyond narrow definitions of adulthood by reproducing problematic constructions of children that play a role in robbing them of their agency. This is evident in how community discourse often does not question the construction of children as asexual and as unrealized adults in need of discipline and punishments. In both studies, notions of innocence were based on white and middle-class values. So on the one hand, while age players benefit from these constructions to access certain sexual and asexual experiences, sanism–adultism and the adult–child binary mostly go unchallenged. On the other hand, participants from the les-bi-trans-queer interview study and some individuals from the forum study question the assumptions of childhood (sexual) innocence and assert children's (limited) agency. Further research could investigate similarities and differences between age play communities in other geographical contexts and how these relate to various BDSM practices and communities. Furthermore, it would be interesting to see how other age play communities are invested in constructions and deconstructions of childhood (sexual) innocence or other constructions of childhood and authenticity.

Notes

1. Because my definitions here are in part already based on the studies, I used quotes to illustrate some of my points made here. Please refer to the methods section for information on the studies and the data presented here.
2. Despite these constructions, children are in reality subject to various forms of abuse, which a shift in discourse from protection to children's rights is trying to address (e.g., MacNaughton & Smith, 2009).

References

Bauer, R. (2007). "Daddy liebt seinen Jungen"—Begehrenswerte Männlichkeiten in Daddy/Boy-Rollenspielen queerer BDSM-Kontexte. In R. Bauer, J. Hoenes, & V. Woltersdorff (Eds.), *Unbeschreiblich männlich. Heteronormativitätskritische Perspektiven* (pp. 170–180). Männerschwarm Verlag.

Bauer, R. (2014). *Queer BDSM intimacies. Critical consent and pushing boundaries.* Palgrave Macmillan.

Bauer, R. (2018). Bois and grrrls meet their daddies and mommies on gender playgrounds: Gendered age play in the les-bi-trans-queer BDSM communities. *Sexualities, 21*(1–2), 139–155. https://doi.org/10.1177/1363460716676987

Brame, G., Brame, W. D., & Jacobs, J. (1993). *Different loving. An exploration of the world of sexual dominance and submission.* Villard Books.

Davis, R. A. (2011). Brilliance of a fire: Innocence, experience and the theory of childhood. *Journal of Philosophy of Education, 45*(2), 379–397. https://doi.org/10.1111/j.1467-9752.2011.00798.x

Freud, S. (1968). *Gesammelte Werke* (Vol. 5, 4th ed.). Fischer.

Gittins, D. (2009). The historical construction of childhood. In J. M. Kehily (Ed.), *An introduction to childhood studies* (2nd ed., pp. 35–49). Open University Press.

Hawkinson, K., & Zamboni, B. D. (2014). Adult baby/diaper lovers: An exploratory study of an online community sample. *Archives of Sexual Behavior, 43*(5), 863–877. https://doi.org/10.1007/s10508-013-0241-7

Jenks, C. (2009). Constructing childhood sociologically. In J. M. Kehily (Ed.), *An introduction to childhood studies* (2nd ed., pp. 93–111). Open University Press.

Keating, F. (2016). Racialized communities, producing madness and dangerousness. *Intersectionalities: A Global Journal of Social Work Analysis, Research, Polity, and Practice, 5*(3), 173–185. https://journals.library.mun.ca/ojs/index.php/IJ/article/view/1664/1336

Kehily, M. J. (2009). Understanding childhood. An introduction to some key themes and issues. In J. M. Kehily (Ed.), *An introduction to childhood studies* (2nd ed., pp. 1–16). Open University Press.

Kehily, M. J., & Montgomery, H. (2009). Innocence and experience. A historical approach to childhood and sexuality. In J. M. Kehily (Ed.), *An introduction to childhood studies* (2nd ed., pp. 70–89). Open University Press.

Lasala, A., Francesco, P., Senese, V. P., & Perrella, R. (2020). An exploratory study of adult baby-diaper lovers' characteristics in an Italian online sample. *International Journal of Environmental Research and Public Health, 17*(4), Article 1371. https://doi.org/10.3390/ijerph17041371

LeFrancois, B. A., & Coppock, V. (2014). Psychiatrised children and their rights: Starting the conversation. *Children and Society, 28,* 165–171. https://doi.org/10.1111/chso.12082

Lewis, A. (2011). Ageplay: An adults only game. *Counselling Australia,* 19–22.

MacNaughton, G., & Smith, K. (2009). Children's rights in early childhood. In J. M. Kehily (Ed.), *An introduction to childhood studies* (2nd ed., pp. 161–176). Open University Press.

Newmahr, S. (2011). *Playing on the edge. Sadomasochism, risk and intimacy.* Indiana University Press.

Piaget, J. (1977). *The language and thought of the child.* Routledge & Kegan Paul.

Piper, C. (n.d.). Historical constructions of childhood innocence: Removing sexuality (pp. 1–33). https://bura.brunel.ac.uk/bitstream/2438/673/3/19thc%2Bsex.pdf

Rand, E. J. (2019). PROTECTing the figure of innocence: Child pornography legislation and the queerness of childhood. *Quarterly Journal of Speech, 105*(3), 251–272. https://doi.org/10.1080/00335630.2019.1629001

Robinson, K. H. (2012). "Difficult citizenship": The precarious relationships between childhood, sexuality, and access to knowledge. *Sexualities, 15*(3–4), 257–276. https://doi.org/10.1177/1363460712436469

Rodham, K., & Gavin, J. (2006). The ethics of using the internet to collect qualitative research data. *Research Ethics Review, 2*(3), 92–97. https://doi.org/10.1177/174701610600200303

Rousseau, J. J. (1889). *Emile; or, concerning education.* Heath & Company.

Speaker, T. J. (1980). *Sexual infantilism in adults: Causes and treatment* [Unpublished master's thesis]. Southern Oregon State College. https://understanding.infantilism.org/surveys/ts_masters_thesis.pdf

Strauss, A. L., & Corbin, J. (1990). *Basics of qualitative research. Grounded theory procedures and techniques.* Sage.

Tiidenberg, K., & Paasonen, S. (2018). Littles: Affects and aesthetics in sexual age-play. *Sexuality & Culture, 23*, 375–393. https://doi.org/10.1007/s12119-018-09580-5

Walkerdine, V. (2009). Developmental psychology and the study of childhood. In J. M. Kehily (Ed.), *An introduction to childhood studies* (2nd ed., pp. 112–123). Open University Press.

Wall, J. (2019). From childhood studies to childism: Reconstructing the scholarly and social imaginations. *Children's Geographies*, 1–14. https://doi.org/10.1080/14733285.2019.1668912

Weiss, M. (2011). *Techniques of pleasure: BDSM and the circuits of sexuality.* Duke University Press.

PART III

RELATIONSHIPS AND COMMUNITIES

6

Navigating Dissonant Desires

Kink (In)Compatibility in Romantic Relationships

Daniel Cardoso, Patrícia M. Pascoal, and Rita Quaresma

Introduction

In adults, "major developmental tasks involve attempts to integrate one's gender identity, sexual orientation and sexual expression with partners" (DeLamater & Hyde, 2005, p. 8). Therefore, relationships are crucial for identity integration, and identity influences relationships in a mutual, bidirectional process throughout one's life. Relationship quality and well-being are important correlates of global and mental health (Whitton & Kuryluk, 2012), and factors that negatively impact relationships—for example, a lack of sexual compatibility and subsequent sexual conflict about sexual preferences (La France, 2019)—are associated with higher levels of negative emotions, poorer mental health (Florean & Păsărelu, 2019), and lower relationship satisfaction. Given the importance of sexual compatibility, the differences between sexual identities (e.g., a person who identifies as kinky and a partner or partners who do not) might translate into interpersonal conflict or tension or generate dissatisfaction in the relationship (Lawrence & Love-Crowell, 2007). We use *kinky* as an umbrella term that encapsulates both BDSM and fetishism (sexual arousal from or desire for non-living objects); as we detail in the methodology section, this approach is informed by the specific debates and positionings of the communities that we focused on when undertaking the survey, and any specific deviation from this terminology is only meant to remain true to the context in which other terms are used.

In the specific context of sexual identity, relationship difficulties can also impact the way people experience their own kink identities or the types of experimentation they engage in. However, the potential for partner dissatisfaction or conflict arising from role or interest incompatibility is not the

Daniel Cardoso, Patrícia M. Pascoal, and Rita Quaresma, *Navigating Dissonant Desires* In: *The Power of BDSM.*
Edited by: Brandy L. Simula, Robin Bauer, and Liam Wignall, Oxford University Press. © Oxford University Press 2023.
DOI: 10.1093/oso/9780197658598.003.0007

sole issue that might emerge. Such stressors should be understood within a wider context of other potential difficulties that kinksters face. These include being afraid to disclose their interests (especially to prospective partners), having difficulty finding a partner whose interests are compatible with theirs, finding partners deemed safe and responsible, engaging in activities outside of their comfort zone, and internalizing shame (Damm et al., 2018; Pascoal et al., 2015). These difficulties not only exist as part of the intrapsychic landscape of a person but also fuel relationship-specific problems.

Identities and practices are sometimes at odds with each other. In the study by Coppens et al. (2020), many respondents who routinely engaged in BDSM practices still did not consider themselves as BDSM-identified; furthermore, practitioners with more experience, including more experience of playing in social contexts, tended to more often perceive and organize their experience in accordance to identities and how those identities were socially perceived (e.g., in BDSM clubs).

Massively mainstream representations of BDSM—with a particular emphasis on the *Fifty Shades of Grey* books and movies—are another way in which personal and relationship problems might arise. As research shows, the way communities and practitioners of BDSM perceive themselves stands mostly at odds with how they are portrayed (Barker, 2013; Drdová & Saxonberg, 2020; Tsaros, 2013). Dymock (2013) notes that the *Fifty Shades* series brought heightened awareness of kink to mainstream audiences (the "*Fifty Shades* effect") and that it resulted in an influx of newcomers who were grossly misinformed about kink and consent, thereby increasing the potential for relationship conflicts and misunderstandings.

Previous research has revealed that having multiple sexual partners (either consensually or covertly) is a strategy adopted by people when their interests do not match their partners' (Bauer, 2014, 2019; Pascoal et al., 2015). However, there still exists a paucity of research on how relationship dynamics play out and are impacted by incompatible interests in kink (i.e., when one person is interested in kink and the other one is not or when people interested in kink consider their interests to be relationally incompatible), namely outside of queer and consensually non-monogamous contexts. (For those contexts see, e.g., Bauer [2014].)

Qualitative research has indicated that those with queer sexualities and gender identities tend to maintain a more flexible approach to their BDSM identities and practices (Martinez, 2018) and that BDSM roles are typically heavily connected to the sexual and gendered scripts prevalent in Western society. The expression of a BDSM identity also seems to be very gendered and along mostly normative lines, more so in mostly cis-heterosexual communities, both in the identities that people take on themselves and in the way that they conceptualize those identities as intrinsic or extrinsic, with men reporting the former more and women the latter more (Yost & Hunter, 2012).

This study follows up on that issue and seeks to address multiple experiences with relationship challenges—and participants' perceptions of those challenges—when it pertains to the kink-related dimension of their relationships, focusing specifically on kink-identified participants and their romantic relationships. While we acknowledge that focusing on romantic relationships carries with it the risk of reinforcing amatonormativity (De las Heras Gómez, 2018)—that is, the belief that the need for romantic relationships is a universal experience and the best form of intimate relationship—research suggests that romantic relationships are still highly valued in contemporary Portugal (Poeschl et al., 2015).

We intend to improve knowledge about the perception of the relationships of people with interest in, or who self-identify with, kink. In this aspect, our study advances knowledge about BDSM and kink by exploring the connection between the social situatedness of kink in regard to normative sexuality and specific relationship challenges and by providing a possible typology of different challenging areas in kink relationships, either in situations where one of the partners is not kinky or where all partners are but the respondent still considers that there are kink-specific challenges.

In the current study, we gathered responses from a sample of people practicing, or having an interest in practicing, BDSM/fetishism; and we explored their perception of challenges encountered at the intersection of their putative or actual romantic relationships and kink.

Method

The survey from which this study and its results were derived is comprised of a series of sociodemographic (age, gender, education, residence, sexual orientation, kink self-identification, and relationship status) and qualitative survey questions. The online survey was developed in LimeSurvey, and the link was circulated in 2018 through theme-specific social networks, such as FetLife, mainly through posts in groups dedicated to the Portuguese community at large. In total, 189 partial or incomplete survey responses were logged by the platform, but only 87 participants completed the survey.

In the current study, we focus on the only open question that addresses perceptions of relationship challenges faced by kinksters:

Do you consider that there are specific challenges that are posed to people with interest and/or practice in BDSM and/or fetishism when they estab- lish romantic relationships with other(s) (e.g. boyfriend/girlfriend) and this person(s) is (are) or is (are) not interested in BDSM and/or fetishism? Which ones, and can you give examples?

Participants

Among the 89 people who answered the question we are analyzing, two answers were eliminated because they were blank or unintelligible, resulting in 87 valid answers. The participants' age varied from 18 to 57 years old ($M = 33.02$, $SD = 9.63$). There were 38 people who identified themselves as men and 45 as women, and four participants made use of an open text box option to specify their gender as neither man nor woman. One person self-identified as agender. One person identified themselves as genderqueer. One person identified themselves as "transgender/bigender," and one person identified themselves as another gender without giving more specific information. Most participants had a university degree, and the next largest group of participants had university attendance. There was a greater representation of the districts of Lisbon, Porto, and Setúbal (which was expected as these are among the most densely populated areas of the country). People identified mostly as heterosexual (56), followed by bisexual (17), undefined orientation (3), and lesbian (2); eight people re- ported other sexual orientations such as heteroflexible (4), pansexual (3), and homoflexible (1). Regarding relationship status, 36 people reported being in a monogamous relationship, followed by 20 in non-monogamous consensual relationships and 16 who were not in a romantic relationship. About 75 people mentioned having practiced something that they consider BDSM/fetishism, and the remainder, due to their interest in kink, had con- tact with the kink community even if they considered themselves as not having engaged in kink practices.

Although this has been the subject of a heated national debate, the Portuguese constitutional framework does not allow for the collection of data on race or ethnicity except in highly specific circumstances and solely under the supervision and authorization of the National Committee for Data Protection. Indeed, not even the national census collects this information (Henriques, 2019; Matos, 2019).

Procedure

This work follows a participatory research approach (Cornwall & Jewkes, 1995); that is, members of the part of the Portuguese kink community that congregates in virtual spaces (internet forums, newsgroups, and closed groups on social media) were contacted and assessed the relevance and adequacy of the survey questions in line with what they felt to be relevant to the community overall. Some community members also reviewed the questionnaire in an effort to ensure that it had clear and inclusive language. The IP addresses of the participants were not kept, and the data was only accessible to people related to the study. The informed consent procedure contained information regarding the voluntary and anonymous nature of the study, the absence of financial compensation, the names of the researchers and their emails, the purpose of the study, and the inclusion criteria: being over 18, having a native-speaker level of understanding of written Portuguese and of writing in Portuguese, living in Portugal, and being interested in kink or self-identified as a kinkster.

Regarding Portuguese mastery, this criterion was discussed among the research team. We decided to make it a requirement for respondents to have an assumed ability to fully comprehend the wording of the questions for our ability, as researchers, to be able to parse the nuance of their responses. This is particularly relevant considering that, in an online survey, there is no possibility for clarification or communication between respondents and researchers. Due to Portugal's colonial history, Portuguese is an official language in 10 different countries; and the majority of migrants coming to Portugal are from these countries, which means that many of them possess a native-speaker level of Portuguese.

Participants were asked to answer a set of sociodemographic questions and a set of open-ended questions. The study was approved by the Ethics and Deontology Commission for Scientific Research from the School of Psychology and Life Sciences (Escola de Psicologia e Ciências da Vida) of the Lusophone University of Humanities and Technologies (Universidade Lusófona de Humanidades e Tecnologias).

Answers to the open-ended question of the current study were processed using NVivo (Bazeley & Jackson, 2007). We followed the method of qualitative data analysis proposed by Braun and Clarke (2006), using an inductive, semantic, and (critical) realist approach. That is, we looked for semantic themes according to the meanings presented in the entire data set. The organization of the data was structured hierarchically into three levels of analysis. The first level consists of codes identified throughout the data set. The second level consists of subthemes that aggregate meaningfully associated codes. The third level encompasses the main themes with more global meanings (Braun & Clarke, 2006). In the current study, the first and third authors coded the data set autonomously. The main themes, subthemes, and codes were found after repeated reading of the answers provided and after a careful understanding developed not only of the patterns of the themes but also of the contradictions and inconsistencies to aggregate the patterns of meaning. Subsequently, the authors compared their versions of the thematic map until a final consensual version was achieved. Coding congruence and consensus, and therefore validity, were achieved after several adjustment discussions among the researchers. Finally, following previously described procedures (Pascoal et al., 2019), the second author reviewed the information, codes, subthemes and themes. This allowed for a more diverse and insightful exploration into the topics previously identified and increased the reliability of the results.

Results

We have identified challenges and coping strategies. The replies given were organized into three main themes: intrapersonal, interpersonal, and societal. A fourth theme emerged to encapsulate the responses that denied the existence of any challenges: absence of challenges (Table 6.1).

Intrapersonal

The responses gathered under this theme point toward difficulties that the respondents felt in regard to themselves as kinksters. The subthemes included here are self-disclosure, negative emotions, and personal transformation. Self-disclosure deals mainly with fear of rejection or self-perceived

Table 6.1 Hierarchic Organization of the Thematic Map with Themes, Subthemes, and Codes

Themes	Subthemes	Codes
1. Intrapersonal	1.1. Self-disclosure	1.1.1. Negative expectations about partner's reaction
		1.1.2. Difficult to expose desires
	1.2. Negative emotions	1.2.1. Emotional or sexual frustration
		1.2.2. Internalized kink-phobia
	1.3. Personal transformation	1.3.1. Fulfillment
		1.3.3. Sexual epiphany
2. Interpersonal	2.1. Relationship dynamics	2.1.1. Interest incompatibility
		2.1.2. Mononormativity
		2.1.3. Partner's positioning
		2.1.4. Feelings of safety
		2.1.5. Inviable relationship
		2.1.6. Relationship transformation
		2.1.7. Difficulty finding a romantic partner
		2.1.8. Kink as a prerequisite
	2.2. Erotic dynamics	2.2.1. Practice rejection
		2.2.2. Diverse practices
		2.2.3. Difficulty in finding an erotic partner
		2.2.4. Kink conversion
		2.2.5. Kink pedagogy
		2.2.6. Non-monogamous strategies
		2.2.7. Communicating and negotiating practices
3. Societal	3.1. Societal representations	3.1.1. Rejection of the *50 Shades* model
		3.1.2. Negative social perceptions about kink
	3.2. Lack of information	
4. Absence of specific challenges		

lack of skill when wanting to communicate one's preferences. For example, one participant replied, "issues might arise around fear of telling or sharing one's interest in BDSM or fetishes, which might wear out the relationship" (woman, 27 years old, BDSMer, monogamous relationship); and another stated, "You can't just go up to someone and say 'I'd like to treat you like a pet'" (man, 46 years old, BDSMer, no relationship). This shows how, even outside the scope of any given relationship, kinksters will sometimes feel that the stigma around kink creates negative emotions and how the expectation or likelihood of an expression of interest in kink being met with negativity might result in negative emotions for them.

The negative emotions subtheme pertains to participants' feelings of internalized kink-phobia and how they say one might feel with incompatible interests, namely, frustrated and/or dissatisfied: "when the sexual behaviours aren't compatible, the romantic relationship ends up making its participants feel frustrated" (woman, 26 years old, interested in BDSM, casual relationships). Personal transformation pertains to the fact that some participants consider BDSM as having been a transformative experience in their lives. This means that BDSM became a fundamental part of their identity, with several describing it as a sexual epiphany. Both framings make it harder to navigate a potential connection with someone who has not experienced those same things or had the same response to them. For instance, a participant said, "the relationship wouldn't even exist without the BDSM component, since it's fundamental to me and to my partner" (man, 23 years old, BDSMer, no relationship), thus noting how the dynamic is not just a component of the relationship but the basis for its existence.

Interpersonal

Here, the focus is on the interaction between partners or potential partners. While arguably some of the responses coded above could be perceived as being interpersonal, we have chosen to code them according to how participants demarcated their focus, whether internally (i.e., intrapersonal) or in their connection to their putative or actual partners (i.e., interpersonal). The replies coded for this theme focus on two different subthemes: relationship dynamics and erotic dynamics. Within relationship dynamics, we find two main types of responses. On the one hand, there are issues that arise in the interaction between people, like interest incompatibility, difficulties finding partners, prejudice from partners, mononormativity (Pieper &

Bauer, 2005)—which is to say, the belief, and incumbent social systems and structures, that posits monogamy as the only valid or healthy way of having intimate relationships—or unmet needs for safety. As one of the respondents said, "There's sometimes risky behaviours that can lead to manipulation or emotional blackmail, when people vent their frustrations through Domination/submission rules, or when they use their knowledge of our desires to make us stay in a relationship with them" (genderqueer, 30 years old, switch, casual relationships). This response shows how kink might introduce an axis of vulnerability and blur the lines between consensual dominance and submission play and psychological manipulation in a way unique to those relationship structures.

On the other hand, there are also references to changes in dynamics that account for, and engage with, those problems (e.g., breaking up the relationship, transforming the relationship by introducing kink dynamics into it, or not even entering into a relationship unless kinky dynamics are present). The subtheme of erotic dynamics has some similarities but collects responses that pertain directly to the erotic or sexual dimension rather than focusing on an overarching romantic relationship. Here, the emphasis falls much more on strategies to cope with potential incompatibilities rather than on the incompatibilities themselves. As can be seen in Table 6.1, the main hurdles mentioned were finding kinky partners or having a partner who totally rejects any kind of kink practices; however, the multitude of kinky identities that exist, and how they might clash, was also seen as a potential problem rather than an opportunity. We also observed that participants have a multitude of ways to cope with such situations: from negotiating roles and trying to find a "middle ground" to deploying the logics of pedagogy or conversion to kink, as we can see when a respondent said that "Introducing the partner to the topic and educating them on it" (woman, 50 years old, BDSMer, casual relationships) was a form of addressing a partner's potential ignorance about kink or engaging in consensual non-monogamy as a way to explore their interests with other partners.

Societal

Under this theme, we have gathered responses that deal with the role society plays in how kinky relationships are perceived and how public representations, such as in movies or books, then become resources that can hinder or boost kink connections and relationships. A specific topic that arose was the lack of information or literacy that non-kinky people are perceived to have on the topic: "Since there's not a proper sexual education system to teach youngsters to explore their sexuality ... prejudice and stigma just accumulate until adulthood, and then it's harder to develop those tools" (man, 31 years old, kinkster, no relationship data provided), which brings to the fore the need for timely and inclusive sex education. Besides this, social representations emerged as a subtheme, split between issues caused by common misconceptions about kink (which contribute to several of the problems seen above) and issues brought about by the popularization of *Fifty Shades of Grey* specifically. This seems to represent, for a number of participants, a paradigm that encapsulates all of the problems with media representations of kink and a phenomenon that altered sociability around this topic.

Absence of Challenges

Lastly, some participants clearly stated that they did not consider that there are any specific challenges to relationships between kinky and non-kinky people. Several respondents just typed "No"; another noted how desire mismatch in kink is "just like with everything else" (woman, 24 years old, sub/switch/brat,[1] non-monogamous relationship), thereby claiming that no difference exists between kink and non-kink contexts when it comes to relationship difficulties. This is not to say that they believe these relationships to be free of any difficulties but that, in their perspective, the relationship difficulties faced by kinksters are equivalent to those found in any other type of romantic relationship. However, these responses tended to be extremely short, and it was therefore impossible to draw more conclusions from the existing data.

Discussion

Othered Sexualities as a Transpersonal, Societal Experience

Our research shows that the individual, interpersonal, and societal aspects of relating are inextricable from one another and that kinksters face specific challenges as a minority.

Two of the subthemes of the intrapersonal dimension demonstrate this. The need for self-disclosure (Bezreh et al., 2012) has to contend with mostly negative expectations about what the reaction of the partner(s) will be and even the difficulty of making oneself understood in the context of a conversation about sexual preferences. Another aspect to this pertains to internalized kink-phobia. This is to say, feelings of shame or uncertainty about whether the participants' sexual interests are somehow "wrong" create an added layer of difficulty in terms of the perception of how communication might happen around kinky desires. Moreover, the lay idea that sexual incompatibility in general may compromise a relationship might contribute to negative expectations (e.g., conflict) about the consequences of self-disclosure of a kinky identity (Maxwell et al., 2017) and to more negative emotions.

Many participants linked these perceptions to societal factors, and these issues can be seen in the theme of the same name. Respondents who mentioned them criticize what they call the "*Fifty Shades* model," in line with extant academic criticism of it (Barker, 2013; Drdová & Saxonberg, 2020; Dymock, 2013; Tsaros, 2013), and mentioned that there is a lack of socially available information about kink. This, in turn, promotes negative social perspectives about kink, according to participants, as is evident by the fact that *prejudice* was a word often used. The "*Fifty Shades* effect" (i.e., the influx of new people into kink communities) has established itself as a linchpin moment within contemporary representations of kink and with far-reaching impact in the kink community (Dymock, 2013), and our findings echo this for the Portuguese kink community, further demonstrating the importance of international media phenomena and how important it is for those phenomena to be congruent with minorities' self-perception.

All of the aforementioned issues contribute to one of the major topics raised: the difficulty in finding a partner with whom to develop a kinky relationship, be it a more romantic or more casual and erotically centered one, as not all kink preferences are understood or experienced as being mutually compatible.

For our participants, being part of a minority group defined by an othered form of living or that defines one's sexuality is an experience that inextricably implies interpersonal, intrapersonal, and societal challenges. What happens at the social level sets the stage on which kinky relationships take place and at least partially defines or constrains even the possibility of those relationships happening, creating hurdles which are not felt by those whose lives and experiences are normatively aligned. People who identify with, or fear that they are perceived as belonging to, a marginalized sexual minority usually worry about being discovered and rejected (Derlega et al., 2002), creating negative feelings and expectations around self-disclosure to a potential partner.

Navigating Multiple Desires

The difficulties in communicating desires are not the only potential hurdle that participants identified. Communication as a relationship tool can even serve to alleviate some of the problems that our participants noted, as per their responses, but can also bring to the fore issues that are harder to overcome.

As is particularly visible in some of the codes under the relationship dynamics and erotic dynamics subthemes, being clear about what one wants can still result in discovering incompatible interests or in the absolute rejection of those same interests by the partner. The fact that there can be multiple ways in which kink desires manifest might result in partners' desires being perceived as incompatible or in someone having an interest in different kinky activities that do not fully match a given partner's interests.

The former point, incompatible interests, can take on several forms. The first is to simply find out that the partner is not interested in kink. Beyond that, the breadth of kinky practices and identities[2] seems to constitute, for the participants, a challenge unto itself. In scenarios where everyone is kinky, the multitude of potential kinky identities or practices and the many ways in which they might be incompatible make it so that having a kinky identity or interest is not the main issue but having specific kinky identities or interests (seen as compatible) is. For a subsection of our respondents, being kinky involved having partners who would, in a broad sense, feel they had compatible proclivities to their own (e.g., someone who is into dominance wanting to partner up with someone who is into submission). Because this allows for a multitude of potential permutations, BDSM-specific communication plays a fundamental role.

Not all respondents, however, seemed to be looking for one specific identity or set of identities in their prospective partners. For some of them, communication was also a way to change and adapt to new realities or interests. Communicating at this stage is referred to as attempting to find a "middle ground," discovering which types of connections and compatibilities might be worthy of exploring in the sense of creating a mutually satisfying connection, which is in line with previous research on markers of sexual satisfaction.

Previous studies have shown that having partners whose identity struggles are, to a point, resolved (e.g., in regard to sexual orientation or sexual identity [Pascoal et al., 2019]) is a key marker of one's sexual satisfaction. This identity work is a cornerstone of these communication processes as being able to express desires, needs, and fantasies requires a degree of self-awareness; and so does exploring potential new interests.

This means creating limits and boundaries in terms of what is and is not included in the relationship, shaping the relationship into a form that creates satisfactory and balanced dynamics capable of holding space for the erotic and/or emotional needs of all those involved. In our study, this is reflected by the code *communicating and negotiating practices*. Part of this process has to do with another potentially problematic element, which we coded as *feelings of safety*, safety both in oneself and in the understanding that existing partners will respect one's limits and attend to their own safety. Communicating can partially expose or alleviate incompatibilities in how people perceive issues around safety, whether there is a perceived lack of rules that might make the relationship or dynamics feel unsafe or differences in how each person holds themselves responsible for proactively advocating for their safety.

As we have seen above, then, communication and dyadic conflict-resolution competences are fundamental not only to relationship management but also to identity management (Lavner, 2017; Martinez et al., 2016), as highlighted by the communication theory of identity (CTI) that advocates the idea that identity is socially constructed, multilayered, dynamic, and communicated verbally and non-verbally and evolves throughout one's life span. CTI highlights that one's identity is acted upon, shaped by, and reshaped by social interaction and posits that all social interaction throughout one's life is meaningful (Shin & Hecht, 2017).

Several participants reported being openly discriminated against by one or more partners. This took the form of judgments of value against participants' kinky preferences or even accounts of abusive behavior. This further illustrates that fear of discrimination is, at least to a point, realistic, inasmuch as there is empirical evidence that points toward discrimination of varying levels against people who express kinky desires (Bezreh et al., 2012).

Landscapes of Relationship Dynamics and Requirements

Because of how fundamental several of our participants feel that kink or fetishism is to their well-being and their personal and relationship fulfillment, it often operates as a gatekeeping system (Mustanski et al., 2014). Many would not consider beginning a relationship with someone who was not kinky and compatible or would have it as at least a central consideration when it came to selecting a partner or falling in love with one. Therefore, it is not only the conscious decision of engaging in a long-term relationship but also the potential for an emotional connection that is made to be dependent upon the existence of a kinky/fetishist compatibility.

There has been a historical shift in romantic relationships toward personal fulfillment (Giddens, 1993, p. 58), and kink/fetish is incorporated into definitions of what personal fulfillment is, be it through the idea of sexual fulfillment or with an integralist approach to kink in regard to one's sense of self. Through this perspective, kink becomes more than just a series of sexual or erotic acts—it is a dimension of interpersonal connection that is fundamental to the mere possibility of an enjoyable life.

However, the configuration of the relationship can be either a mitigating factor or a strategy to cope with the perceived lack of a matching kinky/fetishist. In fact, many participants mentioned how mononormativity (Pieper & Bauer, 2005) is an important issue between kink and non-kink partners or between kinky partners who might have interests that are deemed incompatible. The restriction to be monogamous—be it sexually and/or in a kinky context—can make it more difficult or even impossible for some kinksters to remain or engage in a relationship with someone. This might even occur despite their wanting to be in a relationship and having feelings for that person since some or all of their kinky interests will then be barred to them as that current or potential partner does not want to partake in them.

For some of these participants, at least, one option or management strategy is consensual non-monogamy. This is seen by some participants—especially those who present themselves as having a more varied range of interests in terms of what kinky activities they want to engage in—as a way to address their multiple desires by engaging in kinky play with different people (with whom they establish different dynamics by bracketing out of each interaction the parts deemed incompatible) in ways that feel confluent within each pairing. Therefore, in some respects, our data shows that mononormativity plays a role in how kinksters might consider or disavow certain coping strategies and that relationship configurations are a central element in understanding relationship conflicts and dynamics (Bauer, 2010; Scoats & Anderson, 2019; Willis, 2018). Unlike existing research (Bauer, 2014), resorting to consensual non-monogamy was only seen as a viable option by a very few respondents, while most saw a variety of interests as problematic, making it harder to find a romantic partner who would be seen as compatible.

Personal Identity Fulfillment and the Risk of Interpersonal Ontological Hierarchies

The importance that the exploration of sexual interests has to sexual and global identity development seems to be supported by our results, inasmuch as some of our participants express the feeling that being kinky has made their lives better. In a Foucauldian sense (Foucault, 1994), there are mentions of BDSM being what made it possible for them to be themselves. This places sexuality in a privileged position when it comes to defining one's global identity vis-à-vis other psychosocial markers (Mustanski et al., 2014).

For some of the participants, kink operates as a system of personal realization and as a process through which the field of sexuality itself is transformed. These reported experiences, which we have aggregated under the code "sexual epiphany," see the discovery and/or practice of kink as transcendent regarding what is considered to be non-kinky sexuality. In practice, this creates a hierarchy of different modes of sexuality, where kink is seen as more "authentic" or "liberated" and so "better" or "purer." This can be understood as a reactive process arising from the challenges that kinksters face qua minorities (Mustanski et al., 2014).

Such a perspective can create potentially unbalanced relationship dynamics. Some participants mentioned that sometimes relationships with non-kink-identified persons are possible *because* they present a possibility of transforming the partner into someone who is in fact interested in kink through processes of exposure or intentional persuasion. Rather than allowing for an explicit negotiation of power imbalances and play around those (Bauer, 2019), this means that BDSM becomes another means through which power imbalances are reproduced and naturalized.

As mentioned, identity processes are also intersubjective, and romantic relationships are relevant to such processes as they open up or close down spaces of exploration and relating (Mustanski et al., 2014). We have found differences between responses which emphasized the possibility of making knowledge available to (potential) partner(s)—coded under *kink pedagogy*—and a more instrumentalizing take on how respondents had the tools and occasion to "elevate" the non-kinky partner's sexuality by introducing them to kink. While we acknowledge that even a posture of pedagogy creates a potentially problematic power imbalance between partners (Foucault, 1994, pp. 97–99), we posit here that making available such knowledge is qualitatively different from the more instrumental approach associated with making the relationship dependent upon a form of "conversion."

Such a narrative of transformation (of the other) runs the risk of creating a false dichotomy between "kink" and "non-kink" sexuality as separate and isomorphic, rather than seeing them as socioculturally produced, and contested, arbitrary boundaries between different erotic expressions (Rubin, 2007). While it might contribute to a more self-assured position for the kinky partner in relation to their own sexual expression, it might, contrariwise, provoke feelings of inferiority or unsuitability for the non-kink-identified partner(s), especially if this dynamic presents itself as part of a reactive minority stress response (Simpson & Yinger, 1985), as also evident in other research (Mota & Oliveira, 2012).

Limitations

There are some limitations in our study which need to be considered when interpreting the results and the discussion thereof. While thematic analysis does not rely on large sample sizes, we may not have captured all types of potential relationship difficulties. This is doubly so since our sample lacked diversity: People who were not native-level proficient in Portuguese were excluded, and most respondents were straight, monogamous, and/or cisgender. The geographical distribution of our sample is also mostly focused on more urban areas, which might overly focus on challenges from people who might be more easily capable of accessing kink sociability spaces.

Some of the responses provided were very short and potentially ambiguous. The online data collection method did not allow for the development of ideas by participants, thereby creating difficulties in interpreting and coding some of the responses.

We also had no way to separate the answers according to whether participants had indeed lived through the issues mentioned or not. Even though some of the answers were clearly autobiographical in nature, we did not ask about direct personal experiences, to allow a greater degree of comfort for participants (i.e., to be less intrusive), especially considering that the small dimension of the Portuguese kink community might make participants feel they would be identifiable by their answers.

Conclusions and Future Directions of Study

There are no clear-cut separations between individual, interpersonal, and societal challenges when it comes to constructing and experiencing identity. Sexual and gender minorities face specific hurdles when it comes to how they experience their processes of identity construction and how they are able to live out their lives (Rubin, 2007) and handle self-disclosure. This has potential impacts on their mental and general health and well-being (Ryan et al., 2015; Villicana et al., 2016) and should be a point of consideration in terms of education around sexualities, social policies aimed at combatting discrimination, and specific training for mental and general health professionals (McClelland & Frost, 2014).

When compared to other sociohistorical and geographical settings and communities (Bauer, 2010, 2014), the disruptive potential of BDSM (Bauer, 2019; Cardoso, 2018) seems emptied of power and mononormativity reinstated through it in the largely heterosexual, monogamous, and cisgender composition of our sample (not uncommon for Portuguese-based studies), where attitudes toward consensual non-monogamies are still relatively negative (Cardoso et al., 2020) and where support for marriage is still high and associated with the fulfillment of ideals of love and family building (Poeschl et al., 2015). Alongside such specificities, we also note that many of these topics can help us better understand relationship dynamics in kinky settings, and such lessons might be extrapolated into relating overall. Communication, in particular, appears here as a complex process in which the shared and not-shared literacies between different people impact the possibility of communicating something effectively; and the potential for (symbolic) violence in kink carries implications around self-disclosure, vulnerability, and intimacy.

Conversely, being part of a minority can sometimes be the basis of some potentially problematic relationship dynamics, whereby counteracting stigma will sometimes result in reactive redeployments of potentially aggressive or stereotyping behaviors against those who are not perceived to be from that minority group. This includes situations where those who have been discriminated against will respond with acts of symbolic, individualized aggression against members of the majority group (Simpson & Yinger, 1985).

Considering the above, future research should explore more in depth, with a special emphasis on interpersonal communication and negotiation, what types of problems kinksters face in their relationship dynamics and how they address those issues, namely seeking to identify successful strategies that promote individual and relational well-being. It is also relevant to try and understand what socioeconomic and psychological factors might impact those skills and their deployment.

Other aspects to consider are the potential difficulties that people who are consciously uninterested in engaging with kink experience when faced with a partner(s) who has that interest, what strategies they deploy to cope, and how they impact their relationships. More attention should also be paid to the way consensual non-monogamies operate in articulation with kink-associated identities and practices, as a form of coping strategy applied situationally, rather than framed as an individual relationship orientation.

Acknowledgments

The authors would like to acknowledge all participants for their time and support of our study.

This work is partially funded by national funds from FCT—Fundação para a Ciência e a Tecnologia, I.P, through the Research Center for Psychological Science of the Faculty of Psychology, University of Lisbon (UIDB/04527/2020; UIDP/04527/2020).

Notes

1. A kink identity or role that is associated with bottoming and in which the brat "misbehaves" so that they receive "punishment" by the top.

2. The way kinky identities are understood by participants is diverse: Some consider it to be an intrinsic part of themselves, akin to a sexual orientation but needing an awakening or trigger to come to the fore, while others see it as a set of practices that is more amenable to change.

References

Barker, M. (2013). Consent is a grey area? A comparison of understandings of consent in *Fifty Shades of Grey* and on the BDSM blogosphere. *Sexualities, 16*(8), 896–914. https://doi.org/10.1177/1363460713508881

Bauer, R. (2010). Non-monogamy in queer BDSM communities: Putting the sex back into alternative relationship practices and discourse. In M. Barker & D. Langdridge (Eds.), *Understanding non-monogamies* (pp. 142–153). Routledge.

Bauer, R. (2014). Exploring exuberant intimacies. In *Queer BDSM intimacies: Critical consent and pushing boundaries* (pp. 107–143). Palgrave Macmillan. https://doi.org/10.1057/9781137435026_5

Bauer, R. (2019). BDSM relationships. In B. L. Simula (Ed.), *Expanding the rainbow: Exploring the relationships of Bi+, polyamorous, kinky, ace, intersex, and trans people* (pp. 135–147). Brill | Sense.

Bazeley, P., & Jackson, K. (2007). *Qualitative data analysis with Nvivo* (2nd rev. ed.). SAGE Publications.

Bezreh, T., Weinberg, T. S., & Edgar, T. (2012). BDSM disclosure and stigma management: Identifying opportunities for sex education. *American Journal of Sexuality Education, 7*(1), 37–61. https://doi.org/10.1080/15546128.2012.650984

Braun, V., & Clarke, V. (2006). Using thematic analysis in psychology. *Qualitative Research in Psychology, 3*(2), 77–101. https://doi.org/10.1191/1478088706qp063oa

Cardoso, D. (2018). Bodies and BDSM: Redefining sex through kinky erotics. *The Journal of Sexual Medicine, 15*(7), 931–932. https://doi.org/10.1016/j.jsxm.2018.02.014

Cardoso, D., Pascoal, P. M., & Rosa, P. J. (2020). Facing polyamorous lives: Translation and validation of the attitudes towards polyamory scale in a Portuguese sample. *Sexual and Relationship Therapy, 35*(1), 115–130. https://doi.org/10.1080/14681994.2018.1549361

Coppens, V., Brink, S. T., Huys, W., Fransen, E., & Morrens, M. (2020). A survey on BDSM-related activities: BDSM experience correlates with age of first exposure, interest profile, and role identity. *The Journal of Sex Research, 57*(1), 129–136. https://doi.org/10.1080/00224499.2018.1558437

Cornwall, A., & Jewkes, R. (1995). What is participatory research? *Social Science & Medicine, 41*(12), 1667–1676. https://doi.org/10.1016/0277-9536(95)00127-S

Damm, C., Dentato, M. P., & Busch, N. (2018). Unravelling intersecting identities: Understanding the lives of people who practice BDSM. *Psychology & Sexuality, 9*(1), 21–37. https://doi.org/10.1080/19419899.2017.1410854

DeLamater, J., & Hyde, J. S. (2005). Conceptual and theoretical issues in studying sexuality in close relationships. In J. H. Harvey, A. Wenzel, & S. Sprecher (Eds.), *The handbook of sexuality in close relationships* (pp. 7–30). Routledge.

De las Heras Gómez, R. (2018). Thinking relationship anarchy from a queer feminist approach. *Sociological Research Online*, Article 1360780418811965. https://doi.org/10/gf3spz

Derlega, V. J., Winstead, B. A., Greene, K., Serovich, J., & Elwood, W. N. (2002). Perceived HIV-related stigma and HIV disclosure to relationship partners after finding out about the seropositive diagnosis. *Journal of Health Psychology, 7*(4), 415–432. https://doi.org/10.1177/1359105302007004330

Drdová, L., & Saxonberg, S. (2020). Dilemmas of a subculture: An analysis of BDSM blogs about *Fifty Shades of Grey. Sexualities, 23*(5–6), 987–1008. https://doi.org/10.1177/1363460719876813

Dymock, A. (2013). Flogging sexual transgression: Interrogating the costs of the "*Fifty Shades* effect." *Sexualities, 16*(8), 880–895. https://doi.org/10.1177/1363460713508884

Florean, I.-S., & Păsărelu, C.-R. (2019). Interpersonal emotion regulation and cognitive empathy as mediators between intrapersonal emotion regulation difficulties and couple satisfaction. *Journal of Evidence-Based Psychotherapies, 19*(2), 119–134. https://doi.org/10.24193/jebp.2019.2.17

Foucault, M. (1994). *História da sexualidade 1: A vontade de saber.* Relógio d'Água.

Giddens, A. (1993). *The transformation of intimacy: Sexuality, love and eroticism in modern societies.* Stanford University Press.

Henriques, J. G. (2019, June 17). INE chumba pergunta sobre origem étnico-racial no censos. *PÚBLICO.* https://www.publico.pt/2019/06/17/sociedade/noticia/censos-1876683

La France, B. (2019). The impact of sexual self-disclosure, sexual compatibility, and sexual conflict on predicted outcome values in sexual relationships. *The Canadian Journal of Human Sexuality, 28*(1), 57–67. https://doi.org/10.3138/cjhs.2018-0005

Lavner, J. A. (2017). Relationship satisfaction in lesbian couples: Review, methodological critique, and research agenda. *Journal of Lesbian Studies, 21*(1), 7–29. https://doi.org/10.1080/10894160.2016.1142348

Lawrence, A. A., & Love-Crowell, J. (2007). Psychotherapists' experience with clients who engage in consensual sadomasochism: A qualitative study. *Journal of Sex & Marital Therapy, 34*(1), 67–85. https://doi.org/10.1080/00926230701620936

Martinez, K. (2018). BDSM role fluidity: A mixed-methods approach to investigating switches within dominant/submissive binaries. *Journal of Homosexuality, 65*(10), 1299–1324. https://doi.org/10.1080/00918369.2017.1374062

Martinez, L. V., Ting-Toomey, S., & Dorjee, T. (2016). Identity management and relational culture in interfaith marital communication in a United States context: A qualitative study. *Journal of Intercultural Communication Research, 45*(6), 503–525. https://doi.org/10.1080/17475759.2016.1237984

Matos, A. (2019). *A legitimidade da recolha e processamento de dados relativos à raça e à origem étnica: Impactos na esfera privada dos indivíduos e no combate à discriminação* [Unpublished master's thesis]. Universidade do Porto. https://repositorio-aberto.up.pt/bitstream/10216/126089/2/384586.pdf

Maxwell, J. A., Muise, A., MacDonald, G., Day, L. C., Rosen, N. O., & Impett, E. A. (2017). How implicit theories of sexuality shape sexual and relationship well-being. *Journal of Personality and Social Psychology, 112*(2), 238–279. https://doi.org/10.1037/pspi0000078

McClelland, S. I., & Frost, D. M. (2014). Sexuality and social policy. In D. L. Tolman, L. M. Diamond, J. A. Bauermeister, W. H. George, J. G. Pfaus, & L. M. Ward (Eds.), *APA handbook of sexuality and psychology: Vol. 2. Contextual approaches* (pp. 311–337). American Psychological Association. https://doi.org/10.1037/14194-010

Mota, A. M., & Oliveira, A. (2012, June 19). *Para além da dor: Fantasias de prazer, poder e entrega* [Paper presentation]. VII Congresso Português de Sociologia: Sociedade, Crises e Reconfigurações, Porto, Portugal. http://associacaoportuguesasociologia.pt/vii_congresso/papers/finais/PAP1418_ed.pdf

Mustanski, B., Kuper, L., & Greene, G. J. (2014). Development of sexual orientation and identity. In D. L. Tolman, L. M. Diamond, J. A. Bauermeister, W. H. George, J. G. Pfaus, & L. M. Ward (Eds.), *APA handbook of sexuality and psychology: Vol. 1. Person-based approaches* (pp. 597–628). American Psychological Association. https://doi.org/10.1037/14193-019

Pascoal, P. M., Cardoso, D., & Henriques, R. (2015). Sexual satisfaction and distress in sexual functioning in a sample of the BDSM community: A comparison study between BDSM and non-BDSM contexts. *The Journal of Sexual Medicine, 12*(4), 1052–1061. https://doi.org/10.1111/jsm.12835

Pascoal, P. M., Shaughnessy, K., & Almeida, M. J. (2019). A thematic analysis of a sample of partnered lesbian, gay, and bisexual people's concepts of sexual satisfaction. *Psychology & Sexuality, 10*(2), 101–118. https://doi.org/10.1080/19419899.2018.1555185

Pieper, M., & Bauer, R. (2005). Polyamory und mono-normativität. Ergebnisse einer empirischen studie über nicht-monogame lebensformen. In L. Méritt (Ed.), *Mehr als eine liebe: Polyamouröse beziehungen* (pp. 59–69). Orlanda.

Poeschl, G., da Silva, B. P., & Cardoso, F. T. (2015). Casamento, casamentos? Representações sociais do casamento heterossexual e do casamento homossexual. *Análise Psicológica, 33*(1), 73–87. https://doi.org/10.14417/ap.886

Rubin, G. (2007). Thinking sex: Notes for a radical theory of the politics of sexuality. In R. Parker & P. Aggleton (Eds.), *Culture, society and sexuality: A reader* (2nd ed., pp. 150–187). Routledge.

Ryan, W. S., Legate, N., & Weinstein, N. (2015). Coming out as lesbian, gay, or bisexual: The lasting impact of initial disclosure experiences. *Self and Identity, 14*(5), 549–569. https://doi.org/10.1080/15298868.2015.1029516

Scoats, R., & Anderson, E. (2019). "My partner was just all over her": Jealousy, communication and rules in mixed-sex threesomes. *Culture, Health & Sexuality, 21*(2), 134–146. https://doi.org/10/gdcfht

Shin, Y., & Hecht, M. L. (2017). Communication theory of identity. In Y. Y. Kim (Ed.), *The international encyclopedia of intercultural communication* (1st ed., pp. 1–9). Wiley. https://doi.org/10.1002/9781118783665.ieicc0008

Simpson, G. E., & Yinger, J. M. (1985). Types of response to prejudice and discrimination. In *Racial and cultural minorities: An analysis of prejudice and discrimination* (5th ed., pp. 137–154). Plenum Press.

Tsaros, A. (2013). Consensual non-consent: Comparing EL James's *Fifty Shades of Grey* and Pauline Réage's *Story of O. Sexualities, 16*(8), 864–879. https://doi.org/10.1177/1363460713508903

Villicana, A. J., Delucio, K., & Biernat, M. (2016). "Coming out" among gay Latino and gay white men: Implications of verbal disclosure for well-being. *Self and Identity, 15*(4), 468–487. https://doi.org/10.1080/15298868.2016.1156568

Whitton, S. W., & Kuryluk, A. D. (2012). Relationship satisfaction and depressive symptoms in emerging adults: Cross-sectional associations and moderating effects of relationship characteristics. *Journal of Family Psychology, 26*(2), 226–235. https://doi.org/10.1037/a0027267

Willis, A. S. (2018). "One among many"? Relational panopticism and negotiating non-monogamies. *Sexualities*, Article 136346071875656. https://doi.org/10/gf3snq

Yost, M. R., & Hunter, L. E. (2012). BDSM practitioners' understandings of their initial attraction to BDSM sexuality: Essentialist and constructionist narratives. *Psychology & Sexuality*, 3(3), 244–259. https://doi.org/10.1080/19419899.2012.700028

7

Dispelling the Negative Perception of the BDSM Community in Johannesburg, South Africa

Tracey L. McCormick

Introduction

There are no statutory laws in South Africa that outlaw BDSM. In fact, the criminal courts have never been presented with a case involving BDSM in South Africa. However, there is a lingering perception by many people that BDSM is abnormal and depraved (Noyes, 1998; Soni, 2018; Van Reenen, 2014). Prior to the publication of my article "Yes Master! Multimodal Representations of BDSM Bodies on a South African Website" (McCormick, 2018a), there was only one academic article that focused on BDSM in South Africa; however, the author equates BDSM with violence (Noyes, 1998).

In my 2018 article I draw on literature from the Global North that finds that BDSM communities are safe, sane, and consensual; and I question whether BDSM communities in the South African context operate on similar lines. Although I cannot locate an organized BDSM community, this article is a positive reappraisal of BDSM in the South African context. Having established an academic interest in researching BDSM, I managed through word of mouth in my queer networks to locate a key member of this community; and over a period of 2 years, I managed to gain their trust so that they agreed to be interviewed. This chapter depicts the first case study of the BDSM community in Johannesburg using as evidence an insider's knowledge and experience of this community.

My objectives in this chapter are as follows:

1. To explore the Johannesburg BDSM community by drawing on a case study of the experiences of a key member of the community.

Tracey L. McCormick, *Dispelling the Negative Perception of the BDSM Community in Johannesburg, South Africa*
In: *The Power of BDSM.* Edited by: Brandy L. Simula, Robin Bauer, and Liam Wignall, Oxford University Press.
© Oxford University Press 2023. DOI: 10.1093/oso/9780197658598.003.0008

2. To show how the growth of the internet in South Africa in the late 1990s enabled loosely connected BDSM individuals to form a sexually organized community based on the principles of safety, sanity, and consent.
3. To dispel the negative myths that surround BDSM in South Africa that equate it with pornography and depravity and show instead a close-knit community that has a proud history, with long-standing members and where knowledge about BDSM is prized.
4. To show that although this community is sexually progressive, there are contestations around gender and race.

I begin the chapter with a brief background and a review of the two published articles on BDSM in South Africa (Noyes, 1998; McCormick, 2018a). This is followed by a discussion of how I collected and analyzed my data, and then I show how a queer theoretical framework has informed the interpretation of my data. This is followed by the largest section of this chapter, which is dedicated to the configuration of the BDSM community in Johannesburg. My data will show a tight-knit community where members rise through the ranks having shown the ability to adhere to the strictest of rules and protocols around BDSM play. However, despite such closeness, the community is almost exclusively white; and there are major contestations around race. I conclude this chapter with evidence to suggest that the negative perceptions of BDSM as being abnormal and depraved in South Africa are not true.

Theoretical Framework

The lenses that I operationalize to analyze my data are drawn from queer theory, and there is a body of literature dedicated to pinpointing its emergence in the field of critical studies, tracing its genealogy, and describing its usefulness and limitations in both an international and a South African context (David et al., 2005, p. 3; Halperin, 1995, p. 122; Rubin, 1993, p. 28; Seely, 2020, p. 1232; Warner, 1993, p. 11).

Queer theory underpins my research on the BDSM scene in Johannesburg (Berlant & Warner, 1995, p. 343; Butler, 1993, p. 19; David et al., 2005, p. 3). I employ three specific lenses from queer theory to "grasp" and "hold . . . in view" BDSM and to reappraise it positively (Rubin, 1993, p. 9). Firstly, by employing the notion of the sexual hierarchy of value I can examine how sexualities are valued differently in South Africa (Rubin, 1993, p. 13). The default normative sexuality is married, monogamous heterosexual people; and those who veer from this gold standard cascade down the hierarchy of value. BDSM sexualities are at the bottom of this hierarchy, alongside sex workers, men who have sex with men, and porn actors. Queer theorists value this "sexual rabble" as examples of resistance to compulsory vanilla heterosexuality (Rubin, 1993, p. 13). Secondly, for queer theorists the fact that BDSM sex can be detached from sexuality, gender, and the "exclusive localization in the genitals" is a challenge to conventional heterosexual sex, where the norm is for sex to occur between people of the opposite gender (Halperin, 1995, p. 87). In queer theory, BDSM sex is celebrated as an example of non-productive sex that counters the idea that "natural" sex is productive and good (Rubin, 1993, p. 13). Thirdly, for queer theorists, sexual shame is political, and people whose choice of sex deviates from the normal might be "beaten, murdered, jailed [or] stigmatized as deviants" (Warner, 1999, p. 3). Rubin (1993) argues that "sexual variation per se is more specifically policed by the mental-health professions, popular ideology, and extra-legal social practice" (p. 19) and that the stigma against them "derives from medical and psychiatric opprobrium" (p. 11). Queer theorists pay attention to those hegemonic structures which produce pathological others (such as BDSM practitioners) to validate normal subjects (David et al., 2005, p. 1).

Background and Overview of South African Literature

BDSM communities were late to bloom in Johannesburg compared to the Global North, arguably due to South Africa's violent and segregated past. Prior to the advent of democracy in 1994, the media was controlled by the apartheid government and restricted by Afrikaner Calvinistic morality, which forced it to promote the idea of a white, abstemious nuclear family. However, post-1994 these restrictions were relaxed, and the media could for the first time depict all kinds of subcultures that were considered abnormal during apartheid, including BDSM (Merrett, 2001). But the portrayal of this subculture was bookended by stereotypical and sensationalistic ideas, and it was only when the internet became widely accessible in the late 1990s that BDSMers could take control of their own narrative. The freedom to portray BDSM images in the media and for like-minded BDSMers to find each other and form communities was a concern to Noyes (1998), which he voices in an article entitled "S/M in SA: Sexual Violence, Simulated Sex and Psychoanalytic Theory." The first line of his article, "South Africa is one of the most violent places on earth" (p. 135), creates a causal link between BDSM and violence which is maintained throughout the article. Noyes is concerned about the "steady rise [and] general visibility" as well as the "increase in the availability of S/M sex" (pp. 135–136) facilitated by the internet, which is a "perfect medium for the propagation of S/M" (p. 136). Such propagation, according to him, has filtered into mainstream media, such as the Cape Town–based Sunday newspaper *The Argus* as well as two national society magazines of the time, *Die Kat* and *Style*. Noyes calls for empirical studies to be done on BDSM in South Africa that are informed by sociological and psychoanalytic theories; however, he concludes that such a reappraisal will be daunting because of BDSM's "complex relationship to acts of social and sexual violence" (p. 150).

The association of social and sexual violence with BDSM would seem to prevent academics from taking up the call by Noyes, and it would take another 20 years for the subject of BDSM to be broached.

In 2018 I argued that BDSM should not be equated with violence (McCormick, 2018a). I used literature from the Global North that shows that participants are generally "healthy, educated, well-adjusted and successful" (Dahan, 2019, p. 387). Despite the lingering perception by some South Africans that BDSM is abnormal, I identified a "thriving" (McCormick, 2018a, p. 147) BDSM scene organized around the local site Collar Me but whose members might also be part of FetLife, an international social networking site for the BDSM community with more than 10 million members. Collar Me is a discussion forum for people who are interested in BDSM, and any person can join after agreeing to a stringent privacy policy. Once on the forum, a person is given a bronze status, and they must prove their trustworthiness and intentions to move to silver and then gold status. It is only on achieving gold status that a person might be invited to a play party. Yet, all requests for potential research collaboration with the moderators of Collar Me were not answered; and as FetLife is not involved in the physical meetings of the local BDSM community, it was not approached. With no access to the organized BDSM community in South Africa I used instead classifieds from the "domination and fetish" section in Backpage to try and investigate BDSM. Backpage was an international site that offered free classified adverts and was embargoed by the FBI in 2018. I posited that the existence of a "domination and fetish" section in the South African version of Backpage indicates activity and an appetite for BDSM by some of the readers of this site. However, the people who post in this section are by no means an organized or networked community, but they do show a knowledge of consent and different types of play and are able to represent BDSM through recognizable clothing and language (McCormick, 2018a).

Although my study is not empirical or generalizable, it is worth noting for the following reasons. Firstly, although there is evidence of an organized BDSM community in South Africa that is connected through the online site Collar Me, the moderators of the site are not interested at all in making their site available for research purposes. Secondly, although small-scale, my study is positive in its reappraisal of BDSM in South Africa; and I do not use the negative tropes found in the Noyes study.

Data Collection and Analysis

My present study is based on an interview with Neptune, who is associated with both Collar Me and FetLife. They made it clear to me that they did not want to be identified in any way as this could affect their livelihood; therefore, I am refraining from providing sociodemographic data on them. Neptune revealed that they were a founding member of the public BDSM play parties organized through Collar Me in Johannesburg beginning in about 2000. During the interview Neptune reiterated that for them "public play space has always been, *in a public space*, not a private home party" (original emphasis). These public play parties are not public in the way that Warner (2002) would describe "public." They are for invited members who have accrued a certain status in online forums, so they are exclusive, similar to the Catacombs (Rubin, 1998). They are held in different public venues, such as restaurants and clubs, which are closed to the public when there is a party. As Bauer (2014) explains, public spaces where "non-normative sexual expressions" (p. 107) are enacted are "severely restricted and policed" (p. 107), hence the need for exclusivity to provide safety to practitioners. Further, he calls these "contained" spaces because they are semi-contained spaces "distinct from the general public but shared with others with the same intent" (p. 108).

Neptune is no longer associated with Collar Me, but they are now an active member of FetLife. They are vague about dates and whether what they were describing was associated with Collar Me or FetLife, but they say nothing negative about either site or the leadership of these sites.

The Configuration of BDSM Communities
in Johannesburg, South Africa

There are BDSM communities in many of the major urban areas of South Africa, "but the biggest hub," according to Neptune, is in Johannesburg. The rapid growth of the internet in South Africa from 1996 facilitated connections between like-minded BDSMers in chat rooms and online forums, and in about 1998 collarme.co.za (Collar Me) was established, which was dedicated to the BDSM community. The BDSM communities in South Africa are very secretive, and members communicate through Collar Me or FetLife. Collar Me was, until the arrival of FetLife, the nexus of the BDSM community, organizing members-only educational and public play events in Johannesburg. Neptune speaks of the need for the BDSM community to operate in secret and under the radar because of the popular perceptions associating BDSM with violence and pornography: "There are a lot of closeted people because of the fear of judgment . . . [and because] people see [BDSM] as violence [and] as non-consensual sadism."

This community is organized around the "original" core values of safety, sanity, and consent that have been developed in international communities and prides itself on its education in these values (Simula, 2019). I did not locate any evidence from Neptune of any engagement with the notions that have been debated now for nearly 10 years in the Global North of risk-aware consensual kink (RACK) or the 4Cs (caring, communication, consent, and caution) (Simula, 2019). Rather, Neptune spoke of best prac-tice within the Johannesburg scene: "Our creed in BDSM is safe, sane and consensual, so we only engage once we have consent and for as long as it is safe and sane." Training in various or all of the aspects of BDSM play is central to this community. "You can't just give someone a spanking," Neptune notes, and a person needs to "earn their chips." The training stage starts in a person's 20s and is characterized by "curiosity and exploring"; for example, learning the art of spanking is something that "you build one spank at a time." When I asked Neptune about their training, they replied as follows:

> I trained under a master for two years and I trained in every discipline in BDSM that was available to me and that I could dig up. Everything that I ad-minister I have lived and experienced and I know what it feels like, I know what it does to you.

Neptune's intensive training under a master is reminiscent of what has been described in the American context as an "Old Guard" approach to BDSM, which prizes discipline, etiquette, hierarchy, and formality (Rubin, 1998, p. 2). The disagreement between participants, activists, and academics in the Global North about "Old Guard" and "New Guard" approaches has yet to be solved; however, in the South African context there is no documentation of this in the literature or by my participant. From Neptune's explanations I would surmise that the Johannesburg BDSM scene can be classified as "Old Guard" as there is a strict hierarchy and specific formalities that need to be observed. Such an "Old Guard" approach to BDSM, I would argue, is both liberating and constraining: liberating in that BDSMers can practice their desires freely knowing that there are structures in place to protect them inside and outside the community; constraining in that the hierarchical structure means that potential new BDSMers must proceed through the ranks to be allowed to participate in play parties. And, as I will show below (see "Race in the BDSM community"), the emphasis on having to prove your BDSM credentials is often used as a gatekeeping mechanism to keep out and limit the participation by Black BDSMers. The exact size of this community is not public knowledge, but it is big enough to organize members-only moots and play parties that take place in a public space and that are attended by people from the above-mentioned city.

Moots and Play Parties

According to Neptune, *moots* are "little pub get togethers . . . for discussion on a specific topic, for networking and getting to know the people in the community." Moots are similar to the Global North's *munches*; however, they are not purely social but are based around educating the local community, which has been a priority for the leaders since 2000. "In the earlier days," Neptune recalls, "we made a very big effort to get people to moots and get them informed and get them educated." The growth of the internet made "infinite material available."

As people got to know each other at the moots, parties started to be organized "because people were interested in having a communal area to play in." A party is a "gathering arranged by like-minded BDSM people" and is advertised on Collar Me (or FetLife). Although these parties are held in a public space that the community rents, they are not open to the general public but "open to invitees only"; and in order to be invited, a person needs to be "known by someone and be met and vouched for." When the attendees arrive at the party, "we have equipment ready" with all "different sort of play stations."

There are specific rules of engagement at public play parties. Firstly, people who arrive at the party together must have consented to specific plays prior to the beginning of the party. Secondly, if a person wants to play with another a person who is not their partner, they have to obtain "permission strictly from the person they arrived with." Neptune makes clear that they "wouldn't go ahead with any kind of play scenario without consenting to it." Thirdly, hygiene is of the utmost importance; and "before you move on from your play station you need to clean and sanitise [it], so the next person takes over a clean, safe space." Finally, the shedding of blood (i.e., edge play), the emission of bodily fluids, and sex are not allowed. This is, Neptune clarifies, "not a sex positive society, it is a BDSM society" and there are many things that can be "easily expressed . . . through many acts of BDSM without it turning into a sex act. . . . BDSM isn't sexual at all, it is simply mental, it is an intellectual exchange." The prohibition of sex when public play parties were established in about 2000 was a response to laws that regulated sex in public as public indecency.

And it seems in the contemporary setting that the evacuation of sex has led local BDSMers to experiences of elation connected to the intellect rather than the genitals. This would be consistent with a strain within the literature which details BDSM as transcendent and spiritual (Baker, 2018, p. 440; Carlström, 2020, p. 749; Charles D'Avalon, 2020, p. 1). However, sex is not completely off limits, and Neptune reveals that "at a private home party if we have say 3, 4, 5, 6 couple groups together, I would let play go into sex with my partner or allow it to go with other couples as well." But in a public space BDSM continues to be a sexless practice, and the leadership seems to be unaware (or ignores) debates in the Global North about whether BDSM is sex or not (cf. Bauer, 2014, p. 241; Newmahr, 2010, p. 313; Simula, 2019, p. 209). This might have to do with the Old Guard structure of the scene, which uses as proof of the success of the community the founding principle of no sex in public.

When I questioned Neptune about a possible link between BDSM and having access to capital, they used the emphatic South Africanism "No man" and continued "you certainly don't need cash to practice BDSM . . . BDSM can be done with chopsticks and an elastic band." They mention further the ingenuity of the local scene: "You don't you know need to go and buy, let's go something basic like a pair of nipple clamps . . . you can literally use wooden chopsticks that you get from a takeaway sushi place or a Chinese restaurant." Frugality and ingenuity are also the trademarks when it comes to the clothing worn by members of the Johannesburg BDSM scene. Neptune emphasizes that "many people are into nylon stockings, the pair of nylon stockings that you buy for R5.99."[1] The equipment used at play parties is neither imported from international suppliers nor bought at local suppliers as there are none. "You certainly don't need to go and buy equipment"; rather, Neptune urges people interested in BDSM to "use stuff from your bathroom, from your kitchen [or] from your bedroom." When it comes to equipment, "we have very crafty people in the community [laughs], a load of crafty people." The community has built up a supply of equipment since the first play party in 2000 which they share and maintain. This finding contrasts with that of Weiss (2011, p. 5), who argues that BDSM is a capitalist consumer sexual practice. Rather, where there is not the capital for expensive equipment purchases or attire, inventiveness and creativity are the order of the day in the Johannesburg BDSM scene. In the Global North, Bauer's (2014, p. 15) research located a similar "thrift store" approach to BDSM when there is a lack of capital.

Demographic and Gender Composition in the BDSM Community

The biggest age range of participants in the Johannesburg BDSM scene is, according to Neptune, "between 30 and 40 . . . and then there is a group of older people now between 40 and 50 that sort of established the scene [and that are] sort of handing [it] down to the next generation." There are more submissives than dominants, and the reason for this, Neptune observes, is that "people like to give up power more than they like to take control." Although Neptune does not mention if participants switch from the role of submissive to dominant, the Old Guard character of the scene would suggest that to switch roles would mean to be retrained and might not be desirable because a potential switch to, for example, a submissive would mean a cascade down the hierarchy and the loss of symbolic and real power within the community.

In the Global North there is a growing body of literature which is putting gender firmly on the BDSM map (cf. Barker, 2013, p. 20; Bauer, 2014, p. 194,

2018, p. 139; Simula, 2019, p. 210). However, the scene in Johannesburg is lagging when it comes to gender equity. When I asked the question about the gender composition of the Johannesburg scene, Neptune answered that it's "very difficult to say but, there are more men than women." This is because "historically . . . guys are more inclined to show their devious side or [are] less shy, women were still very much stuck in a mind-set of don't tell until fairly recently." Neptune's stereotypical answer about the historical devious-ness of men and the shyness of women as the reason for the greater partici-pation by men in the contemporary setting perhaps reflects the sentiments of the community at large. However, what Neptune did take pride in reiterating is the pansexual composition of the community that is "*all* gender tolerant in fluidity": "We have pretty much something of everything. We have cross dressers that are gay, crossdressers that are straight, we have transgender straight people, transgender gay people, we have bisexual people, we have asexual people." Issues of gender composition are not pressing for Neptune because pansexuality indicates a sexually progressive and non-judgmental community. This compares negatively to the issue of race, to which, without prompting, they returned throughout the interview and which I will explain in greater detail in the following section.

Race in the BDSM Community

Neptune revealed that the public play parties held in Johannesburg are attended exclusively by white BDSMers and that, despite the scene being es-tablished in the late 1990s, it was only in 2014 that an interest was shown in the online forums by potential Black BDSMers. Initially confined to Black men, after a short while, according to Neptune, two or three Black women "made their arrival but they are unfortunately few and far between." Neptune describes the low participation by Black BDSMers as "unfortunate," and they have "no idea what stopped them from coming on the scene before." When I asked if Black members had their own scene, they replied "I don't know, I don't think so."

In the early 2000s there was a thriving leathermen scene in South Africa with a strong participation by Black leathermen, and the co-winner of the combined male and female leather pageant in 2015 was a female Black BDSMer (McCormick, 2018b, p. 83). So, there is evidence that Black

BDSMers existed and that, rather than being organized in a recognizable and coherent community, they might have been dispersed among other radical sexual subcultures in Johannesburg or other parts of South Africa. However, there is no evidence to suggest that when the BDSM scene was being melded the leadership tried to recruit or enter into alliance with Black BDSMers, and the scene was carved out as a white-only space. The few articles that directly address the lack of Black participation in the BDSM scene in the Global North suggest that, although the exclusion of Black BDSMers might seem unintentional, this exclusion is far from neutral and is an extension of white privilege where BDSM spaces are naturalized as white-only and where "the perverted body" is inscribed with whiteness (Bauer, 2008, p. 238; Cruz, 2015, p. 433; Martinez, 2021, p. 733; Sheff & Hammers, 2011, p. 200; Simula, 2019, p. 2109). Neptune postulates that the lack of participation by Black BDSMers is linked to the shame they might feel if they came out as a BDSMer to their cultural communities.

> Look it's still very much taboo to be out as gay can you imagine coming out as a BDSM practitioner in a world where they can't even accept that people could love each other regardless of gender? And now you want to bring a flogger into the situation or tie someone down.

Recent research in South Africa indicates that while homosexuality might be a taboo in many Black communities, it is certainly not a taboo in all Black communities; and there is evidence to suggest that there is a tolerance and even acceptance of dissident sexualities in both urban and rural areas (Morgan & Wieringa, 2005, p. 22; Ratele, 2014, p. 118; Reid, 2013, p. 5). However, there is a lingering popular perception that homosexuality is shunned in Black communities, and the discourse of homosexuality as being abnormal and anti-family is often encouraged by powerful and often US-based charismatic churches (McEwen, 2018, p. 142). This enters the popular imaginary via the media, and the perceived abnormality of homosexuality could indeed be a barrier to the coming out of many Black BDSMers as the fear of sanction could be worse or as alienating as coming out as homosexual. Sheff and Hammers (2011) argue that Black BDSMers in the Global North could be reluctant to participate in visible BDSM communities as their perceived perversion could "threaten conventional family structures" (Sheff & Hammers, 2011, p. 198) and increase surveillance of their person.

Although Neptune's optimism that participation by Black BDSMers is "growing and it certainly is something that is more thought of more spoken of," they add that "unfortunately racism still plays a role, it's a very sad reality but there is still racism happening." When I directly asked if the community is racist, they replied "well, there's . . . I wouldn't say the community's racist but there is racism involved in the fear of joining such a community." They recall a

> person who joined the communities strictly because he wanted to be treated like Black boys were treated in the colonial times. It was a Black boy who was looking for a, and I'm going to quote it, a "white madam," who could treat him like a garden boy in the colonial times.

The request from this Black BDSMer is for *race play*, which is defined as "erotic play that explores power exchange within the dynamics of cultural, ethnic, socio-economic, religious and/ or racial differences" (Daddy cited in Cruz, 2015, p. 423). However, the response to this request by white BDSMers, according to Neptune, was so racist and "radical and hardcore" that they cannot utter the "terminology used." As the community prides itself on education and knowledge, the request by the Black BDSMer to be treated as a "garden boy" by a "white madam" was deemed unsophisticated by some members of the community. In the Global North Bauer (2008) argues that white BDSMers create an aura of "high quality" with the attendant qualities and attributes of being "highly educated, intelligent or classy individuals" (p. 238). It would seem that a similar situation prevails in South Africa, and the racism that stems from the garden boy/white madam post is because the Black BDSMer does not possess the perceived high-quality white values of education and class. The local BDSM communities' greatest self-imposed taboo is the request for race play because it would materialize the actual deep-seated racism of some members of a community that sets itself apart from mainstream communities that are homophobic, sexist, and vanilla. Neptune distances themselves from these racist white BDSMers and classifies their responses as being judgmental.

> Who are we to judge other people's kinks . . . you can't judge somebody because they sin differently? And the response [to the Black poster] was of racist nature against someone who was asking to be treated in a racist way, in a very derogatory way. So, it was sad.

Neptune is upset with the racism in the BDSM scene, to which they respond on four occasions with the word *sad*; and on one occasion they recall even "crying tears" and having their heart "shattered." Neptune as a founding member witnessed and experienced the inclusivity and openness found within the community which they are proud of and now which some members have lost sight of. They say that the community is

> tolerant, it is inclusive, it is non-judgemental [and that is] why it made me so sad when the people of colour were shunned so quickly for their being different. I think people have joined the community just for being included and for not being judged.

For example, they talk of a man who goes to every play party but does not dress in any BDSM gear or engage in any BDSM activities and "chats to everyone"; and Neptune "thinks it's because no-one judges him for being odd, there's just, this unconditional inclusiveness." Because he is white, he is not judged for being asexual or not kinky because his friendliness is equated with being non-judgmental of the BDSMers around him. However, the same accepting attitude does not extend to potential Black participants, whose race not only prevents them from attending physical parties but also prevents them from participating in online forums; and Black BDSMers, according to Neptune, "regardless of what their kink is are immediately frowned upon." This is because "they are not asking for it in the right way . . . they come in asking for something like slavery and it gets misconstrued." Neptune identifies the perceived lack of knowledge of BDSM by Black BDSMers and the judgmental attitude to this by white BDSMers as the source of exclusion of Black BDSMers from online sites. They are emphatic when they say, "who are you to judge someone else's kink just because you sin differently, doesn't make your sin a lesser sin or a bigger sin."

The racism shown by some BDSMers operates, I would argue, on four levels. Firstly, it denies agency to Black BDSMers as their participation in the community is not based on their own choice; rather, it is subject to white BDSMers being open-minded. Secondly, the judging of race play is a front for the exclusion of Black BDSMers from online and physical spaces. Thirdly, the community assumes that the kink of all Black BDSMers is race play, which they interpret as racist and which has no place on what they perceive to be enlightened online forums. In the Global North Martinez (2021) argues that "racialized individuals do race play whether they desire or not, because they present as such" (p. 736); and whether race play is a challenge to standard racist narratives or whether it re-enforces existing inequalities is still under debate, but it is not simply racist (Cruz, 2015, p. 433, Martinez, 2020, p. 733).

Finally, according to Neptune, replies to requests for race play from community members were "if you want to be treated with the face of racism then you need to find it in a different space. So, it was treated with racism saying that this isn't the place for racism." South Africa is an incredibly race-sensitive society, and to be exposed using actual racism or racist innuendos results in the guilty party or parties facing legal sanction and relegation to the status of social pariahs. For example, in 2016 a white woman uploaded a post on Twitter likening Black people reveling on a beach in Durban to monkeys and went from "relative anonymity to a hate figure within hours" (Mutiga, 2016). This story made international headlines, and she was found guilty of hate speech and fined R150,000.[2] Yet the absolute privacy and detailed terms of use of online BDSM forums protect the racist users from sanction and exposure and permit users to freely voice prejudicial statements. And, despite their pride in being educated in the BDSM arts, some members of the community seem to have side-stepped current debates on race play where it has been shown to have the potential to "counter standard racist narratives" (Smith & Luykx, 2017, p. 433). Because the community is small and tight-knit, a veil of silence protects this space even if members disagree with other members' racism. Differences of opinion regarding race are erased to achieve a common goal, which is for the community to be perceived by society at large as safe, sane, and consensual. Due to the Old Guard structure of the community, racism is overlooked if it manifests from well-established senior members, even if similar-ranking members such as Neptune call it out.

Conclusion

There are BDSM communities in all the major urban areas of South Africa, but Johannesburg is the hub. Once hidden from public view, the rapid growth of the internet in the late 1990s facilitated the creation of forums where like-minded individuals could openly discuss their hidden desires. Armed with freely shared educational texts and how-to manuals, these individuals formed public communities to share information and to play together. They introduced protocols and followed best practices from international communities based on safety, sanity, and consent. Crafty members started making equipment and attire in their homes, friendships formed, and for the first time people whose desires were hidden found a community where they were not judged or made to feel deviant.

However, these communities are furtive and operate on a rigorous vetted membership system because of the popular perceptions that associate BDSM with non-consensual acts of sadism and masochism. By gaining the trust of a key member of the Johannesburg BDSM scene, I was able to obtain a bird's-eye view of the inner workings of this community. Drawing from a queer theory theoretical framework, I was able to evaluate this community without the heteronormative drivers that associate BDSM with sexual rabble, shame, and medical and psychiatric opprobrium. Like the literature from the Global North, I found a tight-knit, open-minded, pansexual, gender-fluid community where ingenuity, education, consent, safety, and training are prized and where friendships endure. However, as with community formation worldwide, there is also dissent and contestation. The community could be characterized as "Old Guard," with an established hierarchical leadership that is resistant to advances made and debated in the Global North such as RACK, the 4Cs, and race play. Additionally, the Old Guard character affords power to some influential members in the community to exclude Black BDSMers for not using "sophisticated" enough language when requesting plays, which is a thinly disguised tactic to keep the community exclusively white. My study, however, is limited as my frequent requests for input from Collar Me were not answered. Going forward I aim to establish more contacts from my participant and investigate in depth the Old Guard character of the community and whether it constrains or enables the community.

Acknowledgments

Thanks to Brandy Simula for their help in shaping my abstract and Robin Bauer for their expert guidance and advice in the development of this chapter.

Notes

1. Equivalent to 41 American cents or 34 Euro cents.
2. Equivalent to $10,305 or €8466.

References

Baker, A. C. (2018). Sacred kink: Finding psychological meaning at the intersection of BDSM and spiritual experience. *Sexual and Relationship Therapy, 33*(4), 440–453. https://doi.org/10.1080/14681994.2016.1205185

Barker, M. (2013). Gender and BDSM revisited. Reflections on a decade of researching kink communities. *Psychology of Women Section Review, 15*(2), 20–28.

Bauer, R. (2008). Transgressive and transformative gendered sexual practices and white privileges: The case of the dyke/trans BDSM communities. *Women's Studies Quarterly, 36*(3/4), 233–253.

Bauer, R. (2014). *Queer BDSM intimacies: Critical consent and pushing boundaries.* Palgrave Macmillan.

Bauer, R. (2018). Bois and grrrls meet their daddies and mommies on gender playgrounds: Gendered age play in the les-bi-trans-queer BDSM communities. *Sexualities, 21*(1–2), 139–155. https://doi.org/10.1177%2F1363460716676987

Berlant, L., & Warner, M. (1995). Guest olumn: What does queer theory teach us about X? *Publications of the Modern Language Association of America, 110*(3), 343–349.

Butler, J. (1993). Critically queer. *GLQ: A Journal of Lesbian and Gay Studies, 1*(1), 17–32.

Carlström, C. (2020). Spiritual experiences and altered states of consciousness—Parallels between BDSM and Christianity. *Sexualities, 24*(5–6), 749–766. https://doi.org/10.1177%2F1363460720964035

Charles D'Avalon, A. (2020). Pain and power: BDSM as spiritual expression. *Inquiries Journal, 12*(11).

Cruz, A. (2015). Beyond black and blue: BDSM, internet pornography, and Black female sexuality. *Feminist Studies, 41*(2), 409–436. https://doi.org/10.15767/feministstudies.41.2.409

Dahan, O. (2019). Submission, pain and pleasure: Considering an evolutionary hypothesis concerning sexual masochism. *Psychology of Consciousness: Theory, Research, and Practice, 6*(4), 386–403. https://doi.org/10.1037/cns0000202

David, L., Halberstam, J., & Muñoz, E. (2005). What's queer about queer studies now? *Social Text, 23*(3–4), 1–17.

Halperin, D. M. (1995). *Saint Foucault: Towards a gay hagiography.* Oxford University Press.

Martinez, K. (2021). Overwhelming whiteness of BDSM: A critical discourse analysis of racialization in BDSM. *Sexualities, 24*(5–6), 733–748. https://doi.org/10.1177%2F1363460720932389

McCormick, T. L. (2018a). Yes master! Multimodal representations of BDSM bodies on a South African website. *Southern African Linguistics and Applied Language Studies, 36*(2), 147–160. https://doi.org/10.2989/16073614.2018.1476161

McCormick, T. L. (2018b). Gay leathermen in South Africa: An exploratory study. *Agenda, 32*(3), 74–86. https://doi.org/10.1080/10130950.2018.1498238

McEwen, H. (2018). Weaponising rhetorics of "family": The mobilisation of pro-family politics in Africa. *African Journal of Rhetoric, 10*(1), 142–178. https://hdl.handle.net/10520/EJC-11a5c2ab92

Merrett, C. (2001). A tale of two paradoxes: Media censorship in South Africa, pre-liberation and post-apartheid. *Critical Arts, 15*(1–2), 50–68. https://doi.org/10.1080/02560240185310071

Morgan, R., & Wieringa, S. (2005). *Tommy boys, lesbian men, and ancestral wives: Female same-sex practices in Africa*. Jacana Media.

Mutiga, M. (2016, January 5). South African women faces charges over racist tweets. *The Guardian*. https://www.theguardian.com/world/2016/jan/05/south-african-woman-faces-criminal-charges-racist-tweets

Newmahr, S. (2010). Rethinking kink: Sadomasochism as serious leisure. *Qualitative Sociology, 33*(3), 313–331.

Noyes, J. K. (1998). S/M in SA: Sexual violence, simulated sex and psychoanalytic theory. *American Imago, 55*(1), 135–153. https://www.jstor.org/stable/26304332

Ratele, K. (2014). Hegemonic African masculinities and men's heterosexual lives: Some uses for homophobia. *African Studies Review, 57*(2), 115–130.

Reid, G. C. (2013). *How to be a real gay: Gay identities in small-town South Africa*. University of Kwazulu-Natal Press.

Rubin, G. S. (1993). Thinking sex: Notes for a radical theory of the politics of sexuality. In H. Abelove, M. A. Barale, & D. M. Halperin (Eds.), *The lesbian and gay studies reader* (pp. 3–44). Routledge.

Rubin, G. (1998). Old guard, new guard. *Cuir Underground, 4*(2), 2–4.

Seely, S. D. (2020). Queer theory from the south: A contribution to the critique of sexual democracy. *Sexualities, 23*(7), 1228–1247. https://doi.org/10.1177%2F136346071 9893618

Sheff, E., & Hammers, C. (2011). The privilege of perversities: Race, class and education among polyamorists and kinksters. *Psychology & Sexuality, 2*(3), 198–223. https://doi.org/10.1080/19419899.2010.537674

Simula, B. L. (2019). A "different economy of bodies and pleasures"?: Differentiating and evaluating sex and sexual BDSM experiences. *Journal of Homosexuality, 66*(2), 209–237. https://doi.org/10.1080/00918369.2017.1398017

Smith, J. G., & Luykx, A. (2017). Race play in BDSM porn: The eroticization of oppression. *Porn Studies, 4*(4), 433–446. https://doi.org/10.1080/23268743.2016.1252158

Soni, V. K. (2018). *The end of the rope: The criminal law's perspective regarding acts of consensual sexual violence between adult partners within the South African, English and Canadian legal frameworks* [Unpublished doctoral dissertation]. https://ukzn-dspace.ukzn.ac.za/handle/10413/17198

Van Reenen, D. (2014). Is this really what women want? An analysis of *Fifty Shades of Grey* and modern feminist thought. *South African Journal of Philosophy, 33*(2), 223–233. https://doi.org/10.1080/02580136.2014.925730

Warner, M. (Ed.). (1993). *Fear of a queer planet: Queer politics and social theory* (Vol. 6). University of Minnesota Press.

Warner, M. (1999). *The trouble with normal: Sex, politics, and the ethics of queer life*. Harvard University Press.

Warner, M. (2002). Publics and counterpublics. *Public Culture, 14*(1), 49–90.

Weiss, M. (2011). *Techniques of pleasure: BDSM and the circuits of sexuality*. Duke University Press.

8

Kinky, Swinky, and PolyKink

Reflections on BDSM Influences on Other Sexual Communities

Marla Renee Stewart

Introduction

There are so many opportunities for kinksters to be themselves and engage in play, especially in the US South. Since I moved to the South from California in 2004, I have continued to engage in the kink community and realized that the South had a vast number of people who were committed to a lifestyle that felt fulfilling for them. Whether it is belonging to leather communities, participating in casual play, or something in between, the number of kinksters in the South is a true testament to the power and influence that kink has had on other alternative sexual communities.

Academic Research, Intersectional Identities, and Communities

Being a Black person who has navigated between multiple communities, including LGBTQIA+, swingers, and non-monogamous communities, I've noticed how kink culture has migrated into these communities. In my 2013 master's thesis (Stewart, 2013), where I concentrated on Black folks in the South in these particular alternative sexual communities, I found that there was considerable overlap between these communities, along with certain types of identities that were more prone to occupy multiple communities at once. In my research, I also found that once you identify as a person of a various alternative sexual identity you are more open to being in a part of another sexual identity. For instance, if you are a part of the LGBTQIA+ community, you might be more open to being part of the kink community

Marla Renee Stewart, *Kinky, Swinky, and PolyKink* In: *The Power of BDSM.* Edited by: Brandy L. Simula, Robin Bauer, and Liam Wignall, Oxford University Press. © Oxford University Press 2023. DOI: 10.1093/oso/9780197658598.003.0009 or non-monogamous community. This could be because of previous experience with marginalization, which maybe helps you to develop the coping mechanisms and resilience to be an active member of another community, whether experiential or not.

In my research (and limited sample size) on Black folks in alternative sexual communities, I discovered that Black lesbians were drawn toward kink and polyamorous communities. This was because there were multiple groups and communities, including meetup groups and kink events, that catered to many of their intersecting identities. For instance, they would meet up at queer polyamorous groups and/or go to kink events, exclusively for lesbians. Being in these communities, I found that members did not feel pressure to constantly out themselves because those communities were already self-identifying. Because people were safe in these communities, they also felt that they could carve out new identities and really be innovative. For example, one particular participant who was a Black femme and identified as a femme daddy had submissives address her as "Sir," which was not common in the kink lifestyle during that time.

Kink Research, Kink Fiction, and
the Normalization of Kink

During that time, there was limited academic research surrounding BDSM and even less that had to do with people of color and folks who identified as non-white. Since then, there has been more academic research that has helped people understand the kinky experiences of people of color, which is contributing to the steady narrowing of that research gap. Books such as Ariane Cruz's *The Color of Kink* (2016) have become a great reference for many folks who seek to understand Black kink, particularly from a Black woman's perspective and its relation to pornography over time.

This book was particularly timely because of its relation to the release of *Fifty Shades of Grey*—the book in 2011 and the film in 2015. *Fifty Shades of Grey*'s mainstream popularity intrigued people in all sorts of communities and introduced kink to a population that considered kink to be too taboo, particularly middle- and upper-class housewives. Overall, I would say that it helped to normalize kink as something that is desired and a different way of connecting to your lover(s) to whom kink was unfamiliar territory.

Despite the popularity of the story, kink communities found the fiction to be a poor representation of kink and the BDSM lifestyle. Critiques, such as poor writing, consent violations, and common kink inaccuracies, armed kink communities to do more education and outreach about why the fictional story is just that—fictional and a means of entertainment, not an ideal to emulate. Although it's a good start, many kink communities addressed why the story was problematic and encouraged people who wanted to engage in kink that there's a way to safely enter and to increase their knowledge to ensure a good-quality kinky experience.

Black Kink in the Mainstream

At the same time, and before *The Color of Kink* came out in 2016, more and more people of color, and in particular Black people, were also being introduced to the kink community through mainstream society. Kandi Burruss, a Black American songwriter and singer and one of the stars of *The Real Housewives of Atlanta*, introduced her new pleasure product line in 2011. This included sex toys, lubes, and kink accoutrements. Because of her television presence and her social media presence (almost 9 million followers on Instagram alone), her reach is wide. And because her audience is primarily Black, the things that she says and does have a considerable impact on Black communities as a whole.

Later, in 2019, she led mainstream Black audiences to her "dungeon" and soon went on tour having entertainers glamorize kink. This pushed forward the idea that kink, although previously considered taboo, can be enjoyed by folks who want to try something new and is not for "white people" only.

That same year, Jet Setting Jasmine, King Noire, and I did a national dungeon tour where we taught various kink skills and hosted a play party after each lesson. When we came to Atlanta and hosted our tour at the Sex Down South Conference, many folks in the Black community thought we were copying Kandi's dungeon tour, until they realized that we actually had a real dungeon and that we were actual kinksters and educators. We exposed a crowd to a whole different experience from that of Kandi's tour, and now many of those attendees still follow us and seek advice around kink and BDSM. For example, I currently have a client who went to the Kandi's Dungeon Tour and attended our dungeon tour and realized that kink wasn't about entertainment and celebrities but rather a behavior and lifestyle that could enhance their sexual experiences or tap into other ways of arousal and states of being.

With that said, those folks now have an understanding that Kandi was using kink to titillate her audiences, sell her products, and pique people's curiosity on whether or not she had a dungeon. She has denied that she actually has a dungeon, and unfortunately, there hasn't been any documentation on whether or not she identifies as a kinkster. I highly doubt that she does though. Like many people, my belief is that doing the behavior doesn't necessarily mean that it is a part of your identity.

Being Swinky

Between 2017 and 2019, I noticed that kink was making its way into other sexual communities in the US South. One of those communities was the swinger community. Many of the swinger (or what swingers call "lifestyle") events were now including dungeon play areas and featuring professional dommes to facilitate sessions, as well as educating swingers on kink. If there is an introduction ceremony at these events, it's often known by folks who have been in the swinging lifestyle for many years that folks who are swingers and kinky are called *swinky* (a humorous combination that acknowledges their memberships in both of these communities); and it is a generally accepted way of being. Again, it looks as though if you are introduced to one alternative sexual community, you might be open to being in other sexual communities. In a sense, it would seem that your ability to think and behave "outside the box" can lead to sexual and emotional exploration, whereas someone who isn't in any of these communities would not be able to see how these things can be done quite as clearly. I would love to see more research about these two communities and the crossover that we currently see occurring and the overlapping nuances.

One example of things that I have seen practiced more in swinging communities is consent. Consent in kink has always been prevalent, and with the additional awareness brought on by the #MeToo movement, consent has been a bigger force in these communities and is taken more seriously than it has been in the past. In the swinging communities of the past, people tended to be very assertive with their affection, and consent wasn't something that they even considered. Most people greeted you with a kiss (on the lips) and a hug, and people felt comfortable being able to grab your body parts and flirt as they wish with you. Although respect was always given in this community, especially in terms of rejection, the swinging culture socialized people through those consistent types of affection (hugs, kisses, gentle touches). With the highlights of consent that they have learned from kink communities, most swinging communities are now more conscious about asking for permission to get kisses or touch your body parts. This is a remarkable transition from what was happening before, and I believe that it's made swinging communities more hospitable and fun places.

Consent isn't the only thing that has been beneficially added to the swinging communities. In kink, when we negotiate a scene, we also negotiate whether sex will be a part of the scene or not. Negotiating what you will or won't do sexually is the norm in kink, but often in swinging communities, there isn't this common experience. Unfortunately, in the past, people would go into sexual situations making assumptions of what people will do or what people are open to, which is often fueled by alcohol to lift those inhibitions. However, in many swinging 101 and beginners' classes, the educators are doing their due diligence and making sure that folks understand that they start negotiating what kind of sex they want to engage in when they get involved with another couple or individual. Now, you are able to notice that in swinging communities people "flag" themselves (signs, bracelets, event symbols, or identity-oriented meetups) with what they are into, such as indicating if they are into doing a full swap (couple for couple) or other sexual kinds of acts.

PolyKink

Kink has also had its influence on non-monogamous communities. When I present at non-monogamous conferences, there often seem to be a lot of people who are also kinky, which is shown by folks who are doing educational workshops and is apparent in the entertainment. It's prevalent with attendees, as well, as they share their stories during these events. Even when there are talks about group sex, kink seems to be a focal point as it pertains to play parties. Highlighting kink and BDSM behavior seems to permeate how people behave when it comes to certain non-monogamous communities and how they function in this context and is generally celebrated as something that is acceptable and part of the norm when it comes to polyamorous communities. It simply may come from the lack of judgment and the ability to be open and honest when it comes to communicating their needs.

Kink in the Mainstream

Although I have seen kink and BDSM language and behaviors in these alternative sexual communities, they are also being used in mainstream communities. As a contributor to many articles around sex and sexuality, I have noticed that the concept of aftercare has been floating around as a thing that you should try, even if you are not a part of the BDSM community (Garis, 2020). Aftercare has traditionally been seen as a way to care for a person or person(s) after a scene and is usually negotiated before play. There's physical aftercare, which includes things like hydrating, drinking juice, eating chocolate, or even taking a shower or cuddling with blankets. There's also emotional aftercare, which consists of talking about the experience of what they enjoyed, words of affirmation, or other talk about the experience or future play experiences. The fact that it has worked itself into the mainstream goes to show that the normalization of kink is more present than ever.

I believe that soon enough kink/BDSM won't be as taboo as it once was. We see more of it on mainstream television, and as the language and behaviors start to go beyond the community itself, we see how much kink/BDSM has contributed to the greater good of many people's sexual lives. Once deemed taboo and often hidden because of the shame and stigma attached to being in the kink/BDSM lifestyle, the impact of being kinky or being more sexually liberated is often now celebrated as a way of tapping into our most authentic selves. We also now know that kink/BDSM can be used as a healing modality for somatic practitioners for folks who have experienced trauma, and the need for kink and kink-aware practitioners is on the rise as more and more people get involved in the community.

Whatever community you reside in, know that kink is probably coming your way—if it hasn't arrived already. Whether this changes the communities of kink, only time will tell.

References

Cruz, A. (2016). *The color of kink: Black women, BDSM, and pornography.* New York University Press.

Garis, M. G. (2020). *Sexual aftercare isn't just a BDSM thing—Here's why everyone shoul try it.* Well + Good. https://www.wellandgood.com/aftercare-after-sex/

Stewart, M. R. (2013). *"Getting freaky": Perversion and promiscuity within alternative relationships and sexual modalities among people of color* [Unpublished master's thesis]. Georgia State University. https://scholarworks.gsu.edu/sociology_theses/40

PART IV

REPRESENTATIONS AND PERSONAL REFLECTIONS

9

Examining Representations of BDSM in Undergraduate Human Sexuality Textbooks

Academic and Community Perspectives

*Benjamin C. Graham, Tsolak M. Kirakosyan,
Jessica A. Fox, and Miles Ruvabalca*

Introduction

Within academia, one of the most common ways in which college students in North America and other countries learn about sexual topics is through introductory human sexuality courses. Such classes are popular (King et al., 2017), and both the knowledge sources offered and the instructors who employ them are critical agents in how sexual diversity is framed and represented. Central tools for providing structure and content to such courses are human sexuality textbooks, which we define here as widely circulated, interdisciplinary books used in introductory human sexuality courses within higher education. In the United States human sexuality courses of this nature are most typically taught in psychology, health, and sociology departments (King et al., 2017); and pedagogical norms within higher education in other countries may differ in terms of the structure, content, and frequency of course offerings.

The role of human sexuality textbooks in influencing paradigmatic thought is likely quite substantial. In the broader scientific pantheon, Thomas Kuhn in *The Structure of Scientific Revolutions* (1962) identified textbooks as critical enforcers of dominant paradigms. Within the social sciences, the vital role of textbooks has been similarly acknowledged by authors both before

Benjamin C. Graham, Jessica A. Fox, and Miles Ruvabalca, *Examining Representations of BDSM in Undergraduate Human Sexuality Textbooks* In: *The Power of BDSM.* Edited by: Brandy L. Simula, Robin Bauer, and Liam Wignall, Oxford University Press. © Oxford University Press 2023. DOI: 10.1093/oso/9780197658598.003.0010 (e.g., Herma et al., 1943) and after (e.g., Whissell, 1997) Kuhn's seminal work. Since the (US) civil rights movement, social science researchers have conducted systematic reviews of textbooks to appraise the representation of socially marginalized experiences (Padgett, 2015), including women's contribution to psychology (Unger, 2010), gay/lesbian issues (Weitz, 1982), and disability status (Goldstein et al., 2010). In the domain of sexual expression, another socially marginalized experience whose representation warrants appraisal is that of people who identify with BDSM.

BDSM is an umbrella term for bondage, discipline, dominance/submission, and sadomasochism (described in detail in the introduction of this volume) and, given its relative prevalence (Brown et al., 2020), is regularly mentioned in human sexuality textbooks. Historically, BDSM has been negatively framed in multiple ways, including as an individual pathology (Moser & Kleinplatz, 2006), an expression of past abuse (Sprott & Hadcock, 2018), and, in the case of sadism, a criminally deviant set of behaviors (Nitschke et al., 2009). By contrast, most contemporary research has incorporated a more sex-positive and empowering lens for what BDSM means for those who participate in it (e.g., Dunkley & Brotto, 2020; Graham et al., 2016). New research, including this volume, speaks to the diversity of topics emerging within the field. Despite increases in empowering frameworks for BDSM, studies of practitioners suggest that stigma around BDSM remains (Brown et al., 2020).

Many analyses exist of popular media representations of BDSM (e.g., Khan, 2017; Weiss, 2006). However, no study to date has explored the extent to which current conceptualizations of BDSM are reflected in human sexuality textbooks. There is an important need to describe the current state of BDSM representation in these foundational texts.

In addition to describing representation of marginalized sexual identities, it is worthwhile to consider how the perspectives of actual BDSM practitioners are or are not represented in authoritative sources such as human sexuality textbooks. The cultural knowledge found within BDSM communities has value, agency, and authority in how we understand BDSM; and community practitioners have called for increased involvement in the research process (Community Academic Consortium for Research on Alternative Sexualities [CARAS], 2023; Langdridge & Barker, 2007). Community-based participatory research provides methods for bridging community and academic approaches to knowledge (Koshy, 2005) and, in its various forms, provides community members avenues for guiding research (Wadsworth, 1998). A community-based participatory research study was undertaken by the current author (Graham et al., 2016), resulting in a taxonomy of terms BDSM practitioners use to describe the role of the community. This window into BDSM member experience is one example of participatory structures that can be utilized to inform research and empower members in how their experience is represented within human sexuality courses.

In sum, in addition to the need to describe the way academia represents BDSM in human sexuality textbooks, there is a need to assess such representation through a community-based participatory research framework based on features that practitioners themselves value. The current study aimed to address these twin concerns.

An Overview of the Kink Representation Outreach Project

The Kink Representation Outreach Project is an ongoing participatory research program that seeks to empower community voice around BDSM experience and analyze the representation of BDSM within human sexuality textbooks. The project is built around three studies, the second of which is the focus of this chapter: (1) a prior study of BDSM community member experience (Graham et al., 2016), (2) a content analysis of BDSM representation in top-selling human sexuality textbooks, and (3) a forthcoming participatory appraisal of current textbook representations by BDSM community members. Participants from the first study as well as distribution markets of textbooks reviewed here were geographically based in North America.

Study 1 examined the role, meaning, and function of BDSM communities from the perspective of practitioners. Seven workshops were conducted with 48 BDSM community members. Qualitative coding resulted in the identification of three overarching domains of social features, personal development, and functional resources. Each domain was subdivided into four to six categories, including themes such as acceptance, sexual expression, friendship, and safety. The results provided a member-derived inventory that was used to inform our second study, specifically in structuring the deductive coding rubric. A full description of the method and results is given in Graham et al. (2016). Study 2 consists of a content analysis of undergraduate human sexuality textbooks and is described herein. Study 3 is a future project that will involve direct member appraisal of and recommendations for textbook descriptions of BDSM.

Goals of the Current Study

The current study explores representations of BDSM found in human sexuality textbooks from academic and community perspectives. The first goal was to systematically review popular textbooks and describe BDSM descriptions. The second goal was to assess the way community experience was represented in the current texts. These goals are reflected in the following research questions:

RQ1: How are descriptions of BDSM currently structured within human sexuality textbooks?

RQ2: What are the scope and frequency of themes found in descriptions of BDSM in human sexuality textbooks?

RQ3: How are member-defined BDSM community experiences reflected in human sexuality textbooks?

Method

Textbook Selection

The project targeted English-language undergraduate human sexuality textbooks that provide an introduction to the field of human sexuality, in circulation primarily in North America. This book type was selected as it is typically the foundational structure of introductory human sexuality courses and regularly includes BDSM in its content. The books reviewed were the most recent editions available in the spring of 2019 and included publication years between 2017 and 2019. Our search excluded edited volumes, workbooks, and other books addressing sexuality but not written to serve as a primary introductory text. We used a three-method approach to identify a representative sample of the most widely used textbooks. Sales data were collected from (1) a literature review of published textbooks using university library search engines, (2) sales reported on Amazon.com, and (3) an online faculty resource (www.facultycenter.net) which rates textbook sales at over

2000 North American universities/colleges. While the implications for the study's findings apply to future open-source textbooks, no such books were found at the time of the study.

Our review resulted in an original list of textbooks meeting the criteria. We then rank-ordered the titles based on Amazon.com sales. Because reported sales expressed the total sales since publication, a textbook may have higher sales simply by being on the market for a longer period. To validate the rankings, we compared the lists with an online faculty resource (www.facultycenter.net) which rates sales over the past 12 months. From this triangulated procedure we identified a set of textbooks to review for the study, selecting five for our analysis. Title, author(s), and publication years are listed in Table 9.1.

The textbooks selected should not be construed as a definitive top five list; rather, our process validates that these five are among the top-selling books and therefore represent an approximation of the most popular introductory human sexuality textbooks in circulation in North America at the time of the study.

Procedure

Mentions of BDSM were identified by searching a set of related keywords (e.g., *kink*, *S/M*, *masochism*, *dominance*) in the index, table of contents, and glossary of each textbook. We found that without exception each book listed BDSM as a distinct section or set of subsections within a single chapter. We revisited our review by manually reviewing the full content of each book and confirmed that the sections were the focal point of discussions of BDSM.

Descriptive Features

To determine the structure of BDSM representations, we collected data in the areas of location/space allocation and listing of resources. Uniformly, all books mentioned BDSM in a specific chapter pertaining to statistically non-normative sexuality ("abnormal" sexuality). The word length for each chapter subsection describing BDSM was calculated electronically by transferring the text into word processing software and using the software's word count function. Length was validated by manually counting words for each subsection. Human sexuality textbooks commonly end a chapter's content with a list of resources for further information. These include informational

Table 9.1 Location and Space Allocation of BDSM Descriptions

	Carroll (2019)	Hyde and DeLamater (2017)	LeVay et al. (2018)	Rathus et al. (2018)	Yarber and Sayad (2019)
Book title	*Sexuality Now: Embracing Diversity (6th ed.)*	*Understanding Human Sexuality (13th ed.)*	*Discovering Human Sexuality (4th ed.)*	*Human Sexuality in a Changing World (10th ed.)*	*Human Sexuality: Diversity in Contemporary Society (10th ed.)*
Chapter title	Varieties of Sexual Expression	Variations in Sexual Behavior	Atypical Sexuality	Atypical Sexual Variations	Variations in Sexual Behavior
Section heading(s)	Sexual Sadism and Sexual Masochism Disorders	Sadism and Masochism	Sadomasochism Involves the Infliction or Receipt of Pain or Degradation	Sexual Masochism Disorder; Sexual Sadism Disorder	BDSM, Sexual Masochism, and Sexual Sadism
Subsection heading(s)		Definitions, Sadomasochistic Behavior, Causes of Sadomasochism, Bondage and Discipline, Dominance and Submission		Sexual Sadomasochism	Sexual Sadism Disorder, Sexual Masochism Disorder, Autoerotic Asphyxia
Number of words in section	1588	2492	1857	2587	2208

websites, books, professional organizations, and other sources related to chapter topics. For our study, the resources section at the end of each chapter where BDSM appeared was recorded.

Coding Rubric Development

To create our inductive and deductive coding rubrics, we first assembled a pilot set of five descriptions of BDSM found in similar textbooks not included in the final study. The two coding rubrics were then generated using this set through independent processes.

Inductive Coding Rubric

An inductive coding approach works from the bottom up to develop a coding scheme based on observations of existing sources (Thomas, 2006). We used a two-step process to distill these observations into our inductive rubric. First, three team members using identical BDSM descriptions independently generated proposed themes found across two or more textbooks. Single-occurrence features were noted in a separate list. From this process, three individually derived lists of potential themes were produced. In the second step, the three original coders and two other team members consolidated and refined the three lists of themes by group consensus. From this process a set of 14 inductive themes was finalized and can be found in the first column of Table 9.2.

Deductive Coding Rubric

Deductive coding employs a top-down approach to coding using a predetermined framework (Boyatzis, 1998). Our deductive coding rubric was structured based on BDSM community features articulated by members of the kink community (reported in Graham et al., 2016). It included three overarching domains, each consisting of a set of four to six themes. To test the coding rubric, sample data was produced using two versions: domains only and domains plus themes. Notes were taken on the feasibility of the versions, including challenges to its use. Although the more granular coding structure identified only sparse occurrences within the section descriptions, there was enough diversity between books to warrant the use of the domains plus themes rubric, comprised of 15 themes nested within three domains. The first domain, *social features*, includes the themes of *social network, sense of community, acceptance, having fun, friendship,* and *interpersonal problems within community. Personal development* is comprised of *spiritual/philosophical dimensions, sexual expression, personal growth,* and *therapeutic aspects.*

Table 9.2 Inductive Coding Themes

	Carroll (2019)	Hyde and DeLamater (2017)	LeVay et al. (2018)	Rathus et al. (2018)	Yarber and Sayad (2019)
History of BDSM terms	Y[a]	Y	Y[a]	Y[a]	—
Prevalence rates	Y[a]	Y[a]	Y	Y[a]	Y[a]
Etiology of BDSM interest	Y[a]	Y[a]	Y[a]	Y[a]	—
DSM-5—sadism and masochism	Y[a]	Y	—	Y[a]	Y[a]
Types of activities/role scripts	Y[a]	Y[a]	Y[a]	Y[a]	Y[a]
Role of consent	Y[a]	Y[a]	Y	Y	Y[a]
Case study	Y	—	—	Y[a]	—
First-person narratives	Y	Y[a]	Y[a]	Y[a]	—
Community	Y[a]	Y[a]	Y	Y[a]	Y[a]
Subcommunities	Y	—	Y	—	Y
Money exchange/sex work	Y	Y	Y[a]	Y[a]	—
Empowering perspective	Y[a]	Y	Y	Y	Y[a]
Confluence of BDSM and criminal behavior	—	—	Y[a]	Y	Y[a]
Unintentional injury/death	Y	Y	Y[a]	Y[a]	Y[a]

[a]Multiple occurrences.

The final domain, *functional resources*, includes the themes of *general resources*, *sharing educational knowledge*, *safety*, *support*, and *activism/service*.

Content Analyses

Team members worked in pairs to apply inductive and deductive codes to the BDSM sections. Descriptions were first coded independently, including notes on location and other features. Codes were then discussed by the full research team and recorded in a single spreadsheet. Discrepancies were resolved by an iterative consensus process, where deliberation sharpened the language of the rubric, which was then reapplied to all five textbooks for consistency.

Results

In this section we describe the study's findings across the three areas of (1) descriptive features, (2) inductive themes, and (3) deductive themes.

Descriptive Features of BDSM Representation

We appraised how BDSM descriptions were structured within textbooks by first determining their location and space allocation. Chapter and section titles are listed in Table 9.1, along with the section word length. Most of the sections used headings derived from the *Diagnostic and Statistical Manual of Mental Disorders*, fifth edition (DSM-5; American Psychiatric Association [APA], 2013) and socio-historical terminology used to describe BDSM, namely *sexual sadism*, *sexual masochism*, and *sadomasochism*. The length of each section ranged from 1588 to 2587 words, or about 2.5 to 5 pages. Overall textbook length ranged from 526 to 672 pages.

We then reviewed resources listed at the end of each chapter. Resources included support groups and resource pages pertinent to the chapter topics. Examples include resources for victims of nonconsensual/pathological activities (e.g., the US National Sex Offender Registry, Sexaholics Anonymous) and sex-positive supports (e.g., Tri-Ess heterosexual crossdressers network). Only one book (Carroll, 2019) included a resource for consensual/sex-positive support for BDSM. The book cited CARAS (https://www.carasresearch.org/), an organization dedicated to the support and promotion of community-based research on alternative sexualities.

Thematic Coding

The five BDSM descriptions were coded first for the 14 inductive and then for the 15 deductive themes. For each textbook, themes were coded dichotomously as *present/not present*. Thus, each of the 29 themes was coded as appearing between zero and five times across the set of five books. All occurrences were archived, allowing for multiple mentions within a single book. In the inductive and deductive subsections below, we share the rates of occurrence of themes across textbooks, grouped in order of occurrence frequency (i.e., occurring in five out of five textbooks, four out of five, etc.). As these groupings are shared, we describe and provide examples for individual themes within each grouping.

Inductive Themes

Inductive coding identifies themes commonly found in similar descriptions of BDSM in human sexuality textbooks. Therefore, this assessment represents how comprehensive a given book is in covering the current industry standards of descriptions, as well as how typical any given theme is across five of the most widely circulated textbooks. Each inductive theme was assessed using our dichotomous coding system (see Table 9.2). All inductive themes were found in at least two textbooks. Below we share examples and descriptions.

Six themes occurred in all five of the textbooks. The first was *prevalence rates*, which included studies that attempt to estimate of the number of people who practice BDSM in the general population (often bounded within a given national context). Overall, prevalence studies differed from textbook to textbook. Exceptions included a work by Kinsey et al. (1953), which was mentioned in four of the five books. Other multiple mentions included the DSM-5 (APA, 2013) and a study by Joyal and Carpentier (2017). Notably, almost all studies were drawn from North American, European, or Australian samples.

The second theme found in all textbooks was *types of activities/role scripts*. This included specific behaviors and associated roles that BDSM practitioners engage with, including the process that goes into embodying such roles. For example, Caroll (2019) described "a kind of drama or performance, which is enhanced by both sides knowing their roles and dressing the part" (p. 440).

The third universal theme was the *role of consent*, which pertained to references to the integral feature of consent in BDSM practice, including the use of safe words. An example of this theme was found in LeVay et al. (2018): "Before the scene, perhaps as a part of flirtation or foreplay, the partners negotiate what will transpire and set limits for behavior."

The fourth theme found in all books was *community infrastructure*. This theme referred to physical and virtual spaces that make up BDSM communities (e.g., bars, clubs, social media, and "munches"). While mentions of communities occurred in all textbooks, such descriptions were most often very brief ("There is a distinct D-S subculture, involving DVDs, clubs, and bars" [Hyde & DeLamater, 2017, p. 360]). In a few books a slightly higher level of detail was shared:

There is a subculture—the S&M subculture—in the United States in which sexual sadists and sexual masochists form liaisons to inflict and receive pain and humiliation during sexual activity (Hell & Simons, 2008). It is catered to by sex shops that sell S&M paraphernalia and magazines. . . . People in the subculture seek one another out through mutual contacts, S&M social organizations, or personal ads in S&M magazines. (Rathus et al., 2018, p. 462)

In our descriptive coding section below we share a more nuanced, member-derived appraisal of community experience.

The fifth universal theme was *empowering perspectives*, which was defined as text that asserted (1) the evidence-based notion that BDSM is primarily psychologically healthy; (2) that many experience BDSM as a lifestyle/identity, as opposed to a strictly sexual phenomenon; or (3) a targeted effort to destigmatize BDSM. LeVay et al. (2018) asserted that

> the relationship of power, trust, and dependency that exists between top and bottom represents a condition of heightened intimacy and that a participant in a BDSM scene may enter an altered state of consciousness that amounts to a spiritual experience. (p. 409)

The sixth and final theme found in all textbooks was *the potential for unintentional injury*. This code pertained to the risk of certain behaviors to result in bodily injury when not done safely. For example, Yarber and Sayad (2019) shared, "the acting out of fantasies involves risk such as physical injury" (p. 281).

Five inductive themes occurred in four textbooks. The first was *history of BDSM terms*, which includes references to the origins of terms which comprise the acronym *BDSM*. For example, the literary authors Marquis de Sade and Leopold Ritter von Sacher-Masoch as well as sexologist Richard von Krafft-Ebing were cited in multiple texts.

Etiology of BDSM interest refers to descriptions of where BDSM interest originates. Hyde and DeLamater (2017) shared several theories of etiology, including learning theory:

> A little boy is being spanked over his mother's knee; in the process, his penis rubs against her knee, and he gets an erection . . . the child has learned to associate pain or spanking with sexual arousal, possibly setting up a lifelong career as a masochist. (p. 357)

Notably, several authors cited the limitations of the scientific literature, underscoring that no definitive scientific consensus exists as to the etiology of BDSM.

The third theme to occur in four of the five textbooks is *DSM-5 categorization criteria*, which refers specifically to mentions of the two diagnoses of sexual sadism disorder and sexual masochism disorder found in the DSM-5 (APA, 2013). Two of the five textbooks used the names of these psychiatric disorders as section titles (Carroll, 2019; Rathus et al., 2018), and a third (Hyde & DeLamater, 2017) introduced the topic of BDSM with definitions of a sexual sadist and sexual masochist in terms of DSM-5 criteria. One textbook (Yarber & Sayad, 2019) mentioned the disorders at the end of the section as one- to two-paragraph subsections, and the fifth textbook (LeVay et al., 2018) provided a rich description of BDSM but did not include the two DSM disorders.

First-person narratives were instances where an actual BDSM practitioner is speaking directly about their experience. The four instances of first-person narratives included those of a woman identifying as a submissive (Hyde & DeLamater, 2017, p. 357), a webcam dominatrix (Rathus et al., 2018, p. 260), and a female kinkster (Carroll, 2019), as well as the reflections of a research-practitioner who took part in an immersive BDSM scene (LeVay et al., 2018, p. 409). First-person narratives were most often excerpts from previously published works.

The fifth and final theme to occur in four of the five textbooks was *money exchange/sex work*. This code refers to the exchange of money or other goods for BDSM services/experiences, which did not have to explicitly include sex. One book integrated sex work into a description of a pathological case of sexual masochism disorder: "This man could never save money or concentrate sufficiently to climb the ladder of success because of his investment of money and time in dominatrix prostitutes" (Rathus et al., 2018, p. 461).

Two inductive themes were found in three out of the five textbooks. The first, *subcommunities within BDSM*, refers to subgroups such as gay leather, pup, latex, and other groups or "scenes." Such descriptions were brief and nonspecific; for example, "there is a small but flourishing lesbian BDSM community, as well as communities in which gay and straight men and women mingle freely" (LeVay et al., 2018, p. 408). *Confluence of BDSM and criminal behavior* refers to mentions of criminal cases where sexual sadism disorder was involved. "Some sexual sadists hurt or humiliate willing partners, such as prostitutes or masochists. Others—a small minority—stalk and attack nonconsenting victims" (Rathus et al., 2018, p. 261).

One code, *case studies*, occurred in two of the five textbooks. This code consisted of individual case studies of a person's experience of BDSM narrated by the textbook author(s). For example, a heterosexual relationship involving a man interested in cross-dressing while in a submissive role was described in Rathus et al. (2018, p. 459). Of our inductive themes, none occurred in one or fewer textbooks.

Deductive Descriptions of BDSM Community Representation

The presence of psychosocial aspects of BDSM community membership was assessed with 15 deductive codes across three overarching domains: (1) social features, (2) personal development, and (3) functional resources (e.g., educational resources, service to the community). Within each of these domains were four to six themes. Operational definitions for each categorical term can be found in the original Graham et al. (2016) article.

Of the three overarching domains, *social features* was found across all five textbooks, while *functional resources* was found in four and *personal development* in only two. Findings for composite themes are discussed below by domain and summarized in Table 9.3.

Social Features

While the *social features* domain was found across all five textbooks, only the *social network* theme occurred with regularity (5/5). For example,

> A sadomasochistic (or 'kink') subculture exists for those who have adopted BDSM as a lifestyle. A variety of organizations cater to consensual BDSM . . . and partners can meet at conferences and learn more in various BDSM newsletters and magazines. (Carroll, 2019, p. 440)

The remaining themes within the *social features* domain did not occur with any regularity. *Sense of community, acceptance,* and *having fun* were mentioned once each across the five textbooks; and *friendship* and *interpersonal problems* were not mentioned at all.

Functional Resources

Similar to the other two domains, the themes comprising *functional resources* were rarely mentioned. *Sharing educational knowledge* and *resources* were mentioned three times and *safety* twice. None mentioned *activism and service* or *support* within sections. Examples of *sharing educational knowledge* include places where "partners can meet at conferences and learn more in various BDSM newsletters and magazines" (Carroll, 2019, p. 440).

Table 9.3 Deductive Coding Domains/Themes

	Carroll (2019)	Hyde and DeLamater (2017)	LeVay et al. (2018)	Rathus et al. (2018)	Yarber and Sayad (2019)
Domain 1: Social features					
Social network	Y	Y[a]	Y[a]	Y[a]	Y
Sense of community	—	—	—	Y	—
Acceptance	—	—	—	Y	—
Having fun	—	Y	—	—	—
Friendship	—	—	—	—	—
Interpersonal problems within community	—	—	—	—	—
Domain 2: Personal development					
Spiritual/philosophical dimensions	Y	—	Y	—	—
Sexual expression	Y	—	—	—	—
Personal growth	—	—	—	—	—
Therapeutic	—	—	—	—	—
Domain 3: Functional resources					
Resources	Y	Y	—	—	Y[a]
Sharing educational knowledge	Y	Y	Y	—	—
Safety	—	Y[a]	Y	—	—
Support	—	—	—	—	—
Activism and service	—	—	—	—	—

[a]Reference in multiple areas.

Referring to scripts provided by the BDSM community to its members, Hyde and DeLamater (2017) reflected the theme of *resources* in descriptions such as "Thus, as two people enact the master–slave script, the master is not in complete control and the slave is not powerless" (p. 361). In contrast to the universal mention of the *role of consent* as an inductive theme, the role of the BDSM community in promoting consent and other issues of *safety* was rarely mentioned. It occurred in only two books, including LeVay et al. (2018): "In S-M clubs there are often rules governing the social and S-M interaction, particularly the creation and enactment of scenes" (p. 357).

Personal Development

Themes within the *personal development* domain occurred least frequently in comparison to those of the other two domains, with only three total occurrences across the set (compared to eight for both *social features* and *functional resources*). The *spiritual/philosophical* theme was present in two texts, represented by the earlier quote from LeVay et al. (2018, p. 409) describing how a BDSM scene can "amount to a spiritual experience."

Sexual expression was operationalized as people's ability to find ways to enact their sexuality, including improving how it is expressed. Only the Carroll (2019) text was found to address this theme, describing BDSM exchange as "a kind of drama or performance, which is enhanced by both sides knowing their roles or dressing the part" (p. 440).

Personal growth and *therapeutic benefits* were not mentioned in any textbook.

Discussion

Introductory human sexuality textbooks are powerful tomes of knowledge encompassing the multidisciplinary expanse of what is known about the complex and personal topic of sex. Representations of BDSM within these texts can have far-reaching impacts on the college students who read them. This study contributes to the research on BDSM by describing how this form of sexuality is represented. Additionally, it assesses how member perspectives on a specific aspect of practitioner experience—that of community—are portrayed (or, as we have seen, *not* portrayed).

Editors of human sexuality textbooks face a challenge both Herculean and Sisyphean: The sheer effort required to summarize such a body of research is massive, and the constant emergence of new research amidst shifting cultural norms requires perpetual revision. Scientific and social understandings of BDSM are but one piece within this larger undertaking. This study contributes to the body of research on BDSM by providing a window into how it is presented and recommendations for future representations.

By employing an inductive approach, we assessed the extent to which individual textbooks reflected the range of information commonly found in human sexuality textbooks. The results suggest a general uniformity in terms of content areas; all of the inductive themes occurred in at least two or more of the textbooks, with the majority (11 of 14) of themes occurring in four or more texts. Additionally, each individual book contained between 10 and 13 of the themes. Closer examination of inductive themes, however, allowed for a more nuanced appraisal of the substance and framing of each, highlighting important distinctions and areas for potential development.

Given the call for increased participatory voice in how the social sciences approach BDSM, we included a deductive rubric based on BDSM community member experiences to see whether or not those features were discussed. Compared to inductive findings, deductive domains/themes were far sparser for all five books. From the deductive analysis we can identify several areas offering further discussion and implications for enhancing descriptions.

Following the appraisal of summaries of BDSM found in a representative sample of the major human sexuality books presented here, we now share a set of recommendations for enhancing BDSM descriptions and amplifying community perspectives.

Recommendations

In considering both inductive and deductive analyses, the three areas emerge (*content, community representation,* and *community input/process*). Across these areas we offer a set of nine recommendations for strengthening how BDSM is depicted in human sexuality textbook revisions, new textbooks, and other publications that wish to accurately/succinctly summarize BDSM. Note that many textbooks, including those reviewed here, are already enacting a portion of these recommendations; this list is intended as a checklist/resource as sections are updated or new sections authored. Readers may conclude other implications from the results; we encourage this and wish to recognize the monumental work of textbook editors in crafting language for BDSM and other experiences.

Content Recommendations

Recommendation 1: Highlight the centrality of consent to BDSM, with inclusion of the role communities play in its articulation. BDSM practitioners have long articulated the centrality of consent (Bauer, 2020; Galilee-Belfer, 2020). It is laudable that all of the textbooks reviewed mentioned this core feature. Descriptions ranged from a short mention to a multidimensional discussion, such as LeVay et al.'s (2018) description that included community adages, the role of communication, the iterative nature of consent within BDSM, and some of the paradoxes ("'Stop, stop!' may mean 'More, more!,'" p. 408) in ensuring consent.

Given the important discussions of sexual consent in current academic discourse (Muehlenhard et al., 2016), the centrality of consent to BDSM benefits from thick, multidimensional descriptions and linkages to the way communities help define and enforce consent. While consent was mentioned in all five textbooks, only two mentioned the role of BDSM communities in providing physical and emotional safety for its members. The cultural norms found within BDSM communities have been highlighted as potential models for sexual consent (Galilee-Belfer, 2020). By including multiple dimensions and the role of BDSM communities in promoting consent, textbooks can situate BDSM within broader efforts to end sexual violence such as Title IX policies, #MeToo, and the proliferation of transformative justice structures.

Recommendation 2: Provide adequate discussion of prevalence rates including operationalization and sampling limitations. It is widely recognized that many attempts to generate BDSM prevalence rates have significant sampling, instrumentation, reporting, and other limitations. Some research may have powerful methodological rigor, like the Richters et al. (2008) study of a random sample of 19,307 Australians, but are limited by narrow operational definitions. Other studies, such as Arndt et al. (1985), have richer operationalization but limited generalizability due to sampling. A challenge for textbook editors is to capture an aggregate summary of what can be gleaned from the many published studies. For the books reviewed, each reported prevalence based on only one or a small handful of studies, with very little overlap book-to-book. Of over a dozen studies mentioned, most occurred only once. The only study commonly cited was that of Kinsey et al. (1953), likely included for its historical significance rather than its relevance to modern cultural norms. There is a need for a coordinated summary of rates and more consistent reporting across texts. A summary of prevalence studies has been recently published (Brown et al., 2020), which can serve as a starting point for a more detailed summary of prevalence rates and their limitations.

Recommendation 3: De-emphasize DSM categorization of BDSM as pathology and structure sections using sex-positive framings. Sections describing BDSM were predominantly derived from clinical nomenclature. What this study's findings make starkly clear is that the DSM, and its framing of sadism and masochism as potential (or overt) pathologies, has an immense influence on how most textbooks frame and discuss BDSM. It has become established in the literature that the vast majority of individuals experiencing BDSM are well adjusted and do not meet the criteria for a disorder (Brown et al., 2020). Utilizing long-contested DSM disorders (Moser & Kleinplatz, 2006) whose DSM-5 iterations lack robust empirical support risks misleading readers into viewing BDSM as fundamentally pathological, even when empowering language is included as a qualifier. Following the strong epistemological, empirical, and practical critiques of the DSM-4-Text Revision by Moser and Kleinplatz (2006), fellow advocates for the depathologizing of BDSM pointed out strengths in the changes made to the DSM-5, specifically in preventing the DSM from being misused in child custody cases (Wright, 2018). What the current study demonstrates is that, despite advancements in destigmatization, in the domain of higher education the DSM-5 continues to create far-reaching pathological framing of BDSM for the legions of college students who enroll in human sexuality courses each year.

Three textbooks structured BDSM sections around the DSM-5 diagnoses of *sexual sadism disorder* and *sexual masochism disorder*, while two did not. We recommend the latter two approaches. Yarber and Sayad (2019) provide a discussion of BDSM followed by one or two paragraphs for the DSM disorders; this approach recognizes the rare cases of disorder but situates them in proper proportion to the body of research indicating BDSM as non-pathological. Using an alternate strategy, LeVay et al. (2018) provide a comprehensive description of non-pathological BDSM, eschewing the DSM-5 diagnostic categories entirely.

Recommendation 4: Integrate emerging trends in BDSM research and community discourse. A burgeoning new literature on BDSM, including chapters in this volume, has emerged in the since the early 2000's. While incorporating new research is inherent to revisions, this recommendation is included to stress the value in updating antiquated research; in our review we found many citations from the 1980s–1990s. The constructs found in older studies are often influenced by social norms, which have changed markedly. Important new discussions are emerging, such as the experiences/needs of people of color within BDSM (Cruz, 2016), as well as new identity models (Sprott & Hadcock, 2018). The exponential growth of the literature underscores the need to include such trends.

Recommendations for Community Representation

Recommendation 5: Provide increased detail in describing BDSM communities. While all textbooks mentioned BDSM communities, none included deeper discussion of their role, meaning, or function. While this was likely not the focus of content editors, the analyses presented here as well as contemporary studies of how communities function to provide safety, counter stigma, and promote personal growth should be integrated into descriptions.

Recommendation 6: Offer first-person, non-pathological narratives and consider multiple perspectives/narratives. Four of the textbooks included first-person narratives of actual BDSM practitioners. Such perspectives can help humanize how readers understand BDSM and offer a device for community voice. Given that BDSM practitioners are overwhelmingly no different from the general population in mental health outcomes (Brown et al., 2020), it is imperative that first-person narratives and case studies reflect healthy individuals in similar proportions. Given the diversity of experiences within BDSM, it is worthwhile to consider multiple people's experiences as well.

Recommendation 7: Incorporate research and member narratives on BDSM's role in promoting personal growth. The deductive themes of *personal growth* and *therapeutic aspects* were not found. These features were commonly mentioned by BDSM community members in the Graham et al. (2016) study and have been the foci of several other papers (e.g., Andrieu et al., 2019; Shahbaz & Chirinos, 2016). New research can help buttress and add dimension to the themes of BDSM pertaining to personal development and therapeutic aspects. Moreover, therapeutic resources for clients seeking mental health services have emerged in the form of "kink-aware" therapists (see Recommendation 8). Given the weight of personal growth/therapeutic aspects, it is recommended that textbooks incorporate these dimensions.

Recommendation 8: Include community, academic, and therapeutic resources for learning about BDSM. Given the self-reflection inherent in undergraduate human sexuality courses, resource listings are an opportunity to link students to a wealth of information. In our review, one book mentioned resources pertaining to BDSM. Organizations such as CARAS (https://www.carasresearch.org/) and the National Coalition for Sexual Freedom (https://ncsfreedom.org/) provide a professional and legal face to alternative sexuality and can serve as BDSM-affirming points for further information. Additionally, specific organizations such as the Society of Janus (https://soj.org/) and the Eulenspiegel Society (https://www.tes.org/) offer educational resources for learning more about BDSM. New resources for training therapists in cultural competence around BDSM have emerged, including books (Shahbaz & Chirinos, 2016), articles (Sprott & Hadcock, 2018), and professional guidelines (Kink Clinical Practice Guidelines Project, 2021). Directories for finding "kink-aware" therapists also exist for those seeking mental health services (e.g., Kink Aware Professionals, https://www.kapprofessionals.org/). Listing these resources would be a worthwhile addition and reflect this emerging trend.

Recommendations for Community Review/Input

Recommendation 9: Conduct participatory review processes in partnership with BDSM communities. The last and perhaps most far-reaching recommendation for textbook authors is to involve BDSM community representatives directly in reviewing and shaping textbook narratives. The third study within the Kink Representation Outreach Project will share descriptions with members of organized BDSM communities and systematically gather feedback. Independently, editors and coauthors of textbooks can directly partner with BDSM community organizations to review BDSM sections as part of their regular revision processes for new editions. Community reviewers can serve as valuable advisors, and organizations such as CARAS can play a versatile role in bridging academic and community communication.

Limitations

Several limitations should be noted. First, our review was limited to five books. While we are confident the set ranks among the most circulated, expanding the set may have revealed other important trends, concerns, and/or exemplars. Second, textbooks were English-language, in circulation primarily in North America. Textbooks in other international contexts might have differing BDSM framings or may not mention it at all. Human sexuality textbooks were chosen as they are actively used in freestanding, introductory-level human sexuality courses found at many institutions of higher learning; we did not include critical essays, edited volumes, and books explicitly focused on BDSM. Exploration into other types of sources is certainly warranted, and results from this study can provide a structure for future work.

Conclusion

By including both academic and community perspectives, this study contributes to research on BDSM by critically examining how the current research as well as member experiences are represented in widely used, far-reaching human sexuality textbooks. Future research can bring new participatory approaches to further assessing representation from the perspective of those who practice BDSM. Moreover, the method employed here can offer strategies for assessing representation for a host of identity experiences (e.g., intersex, asexuality, ethical non-monogamy). The findings and nine recommendations shared here can serve as a resource for editors and others for improving the content, including understandings of BDSM based on those who experience it. Community voice contributes to and elevates sex research, which in turn can improve the dissemination of this powerful body of knowledge.

References

American Psychiatric Association. (2013). *Diagnostic and statistical manual of mental disorders* (5th ed.). https://doi.org/10.1176/appi.books.9780890425596

Andrieu, B., Lahuerta, C., & Luy, A. (2019). Consenting to constraint: BDSM therapy after the DSM-5. *L'Évolution Psychiatrique, 84*(2), e1–e14. https://doi.org/10.1016/j.evopsy.2019.02.005

Arndt, W. B., Foehl, J. C., & Good, F. E. (1985). Specific sexual fantasy themes: A multidimensional study. *Journal of Personality and Social Psychology, 48*(2), 472–480. https://doi.org/10.1037/0022-3514.48.2.472

Bauer, R. (2020). Queering consent: Negotiating critical consent in les-bi-trans-queer BDSM contexts. *Sexualities, 24*(5–6), 767–783. https://doi.org/10.1177/1363460720973902

Boyatzis, R. E. (1998). *Transforming qualitative information: Thematic analysis and code development.* SAGE Publications.

Brown, A., Barker, E. D., & Rahman, Q. (2020). A systematic scoping review of the prevalence, etiological, psychological, and interpersonal factors associated with BDSM. *The Journal of Sex Research, 57*(6), 781–811. https://doi.org/10.1080/00224499.2019.1665619

Carroll, J. L. (2019). *Sexuality now: Embracing diversity* (6th ed.). Cengage.

Community Academic Consortium for Research on Alternative Sexualities. (Jan 3, 2023). The CARAS Research Advisory Committee. https://www.carasresearch.org/community-advisory-board

Cruz, A. (2016). *The color of kink: Black women, BDSM, and pornography*. New York University Press.

Dunkley, C. R., & Brotto, L. A. (2020). The role of consent in the context of BDSM. *Sexual Abuse, 32*(6), 657–678. https://doi.org/10.1177/1079063219842847

Galilee-Belfer, M. (2020). BDSM, kink, and consent: What the law can learn from consent-driven communities. *Arizona Law Review, 62*, 507.

Goldstein, S., Siegel, D., & Seaman, J. (2010). Limited access: The status of disability in introductory psychology textbooks. *Teaching of Psychology, 37*, 21–27. https://doi.org/10.1080/00986280903426290

Graham, B. C., Butler, S. E., McGraw, R., Cannes, S. M., & Smith, J. (2016). Member perspectives on the role of BDSM communities. *The Journal of Sex Research, 53*(8), 895–909. https://doi.org/10.1080/00224499.2015.1067758

Herma, H., Kris, E., & Shor, J. (1943). Freud's theory of the dream in American textbooks. *The Journal of Abnormal and Social Psychology, 38*, 319–334. https://doi.org/10.1037/h0055468

Hyde, J. S., & DeLamater, J. D. (2017). *Understanding human sexuality* (13th ed.). McGraw-Hill Education.

Joyal, C. C., & Carpentier, J. (2017). The prevalence of paraphilic interests and behaviors in the general population: A provincial survey. *The Journal of Sex Research, 54*(2), 161–171.

Khan, U. (2017). Fifty shades of ambivalence: BDSM representation in pop culture. In C. Smith, F. Attwood, & B. McNair (Eds.), *The Routledge companion to media, sex and sexuality* (pp. 59–69). Routledge.

King, B. M., Parker, K. S., Hill, K. J., Kelly, M. J., & Eason, B. L. (2017). Promoting sexual health: Sexuality and gender/women's studies courses in US higher education. *Health Behavior and Policy Review, 4*(3), 213–223.

Kink Clinical Practice Guidelines Project. (2021). *Clinical practice guidelines for working with people with kink interests*. https://www.kinkguidelines.com/the-guidelines

Kinsey, A. C., Pomeroy, W. B., Martin, C. E., & Gebhard, P. H. (1953). *Sexual Behavior in the Human Female*. W.B. Saunders.

Koshy, V. (2005). *Action research for improving practice: A practical guide*. Sage Publications.

Kuhn, T. S. (1962). *The structure of scientific revolutions*. University of Chicago Press.

Langdridge, D., & Barker, M. (Eds.). (2007). *Safe, sane and consensual: Contemporary perspectives on sadomasochism*. Palgrave Macmillan.

LeVay, S., Baldwin, J., & Baldwin J. (2018). *Discovering human sexuality* (4th ed.). Sinauer Associates.

Moser, C., & Kleinplatz, P. J. (2006). DSM-IV-TR and the paraphilias: An argument for removal. *Journal of Psychology & Human Sexuality, 17*(3–4), 91–109. https://doi.org/10.1300/J056v17n03_05

Muehlenhard, C. L., Humphreys, T. P., Jozkowski, K. N., & Peterson, Z. D. (2016). The complexities of sexual consent among college students: A conceptual and empirical review. *The Journal of Sex Research, 53*(4–5), 457–487. https://doi.org/10.1080/00224499.2016.1146651

Nitschke, J., Blendl, V., Ottermann, B., Osterheider, M., & Mokros, A. (2009). Severe sexual sadism—An underdiagnosed disorder? Evidence from a sample of forensic inpatients. *Journal of Forensic Sciences, 54*(3), 685–691. https://doi.org/10.1111/j.1556-4029.2009.01038.x

Padgett, G. (2015). A critical case study of selected US history textbooks from a tribal critical race theory perspective. *The Qualitative Report, 20*(3), 153–171. https://scholar commons.usf.edu/etd/4381

Rathus, S. A., Nevid, J., & Fichner-Rathus, L. (2018). *Human sexuality in a changing world* (10th ed.). Pearson.

Richters, J., de Visser, R., Rissel, C., Grulich, A., & Smith, A. (2008). Demographic and psychosocial features of participants in bondage and discipline, "sadomasochism" or dominance and submission (BDSM): Data from a national survey. *Journal of Sexual Medicine, 5*, 1660–1668. https://doi.org/10.1111/j.1743-6109.2008.00795.x

Shahbaz, C., & Chirinos, P. (2016). *Becoming a kink aware therapist.* Taylor & Francis.

Sprott, R. A., & Hadcock, B. (2018). Bisexuality, pansexuality, queer identity, and kink identity. *Sexual and Relationship Therapy, 33*(1–2), 214–232. https://doi.org/10.1080/14681994.2017.1347616

Thomas, D. R. (2006). A general inductive approach for analyzing qualitative evaluation data. *American Journal of Evaluation, 27*(2), 237–246. https://doi.org/10.1177/10982 14005283748

Unger, R. (2010). Leave no text behind: Teaching the psychology of women during the emergence of second wave feminism. *Sex Roles, 62*, 153–158. https://doi.org/10.1007/s11199-009-9740-3

Wadsworth, Y. J. (1998). What is participatory action research? *Action Research International.* Paper 2. http://www.aral.com.au/ari/p-ywadsworth98.html (published online first Nov 1998)

Weiss, M. D. (2006). Mainstreaming kink: The politics of BDSM representation in US popular media. *Journal of Homosexuality, 50*(2–3), 103–132. https://doi.org/10.1300/J082v50n02_06

Weitz, R. (1982). From the closet to the classroom: Homosexuality in abnormal psychology and sociology of deviance textbooks. *Deviant Behavior, 3*(4), 385–398. https://doi.org/10.1080/01639625.1982.9967597

Whissell, C. (1997). Content, style, and emotional tone of texts in introductory psychology. *Perceptual and Motor Skills, 84*, 115–125. https://doi.org/10.2466/pms.1997.84.1.115

Wright, S. (2018). De-pathologization of consensual BDSM. *The Journal of Sexual Medicine, 15*(5), 622–624. https://doi.org/10.1016/j.jsxm.2018.02.018

Yarber, W., & Sayad, B. (2019). *Human sexuality: Diversity in contemporary society* (10th ed.). McGraw-Hill Education.

10

A Record of Violence

The Continuing Criminalization of BDSM Activities

Theodore Bennett

Introduction

A number of Western common law jurisdictions draw a criminalizing line through BDSM activities. BDSM activities that cross this line will be unlawful regardless of the consent of participants, whereas BDSM activities that do not cross this line will generally be lawful. As I have previously described elsewhere (Bennett, 2021, pp. 163–166), this line is broadly equivalent across Australia, Canada, England and Wales, and the United States of America. It is calibrated on the basis of the severity of any injury inflicted during BDSM activities and is currently set to criminalize the infliction of even minor injuries. BDSM activities are criminalized if they involve at least "bodily harm" in many Australian jurisdictions (Bennett, 2013, pp. 557–558), in Canada (Khan, 2014, pp. 246–252), and in England and Wales (*R v. Brown*, 1994). Bodily harm can mean slightly different things across these jurisdictions, but the foundational formulation of bodily harm is "any hurt or injury calculated to interfere with . . . health or comfort" that is "more than merely transient and trifling" (*R v. Donovan*, 1934, p. 509). In the remaining Australian jurisdictions BDSM activities are criminalized if they involve "wounding," meaning a breach of both skin layers so as to cause the flow of blood (*Vallance v. R*, 1961). While the criminal law varies across different parts of the United States, "most states adopt the Model Penal Code (MPG) approach," which provides that "consent is a defense to an offense that causes or risks injury if the injury is 'not serious'" (Kaplan, 2014, p. 121). However, Kaplan observes that injuries resulting from BDSM activities have typically been "exaggerate[d] or mischaracterize[d]" by American courts so as to criminalize "such minor BDSM-related assaults as spanking or light grazing

Theodore Bennett, *A Record of Violence* In: *The Power of BDSM*. Edited by: Brandy L. Simula, Robin Bauer, and Liam Wignall, Oxford University Press. © Oxford University Press 2023. DOI: 10.1093/oso/9780197658598.003.0011 with a crop" (2014, p. 121), and thus practically this threshold can be quite low. Accordingly, inflicting injuries that are more than trivial in the course of fully consensual BDSM activities can expose a BDSM participant to criminal liability within these Western common law jurisdictions.

Legal opinion across these jurisdictions has long supported shifting the criminalizing line drawn through BDSM activities toward further de-criminalization (e.g., Athanassoulis, 2002; Bamforth, 1994; Cowan, 2010; Kaplan, 2014; Khan, 2014; Law Commission, 1996; Pa, 2001), such as by decriminalizing BDSM activities that involve the consensual infliction of minor injuries. This would bring law's treatment of BDSM activities closer to law's treatment of other consensual activities that involve physical injury, such as contact sports, piercing, and tattooing. But for decades the relevant laws have remained effectively unchanged. Indeed, the landmark English criminalizing precedent of *R v. Brown* (1994) was recently reaffirmed by the Court of Appeal in *R v. M(B)* (2018). As Ashford (2010, p. 357) has identified, there has been an "abject failure of the BDSM community to advance the law relating to sadomasochism." This legal standstill is remarkable given that in recent years BDSM's social profile has significantly increased and that the field of "BDSM studies" has grown exponentially (Simula, 2019).

This chapter engages with the continuing criminalization of BDSM ac-tivities across the Western common law jurisdictions, namely Australia, Canada, England and Wales, and the United States. Its goals are to high-light the impact of criminalization, identify the barriers preventing legal change from occurring, and open up pathways to decriminalizing reform. This chapter begins by identifying the negative effects of criminalization on BDSM communities and participants. It then outlines some of the key barriers blocking decriminalizing legal change, focusing on the interlinking of BDSM and violence within legal discourse. The perceived "violence" of BDSM strongly limits the reformatory potential of BDSM identity claims, such as that law should treat BDSM participants as human rights–bearing subjects and that law should treat BDSM as a sexual identity comparable to other already legitimized sexual identities. This chapter seeks to overcome these limits by reconceptualizing the legal understanding of the connection between BDSM and violence. To do this, it charts the key definitions of vio-lence that have emerged across broad academic thought and feeds back into legal discussions a crucial distinction between the descriptive and normative aspects of violence. This distinction separates out the empirical observation that an interpersonal act involves the use of physical force/injury (descriptive violence) from the normative evaluation that an interpersonal act involves the illegitimate use of physical force/injury (normative violence) (Coady, 2008). This chapter concedes that some BDSM activities constitute descriptive violence but contends that these BDSM activities do not constitute normative violence because there is no persuasive rationale for establishing illegitimacy. If the connection between BDSM and violence is properly understood as being merely descriptive in nature, then it should not pose a barrier to decriminalizing reform because it is a neutral observation rather than a substantive basis for prohibition.

Negative Effects of Criminalization

Despite the criminalizing line that Western common law jurisdictions draw through BDSM activities, there is a significant gap between what the law says and what the law does. While injurious BDSM activities may technically be criminalized, it is clear that in recent years there has not been a widespread practical effort to enforce this prohibition. Police raids of BDSM venues have indeed occurred in previous decades, but across these common law jurisdictions there is little evidence of a consistent contemporary practice of kicking in dungeon doors or surveilling people's private play. Cases involving BDSM activities do occasionally make their way to the criminal courts, but these typically involve some special feature that may explain why law enforcement is involved (Bennett, 2015, p. 32). Such features include injuries reported to the police by medical professionals due to suspicions of domestic violence, contested claims by the participants about whether the BDSM activities were actually consensual, dubious claims of BDSM by defendants that appear to be post hoc attempts to excuse non-BDSM abuse, and deaths in a context involving BDSM (Khan, 2014, p. 225). The breakpoint between the technical criminality of BDSM activities and this practical non-enforcement is the "prosecutorial discretion" exercised by legal officials (Baia, 2018, p. 1055). For whatever reason, BDSM "is generally not targeted by police or prosecutors" (Khan, 2014, p. 213), perhaps as a result of policies about only pursuing cases considered to be in the public interest. While it is important for legal officials to be able to exercise discretion in their duties, the very broad scope of discretion around BDSM activities is problematic. It introduces a significant capacity for arbitrariness, inconsistency, and abuse into the criminal law process. Furthermore, because legal officials are not trained in the norms and conventions of BDSM culture, this discretionary power is not necessarily exercised in an informed way.

The criminalization of BDSM activities is problematic despite its lack of consistent enforcement because it subjects BDSM communities and participants to "the shadow of the law" (Weinberg, 2016, pp. 13 and 91–93). That is, the weight of possible legal repercussions—a "fear of prosecution and harassment" (Pa, 2001, pp. 84–85)—hangs over those organizing BDSM events, running dungeons, and playing with others. Criminalization means that BDSM participants "must negotiate . . . uncertain territory" (Herman, 2007, p. 94) because they live with the constant "worry that the police will raid their establishment or come across a videotape or respond to a complaint by a neighbor" (Tanovich, 2010, p. 95). Weinberg (2016, pp. 87 and 97–98) has documented how some American BDSM communities have responded by trying to "fly under . . . the radar" and avoid potential legal attention through secretiveness and insularity. Going "underground" fosters the risk for abuse within BDSM communities and discourages BDSM participants from reporting legitimate complaints to the police (Pa, 2001, pp. 83–84), sharing skills around "safe bondage and other practices" (Doherty, 2012, p. 135), and "seeking medical help when they are injured during a BDSM encounter" (Haley, 2015, p. 649). Weinberg (2016) has also noted how some American BDSM communities have responded to criminalization via overcompensation instead, instituting internal regulations that minimize potential legal risks and that help project an outward image of propriety. This can result in BDSM communities burdening themselves with onerous restrictions, such as play events with organizer-imposed moratoriums on certain BDSM activities ("house limits"), patrolling community members tasked with safety and limit monitoring ("dungeon monitors"), and entry requirements that attendees sign disclaimers purporting to limit the potential legal liability of organizers (Weinberg, 2016; Weiss, 2011). Overcompensation may also make BDSM participants avoid engaging in activities where minor injuries are a possible or definite outcome. Thus, the shadow of the law warps and twists BDSM in significant ways even in the absence of legal enforcement.

The criminalization of BDSM activities is also significant for symbolic reasons that go beyond practical enforcement. Standards set by law, especially criminal law, send strong messages to society: they are a "public affirmation of social ideals and norms" (Gusfeld, 1967, p. 177). Criminalization of an activity signals that it is a form of wrongdoing that the state condemns, and when that activity is closely tied to a specific identity it signals that people who share that identity stand in opposition to the state. Symbolically, criminalization locates BDSM participants outside the bounds of the legitimate community and, in doing so, "reflects and reinforces the perception that BDSM activities are the domain of the perverted and deviant" (Kaplan, 2014, p. 116). This legal messaging adds to the social stigma already suffered by BDSM participants.

Barriers to Decriminalization

For the reasons given above, despite "the rarity of modern BDSM cases," this does not mean "that the need for legal recognition of consensual BDSM is minor" (Onoma, 2017, p. 42). While the technical criminality of BDSM activities is not consistently enforced, the negative effects of criminalization demonstrate that legal change is nonetheless needed. The fact that the law in these common law jurisdictions remains unchanged is not due to there being a compelling policy basis for the current criminal restrictions. Indeed, as noted in the "Introduction," there is a substantial body of legal opinion in favor of the decriminalization of BDSM activities, especially where just minor injuries are involved. Rather than a sound policy justification, there is instead a diverse collection of practical and conceptual barriers that block meaningful law reform from occurring.

One barrier is that the primary legal material dealing with BDSM activities is both limited and unwarrantedly negative. As noted above, the kinds of criminal cases involving BDSM that are pursued by law enforcement typically misrepresent BDSM by virtue of the special features that trigger the exercise of discretion to prosecute. BDSM activities do not typically involve injuries requiring medical treatment, contested claims of consent, blatant abuse, or the death of a participant; yet this is the impression one gets from reading many of the reported cases where BDSM activities are addressed. A common law student, lawyer, judge, or academic who is familiar with this primary legal material but who is not familiar more broadly with the typical practices and conventions of BDSM culture is liable to fundamentally misunderstand BDSM activities. The inaccurate picture of BDSM that emerges from these legal sources needs to be properly contextualized, but detailed information about BDSM is not a typical feature of legal education or legal professional programs (with the exception of certain specialist university electives).

Another barrier is that the criminalization of BDSM activities derives not from a specific BDSM offense but rather from the judicial interpretation of generalized criminal offenses that prohibit assault and injury. Within common law legal systems judges are bound to follow previous decisions made by higher courts within their court hierarchy. This generates a strong force for legal inertia as judges hearing BDSM cases in inferior courts cannot depart from the current criminalizing precedents. While judges in superior courts could decide differently, they may be reticent to do so because the decriminalization of BDSM involves issues of public policy and not just issues of legal doctrine. In the United Kingdom, for example, it appears "that the judiciary are reluctant to tackle the issue, preferring instead to defer to Parliament on the matter" (Kerr, 2014, p. 67; see also Schumann, 2018, p. 1195). Indeed, the Court of Appeal recently adopted just such a hands-off approach in *R v. M(B)* (2018). But it is unlikely that parliaments would legislate to alter generalized criminal offenses in order to carve out exemptions for BDSM activities. This kind of issue is "not on their radar" (Tanovich, 2010, p. 89), and even if it were, due to the social stigma around BDSM, "few lawmakers who value their careers would be willing to sign a piece of legislation designed to create protections for the BDSM community" (Schumann, 2018, p. 1196).

A further barrier is that while widespread advocacy efforts and heightened community awareness are typically powerful methods for generating legal change, the criminalization of BDSM activities is insulated from critical attention by its lack of practical enforcement. *R v. Brown* (1994) spurred on BDSM campaigning and the formation of activist groups and generated significant public awareness (Califia, 1999/2000, p. 146). It had the effect of "politicizing SM, helping to create a shared sense of oppositional unity among practitioners—visibilized, for example, in 'SM Pride' rallies" (Wilkinson, 2009, p. 192). But no other case across these common law jurisdictions has since generated a similar response. The absence of police and prosecutorial actions against BDSM participants has deprived BDSM communities of rallying events around which they could organize and through which they could make the issue of criminalization visible to the general public. At a practical level it has also meant a lack of suitable cases that could be contested and appealed to courts with sufficient seniority to potentially overturn the current criminalizing precedents.

A further key barrier to legal change is a conceptual issue that carries significant practicable implications: the interlinking of BDSM and violence. The conceptualization of *BDSM as violence* appears within "multiple discourses," including popular culture and feminism, but has manifested strongly and consistently within legal discourse (Williams, 2016, p. 69). It is deeply woven into the fabric of legal discourse in a number of ways (Bennett, 2015, pp. 43–46; Khan, 2014). It is implicit in the very nature of BDSM's criminalization as the relevant offenses of assault occasioning bodily harm, wounding, and the like are all offenses of violence. It is also very explicit within law, especially the landmark case of *R v. Brown* (1994) with its "recurring emphasis . . . on the concept of violence" (Giles, 1994, p. 106). Legal commentary in support of criminalizing restrictions on BDSM activities echoes the notion that BDSM is (or is intrinsically connected to) violence (e.g., Edwards, 1993; Hanna, 2001; Herring, 2017), and violence continues to arise in discussions of legal reform. For example, in a 2018 report on consensual assault law the Tasmania Law Reform Institute (2018, p. 22) discussed BDSM under the heading "consensual sexual violence." As another example, current law reform campaigns in the United Kingdom interrelate BDSM and "domestic violence" (Harman & Garnier, 2019). The interlinking of BDSM and violence blocks the pathways to decriminalizing law reform. At a strategic level, given the normative connotations typically attached to violence, if the decriminalization of BDSM is framed as being about "loosening legal restrictions on violence," then any push for decriminalization is less likely to gain traction with the public, courts, or politicians. Furthermore, this perceived violence undercuts the strength of otherwise promising decriminalizing arguments based on claims of BDSM identity.

Instead of being conceptualized as simply an activity, the possibility of BDSM being regarded within legal discourse "as a specifically rights-bearing identity . . . has significance for engaging with claims of rights and recognition as well as issues of visibility, acknowledgement and respect before the law" (Chatterjee, 2012, p. 742). Understanding BDSM participants through the lens of human rights enables demands for better legal treatment of BDSM to be grounded in rights such as privacy and freedom from discrimination. Human rights claims like these can enable legal change in two ways: by requiring the state to not unduly infringe on those rights and by obliging the state to take steps to protect those rights (*Mosley v. the United Kingdom*, 2011, para. 106). But while the "realm of human rights" may seem like a "promising arena for sadomasochist subjectivity" (Khan, 2014, p. 302), it is limited in the area of criminal law. In an appeal from *R v. Brown* (1994), the European Court of Human Rights in *Laskey, Jaggard and Brown v. UK* (1997) rejected the argument that the criminalization of BDSM activities constituted an unjustifiable violation of the right to privacy. The court heard the UK government's argument that states were "entitled to punish acts of violence" and held that the risk of physical harm involved in BDSM activities meant that criminalizing restrictions were valid (*Laskey, Jaggard and Brown v. UK*, 1997, para 40). The issue here is that no person's human rights are absolute; rather, they are checked by the human rights of others and by legitimate countervailing factors such as the prevention of violence (Weait, 2007, pp. 75–76). The right to privacy is not a right to unchecked private violence, the right to freedom from discrimination is not a right to differential treatment on the basis of legitimate factors such as violent conduct, and the right to sexual autonomy is not a right to do sexual violence to others. If BDSM activities are understood to constitute violence, then it is difficult to mobilize human rights claims to argue for their decriminalization.

The claim that BDSM identity is a kind of sexual identity provides a further pathway toward decriminalization. If BDSM is understood to be a sexual identity, perhaps even a sexual orientation, then this enables arguments to be made to extend to this BDSM identity comparative legal treatment to that provided other legitimized sexual identities, such as heterosexuality and homosexuality (Weait, 2007, p. 75). The push here is for the equal recognition, protection, and promotion of BDSM participants as legitimate "sexual citizens" (Chatterjee, 2012; Langdridge, 2006; Langdridge & Parchev, 2018). Equality would involve decriminalization of BDSM activities in the same way that other consensual sexual activities have been decriminalized, as well as further equalizing reforms around legal issues such as pornography, sex work, and anti-discrimination protections. Sexual identity claims also have clear potential to overlap with (and reinforce) the human rights claims discussed above as human rights claims have been key means by which previously marginalized sexual minorities have pushed for better legal treatment.

The claim that BDSM is a sexual identity is problematic because it has the potential to be reductive of the wide variety of motivations and activities involved in BDSM. However, a deeper issue here is that merely claiming a sexual identity does not thereby establish that that sexual identity deserves legal legitimization. There are plenty of potentially claimable sexual identities that law does not, and should not, countenance because various factors distinguish such identities from those already legitimized, for example, sexual identities based on types of sex that lack consent or that involve serious, disabling harm or death. The issue here is that the connection between BDSM and violence works to "prevent the recognition of BDSM as a legitimate sexuality" within law (Williams, 2016, p. 68) because it establishes what appears to be a clear point of justifiable differentiation between BDSM and the other already legitimized sexual identities, namely the presence of violence. If violence is understood to be "constitutive" of any claimed BDSM sexual identity, it is difficult to see how sexual identity claims could be an effective pathway toward the decriminalization of BDSM activities (Weait, 2007, p. 76).

(Dis)Connections Between BDSM and Violence

While a number of barriers stand in the way of the decriminalization of BDSM activities, legal discourse's interlinking of BDSM and violence is a particularly powerful obstacle to change. Realizing this, many legal commentators have attempted to either decouple BDSM from violence or reframe the perceived "violence" of BDSM activities as not necessarily requiring strict criminalization. BDSM has been argued to not constitute violence because it is consensual, pleasurable, and not subjectively understood by BDSM participants as violence (Bamforth, 1994; Pa, 2001). Even if BDSM is violent, it has been argued to constitute a form of "good violence" (Moran, 1995) because the force and injury it involves is consensual, is internally regulated, and only causes desired harm (Kaplan, 2014); is agreed upon, carefully administered, and accepted (Hoople, 1996); and aims to produce pleasure rather than undesired pain (Athanassoulis, 2002). It has also frequently been argued that while BDSM may involve violence, it is nonetheless a form of sex and that the sexual motivations and context of BDSM activities mean that law should treat them the way it treats consensual sexual activities (Athanassoulis, 2002, p. 152; Bennett, 2015, pp. 43–44; Cowan, 2011, p. 71, 2014, p. 150; Kaplan, 2014, p. 127; Khan, 2014; Pa, 2001, p. 77).

As well argued as these efforts have been, the links between BDSM and violence have proven remarkably tenacious and continue to strongly characterize legal discourse in common law jurisdictions. One reason for this is the lack of a clear common understanding of violence. Different commentators seem to mean different things when they use this term and thus talk past one another. Another reason is that if BDSM and violence are only partially decoupled, then a delegitimizing residue of violence nevertheless remains.

That is, BDSM remains characterized by violence even if it can be success-fully established that on balance BDSM activities are more akin to sex.

The connection between BDSM and violence thus remains an obstacle to decriminalizing legal change. While some progress past this obstacle has been made via attempts to guide legal discourse toward a better under-standing of BDSM, this chapter argues that further progress can be made by also simultaneously attempting to guide legal discourse toward a better un-derstanding of violence. If we can better understand the concept of violence itself, then we can better understand the nature of the connection between BDSM and violence and better assess what legal consequences should flow from this connection.

In seeking to better understand violence, it must be recognized that while violence is a concept that is relevant to law, it is not a concept that is relevant only to law. As such, legal academia should be a starting point but not an ending point for where to look for further clarity on violence. Useful insights into violence can be found in other academic fields, such as philosophy; thus, this chapter draws on a broad range of material in order to move legal dis-course forward. In order to justify reaching outside law, it is important to address the fact that "one of the most common ways of defining violence is to only consider forms of *criminal* [emphasis in original] violence and to argue that violence is the use of force that has been prohibited by law" (de Haan, 2008, p. 27). To collapse the concept of violence into criminality would be re-ductive. It is intuitively unsatisfactory as examples such as lawful war and the lawful gladiatorial combat of ancient Rome seem undoubtedly to be violent. It is also academically unsatisfactory as there is a strong line of sociolegal scholarship establishing that violence does not stand solely in opposition to the law but rather that law variously allows, excuses, justifies, authorizes, and even requires the use of various forms of force that can be understood to be violent (Cover, 1986; Moran, 1995; Ramos, 2003; Ristroph, 2011; Sarat, 2001; Sarat & Kearns, 1992). Take, for example, the force threatened and used by police officers, court security, and prison officials in properly carrying out their duties.

If violence cannot be defined simply as criminal uses of force, and thus cannot be defined wholly in terms of law, then what exactly is it? Scholars working across various academic fields acknowledge that there is a funda-mental lack of clarity around violence. Violence "is, frankly, not well under-stood" (Vorobej, 2016, p. 12) and has proven "notoriously difficult to define because as a phenomenon it is multifaceted, socially constructed and highly ambivalent" (de Haan, 2008, p. 28). Given the intractable complexity of this concept, this chapter will not try to develop a unified theory of violence, nor will it argue for the correctness of one definition of violence over all others. Rather, this chapter aims to identify the major definitions of violence and work through how they relate to legal discourse around the perceived "violence" of BDSM activities. Some key groupings emerge from the various definitions of violence found within academia, and these groupings enable the complexity of violence to be approached in a systematic manner. Here, this chapter adopts Coady's (2008, p. 22) taxonomy of the three major types of definitions of violence found within the academic literature.

First is the "restricted" definition of violence (Coady, 2008, p. 22). This defines violence as a "positive interpersonal [act] of force, usually involving the infliction of physical injury" (Coady, 2008, p. 23). This definition links to the origins of the word *violence* in the Latin "*violentia*, meaning 'vehemence', a passionate and uncontrolled force" (Buffachi, 2005, p. 194). This definition is purely descriptive in that the means, ends, and context of interpersonal force are irrelevant to whether it constitutes violence. The focus on force and injury within this definition clarifies why violence is a conceptual category that has social significance: violence "is a concern of human beings because ... [we] are physically embodied, vulnerable, and mortal creatures" (Ristroph, 2014, p. 1024).

Second is the "legitimist" definition of violence (Coady, 2008, p. 22). This defines violence as an "illegal or illegitimate use of force," also typically understood in an interpersonal sense (Coady, 2008, p. 23). This definition links to the alternative Latin word *violare*, meaning "infringement" (Buffachi, 2005, p. 194). Violence here is understood not as vehemence but as a "violation" (Buffachi, 2005, pp. 194–195), perhaps of consent, social standards, morality, law, human rights, human dignity, etc. This definition is normative in that an assessment of the illegitimacy of the means, ends, and/or context of interpersonal force is crucial as to whether it constitutes violence. Violence within this definition partly reflects the embodied fragility of humanity but also functions as a delegitimizing condemnation that serves the political interests of whomever deploys the term (Wolff, 1969).

Third are the "wide" definitions of violence (Coady, 2008, p. 22). These definitions come in a number of different forms, but all stretch the concept of violence beyond interpersonal acts of force. Some forms extend violence to include psychological violence, that is, instances of psychological injury caused by interpersonal acts that need not include physical force. Some forms extend violence beyond interpersonal acts to include systems of meaning, that is, the "symbolic violence" of imposing "ways of seeing and evaluating the world" on others (Ramos, 2003, p. 3), or to include processes and systems, that is, the "structural violence" of the systemic ways in which social institutions inequitably distribute opportunities and resources (Vorobej, 2016, chapter 2).

Having identified the three major definitions of violence, it becomes possible to chart how each definition could connect to BDSM and work through what any such connection would mean for law. Under the restricted definition, for BDSM to be violent it must involve interpersonal acts of force and possibly physical injury. Many BDSM activities do not involve physical force or injury, such as power-based play like service, humiliation, and role-playing. However, some BDSM activities clearly do involve physical force and possible injury, such as impact- and pain-based play like flogging, caning, cutting, needling, and wrestling. Even though certain BDSM activities may constitute violence under this definition, the resulting connection between BDSM and violence carries no clear legal implications. There are plenty of instances of force and injury that are both justified and entirely legitimate and that should be lawful, such as a concerned bystander "who lunges into a child in order to knock him out of the path of a speeding car" (Wade, 1971, p. 370), as well as plenty of instances that are unjustified and illegitimate and that should be criminal, such as a robber who knocks their victim over in order to take their belongings. Because the connection between BDSM and violence established by this definition is merely descriptive, it does not, in and of itself, indicate how BDSM activities should be regulated.

If we were to follow the legitimist definition instead, for BDSM to be violent it must involve illegitimate acts of force. Like the restricted definition, the legitimist definition only partially connects to BDSM because while some BDSM activities involve physical force and possible injury, other BDSM activities do not. But the restricted definition also goes further. The crucial difference here is this definition's element of illegitimacy, an addition that carries with it a requirement that some disqualifying factor—immorality, unjustifiability, social unacceptability, etc.—characterize the physical force involved in BDSM activities. If BDSM were to satisfy this definition of violence, the resulting connection between BDSM and violence would be normative in nature and, as such, would function as an injunction against BDSM activities and a potential factor in favor of criminalization.

Wide definitions of violence are irrelevant to legal discussions about the decriminalization of BDSM activities. Because common law jurisdictions draw their criminalizing line through BDSM activities entirely on a physical basis, it is a moot point whether BDSM activities constitute psychological, symbolic, or structural violence. Only physically forceful BDSM activities are currently criminalized, and this criminalization responds only to the degree of physical injury inflicted and nothing else (not psychological power dynamics, not systems of meaning, not social inequalities, etc.). Accordingly, if the perceived "violence" of BDSM is to be a reason against the decriminalization of BDSM activities, it must be a reason that justifies continuing law's selective criminalization of just those BDSM activities involving physical force and injury. It must, therefore, be based on a definition of violence that focuses on physical force/injury, like the restricted and legitimist definitions, and cannot be based on a definition of violence that goes beyond this.

Having outlined the major definitions of violence and set out their potential connections to legal discussions around BDSM, we can now see why the perceived "violence" of BDSM, when properly understood, should not obstruct decriminalizing legal change. Given the pejorative connotations of the legitimist definition of violence, it is entirely fair that BDSM "participants do not generally use 'violent' as an adjective to describe their play" and that "most would, understandably, vociferously object to its categorization as violence" (Newmahr, 2011, p. 127). However, this chapter argues that some BDSM activities are indeed violent but that this is not legally or normatively disqualifying as they are merely descriptive violence in accordance with the restricted definition. This argument develops in two stages.

The first stage is to disaggregate BDSM into activities that involve physical force and those that do not. BDSM should not be regarded as an undifferentiated whole, and only some BDSM activities are impact- or pain-based or otherwise involve physical force. BDSM activities that do not involve physical force are not violent in any legally relevant sense because they satisfy neither the restricted nor the legitimist definition of violence. While it is important to appreciate this point, we need to go further because criminalization already centers on those BDSM activities that do involve physical force and injury.

The second stage deals squarely with BDSM activities involving physical force and maintains that while these BDSM activities do constitute violence, they only constitute violence in a limited way. The two definitions of violence that are legally relevant here are markedly different from one another: The restricted definition describes empirical fact, while the legitimist definition also assigns normative value. Care must be taken lest the descriptive and normative aspects of violence blur together or "run seamlessly into one another" within legal discussions (Ristroph, 2011, pp. 574–575). Appreciating that "an action may be violent (descriptively) and not be a case of violence (normatively)" (Wade, 1971, p. 370) enables us to concede that BDSM activities involving physical force and injury are descriptively violent according to the restricted definition without also accepting that this force is illegitimate and thus normatively violent according to the legitimist definition. The connection between BDSM and violence should be understood within legal discourse as simply a neutral observation of the physical force inherent to some BDSM activities. This connection cannot be leveraged to do any normative work without further establishing that this physical force is illegitimate. Where BDSM activities involve minor injuries that are inflicted with the full consent of the participants there is simply no compelling basis to establish illegitimacy. Rather, there is an array of potential countervailing rationales that establish legitimacy, including the pleasure taken from the activities, the structure provided by the rules and conventions of BDSM culture, the careful and planned use of force, and the value of sexual autonomy. The argument that the physical force involved in some BDSM activities is illegitimate because it is criminal could be made but would establish nothing of value because if BDSM activities are violent simply because they are criminalized, then the perceived "violence" of BDSM activities cannot be a reason why they should remain criminalized.

Accepting that some BDSM activities are descriptively violent without also accepting the "accompanying and limiting moral problem" of normative violence (Newmahr, 2011, p. 130) strips the pejorative connotations of violence from BDSM. In this way, and contrary to Houlihan's (2011, p. 45) concern, defining BDSM as violence does not necessarily reinforce "criminolegal definitions of s/m as bad or illegitimate violence." Rather, it can challenge the easy conflation of violence with badness or illegitimacy within legal discourse. This limited acknowledgment of the descriptive violence of BDSM seems likely what Hoople (1996, p. 206) had in mind when he observed that "proposing that patriarchal violence and SM violence are both 'genuine' forms of violence *does not render them the same*, [emphasis in original] just as surgery is not the same as a street fight or, for that matter, ritual scarification." Surgery, street fights, and ritual scarification are all indeed descriptive violence; but this tells us nothing about whether they are legitimate uses of physical force, and thus whether they are also normative violence. Some people may be "ideologically troubled" about the potential for diluting "the conceptual potency of violence by including SM in its definition" (Newmahr, 2011, p. 130). But while the potency of normative violence could indeed be threatened by the unjustifiable inclusion of BDSM activities, descriptive violence is a concept that has no potency to dilute, and thus this problem does not arise.

If the true nature of the connection between BDSM and violence is descriptive rather than normative, then the perceived "violence" of BDSM activities should not pose an obstacle to their decriminalization. This is because it is the normative rather than the descriptive aspects of violence that raise meaningful barriers to legal reform. If BDSM is understood as descriptive violence, then even if the decriminalization of BDSM is framed as "loosening legal restrictions on violence," this is not an inherently negative proposition as *violence* here carries no pejorative connotations. Similarly, the mobilization of human rights claims by BDSM participants should not necessarily be limited by concerns about the state's interest in minimizing violence. This is because there are plenty of forms of legitimate force that the state has no interest in preventing, such as that used by medical professionals in the course of surgery/treatment or that involved in police officers properly carrying out their duties. Furthermore, claims that BDSM is a sexual identity that should receive comparable legal treatment to other already legitimized sexual identities should not be dismissed on the basis that violence provides a clear differentiating factor. This is because the presence of descriptive violence does not provide a substantive basis for differentiation. Thus, by better understanding the concept of violence, it becomes clear that the limited nature of BDSM's connection to violence should not bar these promising reformatory pathways.

Conclusion

Across the Western common law jurisdictions of Australia, Canada, England and Wales, and the United States, the continuing criminalization of BDSM activities involving minor injuries is profoundly negative for BDSM participants and communities. While technical criminalization has not been matched with concerted enforcement, it has effects that are nonetheless real. As this chapter has shown, these effects include the granting of excessive discretionary power to underinformed legal officials, the ongoing threat of arbitrary and sporadic enforcement, the warping of BDSM communities and practices by the shadow of the law, and the compounding of social stigma against BDSM. While legal change here is justified and necessary, it has been blocked by a number of barriers including the skewed nature of primary legal material on BDSM activities, the inertia of common law systems, and the fact that the criminal law's failings are insulated from scrutiny by the lack of enforcement. A further significant barrier to legal change is the fact that legal discourse has freighted BDSM with violence. This places significant limitations on the possibility of legal change in this area because the interlinking of BDSM and violence pejoratively loads legal discussions of BDSM and prevents the effective mobilization of decriminalizing claims based on BDSM identity.

In order to move criminal law forward in these common law jurisdictions, this chapter has attempted to better legal discourse's understanding of the nature of the connection between BDSM and violence. It has clarified the ambiguous and contested concept of violence by identifying the three major definitions of violence and showing how each one links back to legal discourse around BDSM activities. By disaggregating BDSM activities, we can see that those BDSM activities that lack physical force and injury do not satisfy any definition of violence that is relevant to legal discussions here. In order to understand the connection between violence and BDSM activities that do involve physical force, it is necessary to draw a crucial distinction between the descriptive and normative aspects of violence. BDSM activities that involve physical force are indeed descriptive violence, but they are not normative violence because there is no compelling reason to regard the force that they involve as illegitimate (and, indeed, there are plenty of reasons to regard such force as legitimate). Given that it is the normative aspects of violence that render the perceived "violence" of BDSM an effective barrier to legal change, this better understanding of violence opens up previously closed pathways for decriminalizing legal change. While other barriers to reform may remain, if we can correct BDSM's record of violence within legal discourse, it is much more likely that we can also correct the continuing criminalization of BDSM activities.

References

Ashford, C. (2010). Barebacking and the "cult of violence": Queering the criminal law. *Journal of Criminal Law*, 74(4), 339–357. https://doi.org/10.1350/jcla.2010.74.4.647

Athanassoulis, N. (2002). The role of consent in sado-masochistic practices. *Res Publica*, 8, 141–155. https://doi.org/10.1023/A:1016069407235

Baia, E. J. (2018). Akin to madmen: A queer critique of the gay rights cases. *Virginia Law Review*, 104(5), 1021–1063. https://www.jstor.org/stable/26525278

Bamforth, N. (1994, September). Sado-masochism and consent. *Criminal Law Review*, 1994(Sep), 661–664.

Bennett, T. (2013). Sadomasochism under the Human Rights (Sexual Conduct) Act 1994. *Sydney Law Review*, 35(3), 541–564. http://www.austlii.edu.au/cgi-bin/viewdoc/au/journals/SydLawRw/2013/22.html

Bennett, T. (2015). *Cuts and criminality: Body alteration in legal discourse*. Ashgate Publishing.

Bennett, T. (2021). A fine line between pleasure and pain: Would decriminalising BDSM permit nonconsensual abuse? *Liverpool Law Review*, 42, 161–183. https://doi.org/10.1007/s10991-020-09268-7

Buffachi, V. (2005). Two concepts of violence. *Political Studies Review*, 3(2), 193–204. https://doi.org/10.1111/j.1478-9299.2005.00023.x

Califia, P. (2000). Antidote to shame. In P. Califia (Ed.), *Public sex: The culture of radical sex* (pp. 139–147). Cleis. (Original work published 1999)

Chatterjee, B. B. (2012). *Pay v UK*, the probation service and consensual BDSM sexual citizenship. *Sexualities*, 15(5–6), 739–757. https://doi.org/10.1177/1363460712446279

Coady, C. A. J. (2008). *Morality and political violence*. Cambridge University Press.

Cover, R. M. (1986). Violence and the word. *The Yale Law Journal*, 95(8), 1601–1629. https://doi.org/10.2307/796468

Cowan, S. (2010). The pain of pleasure: Consent and the criminalisation of sado-masochistic "assaults." In J. Chalmer, F. Leverick, & L. Farmer (Eds.), *Essays in criminal law in honour of Sir Gerald Gordon* (pp. 126–140). Edinburgh University Press.

Cowan, S. (2011). Criminalizing SM: Disavowing the erotic, instantiating violence. In R. Duff, L. Farmer, S. Marshall, M. Renzo, & V. Tadros (Eds.), *The structures of the criminal law* (pp. 59–84). Oxford University Press.

Cowan, S. (2014). Offenses of sex or violence? Consent, fraud, and HIV transmission. *New Criminal Law Review*, 17(1), 135–161. https://doi.org/10.1525/nclr.2014.17.1.135

de Haan, W. (2008). Violence as an essentially contested concept. In S. Body-Gendrot (Ed.), *Violence in Europe: Historical and contemporary perspectives* (pp. 27–40). Springer.

Doherty, S. (2012). Sadomasochism and the criminal law: A human rights approach. *King's Student Law Review*, 3(2), 119–136.

Edwards, S. (1993). No defence for a sado-masochistic libido. *New Law Journal*, 19(143), 406–407.

Giles, M. (1994). R v Brown: Consensual harm and the public interest. *Modern Law Review*, 57(1), 101–111. https://doi.org/10.1111/j.1468-2230.1994.tb01924.x

Gusfeld, J. R. (1967). Moral passage: The symbolic process in public designations of deviance. *Social Problems*, 15(2), 175–188. https://doi.org/10.2307/799511

Haley, D. (2015). Bound by law: A roadmap for the practical legalization of BDSM. *Cardozo Journal of Law & Gender*, 21, 631–656.

Hanna, C. (2001). Sex is not a sport: Consent and violence in criminal law. *Boston College Law Review*, 42(2), 239–290. https://lira.bc.edu/work/ns/c1235e1f-b53d-42d9-8be9-4460f3769000

Harman, H., & Garnier, M. (2019). *Men are using the narrative of women's sexual enjoyment to get away with murder, literally.* HuffPost. https://tinyurl.com/y44gkpf4

Herman, R. D. K. (2007). Playing with restraints: Space, citizenship and BDSM. In K. Browne, J. Lim, & G. Brown (Eds.), *Geographies of sexualities: Theory, practices and politics* (pp. 89–100). Ashgate.

Herring, J. (2017). *R v Brown* (1993). In P. Handler, H. Mares, & I. Williams (Eds.), *Landmark cases in criminal law* (pp. 333–356). Hart Publishing.

Hoople, T. (1996). Conflicting visions: SM, feminism, and the law. A problem of representation. *Canadian Journal of Law and Society, 11*(1), 177–220. https://doi.org/10.1017/S0829320100004634

Houlihan, A. (2011). When "no" means "yes" and "yes" means harm: HIV risk, consent and sadomasochism case law. *Law & Sexuality: Review of Lesbian, Gay, Bisexual & Transgender Legal Issues, 20*, 31–60. https://journals.tulane.edu/tjls/article/view/2842

Kaplan, M. (2014). Sex-positive law. *NYU Law Review, 89*(1), 89–164. https://www.nyulawreview.org/issues/volume-89-number-1/sex-positive-law/

Kerr, A. (2014). Consensual sado-masochism and the public interest: Distinguishing morality and legality. *North East Law Review, 2*, 51–82.

Khan, U. (2014). *Vicarious kinks: S/M in the socio-legal imaginary.* University of Toronto Press.

Langdridge, D. (2006). Voices from the margins: Sadomasochism and sexual citizenship. *Citizenship Studies, 10*(4), 373–389. https://doi.org/10.1080/13621020600857940

Langdridge, D., & Parchev, O. (2018). Transgression and (sexual) citizenship: The political struggle for self-determination within BDSM communities. *Citizenship Studies, 22*(7), 667–684. https://doi.org/10.1080/13621025.2018.1508413

Laskey, Jaggard and Brown v. UK, 24 EHRR 39 (1997).

Law Commission. (1996). *Consent in the criminal law* (Consultation Paper No. 139). Her Majesty's Stationery Office.

Moran, L. J. (1995). Violence and the law: The case of sado-masochism. *Social & Legal Studies, 4*(2), 225–251. https://doi.org/10.1177/096466399500400204

Mosley v. the United Kingdom. European Court of Human Rights, Application No. 48009/08, 10 May (2011).

Newmahr, S. (2011). *Playing on the edge: Sadomasochism, risk, and intimacy.* Indiana University Press.

Onoma, A. (2017). Legal censure of unconventional expressions of love and sexuality; finding place in the law for BDSM. *Hastings Women's Law Journal, 28*(1), 25–44. https://repository.uchastings.edu/hwlj/vol28/iss1/3/

Pa, M. (2001). Beyond the pleasure principle: The criminalization of consensual sadomasochistic sex. *Texas Journal of Women and the Law, 11*(1), 51–92.

R v. Brown, 1 AC 212 (1994).

R v. Donovan, 2 KB 498 (1934).

R v. M(B), EWCACrim 560 (2018).

Ramos, E. R. (2003). Violence and the law: Notes under the influence of an extreme violence. *SELA (Seminario en Latinoamérica de Teoría Constitucional y Política) Papers,* Paper 27. https://openyls.law.yale.edu/handle/20.500.13051/17522

Ristroph, A. (2011). Criminal law in the shadow of violence. *Alabama Law Review, 62*(3), 571–621. https://www.law.ua.edu/pubs/lrarticles/Volume%2062/Issue%203/RISTROPH-Shadow_of_Violence.pdf

Ristroph, A. (2014). Just violence. *Arizona Law Review*, *56*(4), 1017–1064. https://arizo nalawreview.org/ristroph/

Sarat, A. (Ed.). (2001). *Law, violence, and the possibility of justice.* Princeton University Press.

Sarat, A., & Kearns, T. R (Eds.). (1992). *Law's violence.* University of Michigan Press.

Schumann, M. (2018). Pain, please: Consent to sadomasochistic conduct. *University of Illinois Law Review*, *3*, 1177–1205. https://www.illinoislawreview.org/print/vol-2018-no-3/pain-please/

Simula, B. L. (2019). Pleasure, power and pain: A review of the literature on the experiences of BDSM participants. *Sociology Compass*, *13*(3), 1–24. https://doi.org/10.1111/soc4.12668

Tanovich, D. M. (2010). Criminalizing sex at the margins. *Criminal Reports*, *74*, 86–95.

Tasmania Law Reform Institute. (2018). *Consensual assault* (Final Report No. 25). https://www.utas.edu.au/__data/assets/pdf_file/0013/1102630/Consensual-Assault.pdf

Vallance v. R, 108 CLR 56 (1961).

Vorobej, M. (2016). *The concept of violence.* Routledge.

Wade, F. C. (1971). On violence. *The Journal of Philosophy*, *68*(12), 369–377. https://doi.org/10.2307/2024918

Weait, M. (2007). Sadomasochism and the law. In D. Langdridge & M. Barker (Eds.), *Safe, sane and consensual: Contemporary perspectives on sadomasochism* (pp. 63–82). Palgrave Macmillan.

Weinberg, J. D. (2016). *Consensual violence: Sex, sports, and the politics of injury.* University of California Press.

Weiss, M. (2011). *Techniques of pleasure: BDSM and the circuits of sexuality.* Duke University Press.

Wilkinson, E. (2009). Perverting visual pleasure: Representing sadomasochism. *Sexualities*, *12*(2), 181–198. https://doi.org/10.1177/1363460708100918

Williams, J. (2016). Sadomasochism to BDSM: Discourse across disciplines. *Limina*, *22*(1), 67–83. https://www.limina.arts.uwa.edu.au/volumes/volume-22.1-2016/arti cle-williams

Wolff, R. P. (1969). On violence. *The Journal of Philosophy*, *66*(19), 601–616. https://doi.org/10.2307/2024177

11

Dominance, Submission, and Intersectionality

The Liberatory Potential of Authority Exchange

Sinclair Sexsmith

Introduction

I hissed in her ear, "You are such a fucking slut." And that was the kindest name I called her in that scene.

She looked at me with big brown eyes and her mouth open a little in surprise, though she knew we were going there. And then she melted, leaning against me, whispering, "Yes, yes," over and over.

It was later, when I was calling her other things, when we were acting out a scene she had chosen and requested, that I got a flash of something new. She, a friend,[1] had asked me to flog her with a thick, hunter green, deerskin leather flogger; to spit on her; to call her some specific sexist names; and, when the time was right, to hand her the Magic Wand vibrator conveniently and eagerly placed nearby.

She was very sexy, and I trusted her and agreed. I hadn't planned on having a momentary flash of panic, then realization, that calling her certain names had different meanings than when I'd used similar terms in other scenes. I realized, in that moment, that what I was feeling was an embodied sense of what intersectionality means.

Intersectionality

The term *intersectionality* was coined in 1989 by Kimberlé Crenshaw, a legal scholar, in a paper where she was discussing discrimination on both a racial and a gender basis. Crenshaw defined an intersection of multiple social

Sinclair Sexsmith, *Dominance, Submission, and Intersectionality* In: *The Power of BDSM*. Edited by: Brandy L. Simula, Robin Bauer, and Liam Wignall, Oxford University Press. © Oxford University Press 2023.
DOI: 10.1093/oso/9780197658598.003.0012

identities through which disadvantage and marginalization occur. The term caught on in the 2010s, and many people of varying backgrounds use it to describe the complexities of holding multiple identities at once.

We, my friend and I, were on a safe BDSM retreat weekend where we'd been exploring consent, negotiation, desires, asking for what we want, erotic energy, ritual, movement, expression, and so much more. We had good chemistry, had known each other for a few years, and chatted easily about similar interests in our lives. I trusted her agency—I believed that she would tell me what she needed and that I could read her to follow her pacing lead. At the retreat, we generally used the safe words *red*, *yellow*, and *green*, like a stoplight, through the weekend, so I knew she could use those if she needed to. Because we weren't playing with any non-consent, words like *wait* or *slow down* or *hold on* or any kind of communication about what was working or wasn't would do just fine. I knew from past experience with her that she often went deep into a submissive headspace, which often looks like being non-verbal or consenting to everything I asked for, so I stuck with the things we had planned and didn't change anything mid-scene.

I wasn't expecting to have a moment in our play together in which our different intersectional positions became forcefully evident. I was, of course, aware that this submissive friend of mine was an Asian woman and that women of color experience different kinds of discrimination, a particularly racist flavor of sexism that is not the same as the kind of sexism I have experienced, as a masculine nonbinary white person. I knew those things intellectually, even knew them second hand through friends and stories and memoirs. I still didn't see the revelation coming.

Before the scene, we had talked about what it was like for her to submit to a white person and what it was like for me to be dominating a woman of color. We asked each other how it might influence the dynamic. How do real-life power differentials, particularly around these racial identities, influence and affect the practice of dominance and submission? We named the differentials between us, got some clarity and shared language around them, and tried to bring them to our awareness. It isn't a scene about race, we said, but there is an element of that present just because of who we are and what we bring to each other. Ignoring it wouldn't make it go away, so we tried to be conscious.

Years before this particular weekend, I'd studied the concept of intersectionality through a gender studies degree and in my own social justice work and interests, so I thought I understood it. I'd taught classes on dirty talk and arousal and a dozen other things. I'd worked through my internalized shame and come to claim my kink identity[2] unapologetically, and that felt so right and explained so many things about my erotic energy and desires. I'd even used these same words in other play with other women and nonbinary folks.

But when I stood over a woman of color and called her names—as we had negotiated—I felt the meaning of intersectionality in my body in a new way I never had before. In that moment, looking down into her eyes, the naughty, loaded words on the tip of my tongue, I realized that all of the women I'd dominated in previous humiliation scenes were white. I had played with and dated women of color, but my experience with these specific words had exclusively been with white women.

As she looked up at me, I felt a surge of knowing rush in through my upper back, pour its way into my body, and land inside of me. I understood something deep about the difference between her experiences living in her body and mine living in my body. I understood that bringing up sexist terms to use in an erotic context had different layers of meaning for her because of her experience as a woman of color.

I remember clearly thinking, *this doesn't mean what I think it means.*

Complicating Power

In my kink life, and outside of it, I study power in many different forms. In his speech "All Labor Has Dignity," Dr. Martin Luther King wrote, "Power is the ability to achieve purpose, power is the ability to effect change" (2011, p. 177), which is my favorite way to think about what power is and how it functions.

When we use the word *power*, we use it to mean many different things. I like to break it into three levels: personal, interpersonal, and systemic. I think of personal power as empowerment, agency, and an internal sense of power in the world; interpersonal power is between two people, though sometimes more, and is called an *authority exchange* or *power dynamics*, whether conscious or unconscious; and systemic power is the institutionalized systems that define which types of people with which kinds of bodies will benefit and which will be actively suppressed.

There is sometimes some confusion about the BDSM practice of power exchange, or power dynamics, precisely because of the multiple definitions of the word *power*. You might hear phrases like submissives *give up* power.

People can confuse this for giving up their personal empowerment, particularly because BDSM and authority exchange can also play with humiliation and degradation; and some people have the misunderstanding that submissives are unempowered and stripped of agency.

In truth, many people speak about their submission as a way they feel powerful, not powerless. In *The New Bottoming Book*, Dossie Easton writes,

> When I'm being flogged, early on I often come to a place where I need to stretch to take in the intense sensation, where I struggle and wonder if I can take it at all. That struggle seems to make me stronger and soon I feel intense energy running through me, as if all the force with which the whip is thrown at me is injected into me—becomes my energy to play with. While my tops throw the whips at me as hard as they can, I take in their power and dance in the center of the storm. (Easton & Hardy, 2001, p. 23)

I tend to call consensual, conscious, asymmetrical interpersonal relationship structures *authority exchange* rather than *power dynamics* because one person is giving authority over to the other, and the other is exercising authority. Calling it *power exchange* or a *power dynamic* can inadvertently reinforce the idea that the submissive is "giving up" power and is powerless because we use the word *power* to mean multiple things, including personal empowerment. It is a clearer way to describe the arrangement, which is more about authority than it is about power.

In addition to playing with people in kink scenes like the one with my friend above, I have been in authority exchange relationships as a dominant on and off since 2005. While kink scenes might have authority exchange within them, where one person is driving the action and the other is surrendering and submitting, relationships based on these dynamics are different; they can extend outside of bedroom play or scenes and into day-to-day life. There's a wide range of expression within the practice of consensual authority exchange relationships—some people have many areas that they are in control of and in charge of for their partner(s), and some have few. I have full and exhaustive control, authority, and ownership[3] over my submissive, who is also my partner and spouse.

I don't know exactly why authority exchange relationships work for me or why that is what I want so deeply. I do feel as though it is an orientation, that there is some program in my body which is only satisfied when I am in that dominant role. I understand how problematic hierarchies are, and I work to dismantle them in many aspects of my life on systemic levels of power. Interpersonally, I don't just want this—I need it.

Maybe it's precisely because I study systemic power and seek liberation from the many institutionalized power structures that keep marginalized people oppressed that I am fascinated by it in my personal life.

Sometimes outrage and erotic charge go hand in hand.

I spent almost 10 years playing with power in relationships before I understood the extent of the power exchange that I wanted. I wanted so much control and ownership that I thought something was wrong with me. Most of the people I knew were not doing power exchange relationships the same way I was, and I was continually hungry for more, more, more. I tried to get underneath it. I studied attachment theory and early childhood woundings. I read books on and practiced non-monogamy, particularly attempting to unlearn my own tendencies toward jealousy and possessiveness, which many theories and practices of non-monogamy actively investigate. I went to (a lot of) therapy. I went to psychology and domination/submission (D/s) retreats, workshops, and groups to learn as much as I could about power exchange and the different options. There was something I wanted—needed—to figure out inside of my desire for an authority exchange.

I quickly came to understand that relationships without authority exchange are not relationships without power dynamics.

Intersectionality and Authority Exchange

Power dynamics exist within just about every relationship, based on complex social positioning and whether someone holds privilege or is on the margins in different categories. Race, class, religion, age, ability, neurodiversity,[4] nationality—all of these and more affect the dynamics between us. A woman I dated for a while had a significantly different class background from me, and that affected the authority exchange in our relationship as people who have more money are often perceived to be more in charge and to make more decisions. It was difficult to still feel in control and dominant when her money gave her more access to effecting change and achieving purpose than I felt I had. We tried to make it conscious in our dynamic and to name it and compensate for it in other ways, but it was difficult.

Even when I look back at my more egalitarian relationships, I can see the places where one or the other of us held more systemic power or where we didn't. That had both subtle and more obvious consequences within the relationships, much of which I didn't see at the time; but as I grew to understand and embody authority exchange relationships more, it became more obvious.

Being in a conscious authority exchange relationship has made it much more obvious when power dynamics are unconscious or unnegotiated, which happens in many, many aspects of our lives, from relationships with teachers and bosses to social standings and reputation. When I went on a retreat a few years ago, I was told that the facilitator was "quirky" and liked things just so, but people made vague comments, like "you'll see," when I asked them to elaborate. I was so frustrated that people knew there were protocols and guidelines in place but would not clearly communicate them. I really appreciate the comfort, safety, and transparency of conscious authority exchange as it lays out explicitly and verbally the guidelines and protocols someone would need to be successful and respectful.

Kink communities aren't perfect. As much as they feel like safe havens when someone discovers them, and as liberating as it can be to be surrounded by sex-positive folks who are attempting to build consent practices, communication skills, and self-awareness, these spaces are in fact microcosms of the overculture.[5] They have many, many unspoken guidelines that can be difficult to navigate; and they reproduce the same sexism, racism, classism, homophobia, ableism, and many other forms of discrimination. I came into the kink community in Seattle in the early 2000s and have since lived in New York City and in San Francisco, staying heavily involved with BDSM educational organizations, learning from and contributing to the communities. There are subtle differences in different parts of the United States, and even in different club events in the same city, but many of the expectations have been consistent through all of those (similarly coastal, high-population, liberal) cities.

As I became more heavily involved in not just the kink communities but also the authority exchange subculture within it, I faced more discrimination and marginalization than I expected. While I center queer culture in my life, the authority exchange subculture is predominantly heterosexual, with the couples primarily falling into line with the gender role expectations that the man is the dominant and the woman is the submissive in their relationships. That can recreate all kinds of heteronormative, patriarchal values, which are things I generally have done my best to unlearn and from which I have separated, so I often feel marginalized within the authority exchange subculture.

It has been especially challenging to be validated as a nonbinary butch queer dominant in these communities, and at times I don't know if the cold shoulder, rejection, or outright scorn I receive is from being (misgendered and) perceived as a woman, from homophobia, from transphobia—or from simply being in the wrong place at the wrong time. But because I have multiple marginalized identities, I rarely know why I'm being dismissed or outright mistreated. This is a way that I have felt what it's like to be at the intersection of multiple marginalized identities—to be experiencing accidents in an intersection, as Crenshaw described, and not knowing which direction the cars are coming from. "Discrimination," she writes, "like traffic through an intersection, may flow in one direction, and it may flow in another. If an accident happened in an intersection, it can be caused by cars travelling from any number of directions and, sometimes, from all of them" (1989, p. 149).

While I hold marginalized gender identities, I still benefit from masculine privilege. When I have been accepted as a fellow dominant in different groups or clubs, I have heard from dominant friends who are just as skillful and experienced, but who present much more feminine than I do, that they never felt comfortable or accepted in that space. My masculine privilege does occasionally allot me privileges of acceptance in dominant spaces, which are primarily filled with cisgender men.

I do continue to find acceptance in queer-focused or -specific kink spaces, and I have seen the presence of nonbinary and trans folks in the kink community grow in the 20 years I've been involved. I still am frequently misgendered in the kink community, and many people do not use my pronouns (they, them, theirs, themself) accurately or consistently. I continue to offer resources and education on trans and nonbinary issues with the hope that kink communities will continue evolving their gender knowledge. While I am visible in and feel respected by queer, trans, and nonbinary communities because I am seen and validated in my gender, I am not seen for my identity as a dominant in those spaces; and it still feels harder to seek kink acceptance from non-kink folks than it does to seek gender acceptance from kinky folks. Folks in the queer and trans communities understand my gender but not my relationship dynamics, while folks in the D/s community constantly misgender me but understand my relationship orientation. Sometimes it seems as though I can either be validated as a nonbinary queer or be validated as kinky dominant, but not both at the same time. These identities are not in opposition to each other, and indeed I can and do occupy multiple marginalized identities at once; but they are rarely seen or validated as an intersectional whole.

Embodied Intersectionality Through Kink

It's been many years now since that scene with my submissive friend and my flash of embodied insight about intersectionality through kink, D/s, and humiliation. We remain friends, and we still talk about that scene occasionally. For her, it was a powerful reclaiming of terms that had been used against her, non-consensually, for decades. But in that situation, she had control. She knew she could stop me at any time, for any reason. Plus, it was sexy. She told me, later, that her orgasms that weekend were very powerful; but beyond just the pleasure, she shared that she didn't have the same kind of charge with those terms when they came up in her life as they had before. She had knocked some of the power out of them.

For me, it was in service to her, and it was incredibly sexy, and it was also a lesson in humility. Though I was confident in my intellectual knowledge, feeling the insight in my body as the power and energy of the scene built and released in me gave me an embodied knowledge I hadn't had before. That sense of knowing in my body, not just in my mind, changed the way I interact in BDSM scenes when there are differences in the privilege and margins that we occupy—and there are almost always differences. I am more careful to mention those differences as part of the negotiations, and I am more aware of checking in about it and ensuring that we both feel grounded in our own personal empowerment in our aftercare. I want to ensure that we are making these real-life power differentials conscious, as much as possible, so that they do not accidentally come out sideways in a scene. And if they do, somehow, accidentally, I want to be accountable, take responsibility, and hopefully resolve it.

I had been confident in my intellectual understanding of intersectionality and, being at the intersection of identities myself, I thought I understood how intersectionality worked, even in my own body. But in that scene I could feel the differences between us, the ways that certain terms were more loaded for her because of her skin and race than they are for me. It isn't inherently good or bad that certain terms are more loaded—it just is. And, in fact, it's useful to have the added fuel that comes from loaded terms during a kink scene; but it is difficult to actually use the fuel to alchemize the experience, body sensation, and connection into transformation if we aren't somewhat aware of what we're doing. Otherwise, the real-life power differentials between us could create awkward static that could muddle the energy we are building and releasing.

Currently, I've been in an authority exchange relationship for more than 10 years, and it is wildly fulfilling. Something in me that was never before satisfied has curled up on the rug and is napping peacefully, no longer circling to find comfort and meaning. Power, control, and authority of all kinds continue to fascinate me personally, politically, and erotically. I crave the deep insights that can come from the friction of the dance of dominance and submission, of power and surrender; and I want to continue to use the knowledge for empowerment and liberation for myself—and for all of us.

Notes

1. This friend is a fictionalized amalgamated character of multiple scenes with multiple people. All identifying details have been changed to keep them anonymous.
2. See https://sugarbutch.net/2012/06/feminist-butch-top/, where I grapple with feminist values as applied to kink.
3. "Ownership" is often seen as negative in relationships, but as a part of authority exchange dynamics, it can be consensual and desired.
4. *Neurodiversity* is the idea that brain differences are normal, rather than deficits. Judy Singer, an Australian sociologist on the autism spectrum, used the term in the late 1990s in her thesis and was widely noted when her article "Why Can't You Be Normal for Once in Your Life?" was published in the United Kingdom in 1999 in the book *Disability Discourse*, edited by Mairian Corker and Sally French. Neurodiversity often describes attention-deficit hyperactivity disorder, autism spectrum disorder, dyslexia, dyspraxia, and others. If one is not neurodivergent, one is neurotypical.
5. *Overculture* is the dominant culture, including traditions, customs, and biases normally followed in public spaces. If one is not in the overculture, one is in a subculture, multiple subcultures, or a counterculture.

References

Crenshaw, K. (1989). Demarginalizing the intersection of race and sex: A Black feminist critique of antidiscrimination doctrine, feminist theory and antiracist politics. *University of Chicago Legal Forum*, 1(8), 139–167.

Easton, D., & Hardy, J. W. (2001). *The new bottoming book*. Greenery Press.

King, M. L., Jr. (2011). *All labor has dignity* (M. K. Honey, Ed.). Beacon Press.

Singer, J. (1999). "Why can't you be normal for once in your life?" From a "problem with no name" to the emergence of a new category of difference. In M. Corker & S. French (Eds.), *Disability discourse* (pp. 59–67). Open University Press.

PART V

ETHICS AND CONSENT IN THE SCENE AND IN BDSM STUDIES

12

The Politics of BDSM Play

Racial Dynamics and Critical Consent

Amber R. Norman

Introduction

In the formative years of the United States, the institution of a labor system based on skin color transformed the lives of Black, Indigenous, and people of color (BIPOC) living in North America. Racial slavery became a pervasive system of classification relating to power, privilege, and differences in social hierarchy (Bogues, 2012). Explicit boundaries were implemented and enforced through fugitive laws, designating ownership over Black bodies by whites, establishing police and surveillance practices, and using punitive action toward individuals who resisted the social order. The application of property laws to enslave Africans allowed white Americans to own, sell, and buy Black men and women, while disabling their ability to withdraw unilaterally from such an arrangement. As property, enslaved men's and women's reproductive labor was valued for its economic benefit. And without rights to parenthood or autonomy over their sexuality, enslaved Africans were systematically robbed of their humanity and societal worth (Nittle, 2019).

Beyond the legal emancipation of enslaved people in North America, activists in the modern era continue to fight systemic racism across the United States. The concept of liberation for Black people in America, however, begins with an explicit recognition of the impact of racial slavery on present-day power structures, relationships, and identity. In her text *Killing Rage*, bell hooks (1995) resists the notion that individuals can forsake attachment to race or cultural identity and exist as "just humans" within power systems. As individual bodies are embedded within social systems, BIPOC individuals cannot conceptualize themselves without consideration for the structures that influence their behaviors. Therefore, systemic oppression such

Amber R. Norman, *The Politics of BDSM Play* In: *The Power of BDSM.* Edited by: Brandy L. Simula, Robin Bauer, and Liam Wignall, Oxford University Press. © Oxford University Press 2023. DOI: 10.1093/oso/9780197658598.003.0013 as racism, sexism, ageism, homophobia, fatphobia, and other marginalizing structures live within and cannot be separated from personal interactions and relationships. Historically and socially, racial and sexual minorities have experienced systemic regulations on their bodies, and these realities must be considered in BDSM play spaces.

BDSM and the Black Community

In her work *Uses of the Erotic*, Audre Lorde (1978) argues that the historic sexual exploitation of Black bodies has contributed to the suppression of Black sexuality, creating a disconnect between the erotic and personal fulfillment. Rather than considering sexuality as a source of power, Black Americans are often discouraged from exploring their bodies and defining pleasurable experiences in order to subvert enduring stereotypes of hypersexuality and racial fetishism. Under colonialism, African cultures were seen as primitive in comparison to Western cultures. In *Black Sexual Politics*, Patricia Hill Collins (2004) notes how white Europeans were able to justify the exploitation and subjugation of Africans by establishing their cultural values as normal while deeming African culture as abnormal. Black physiology was also labeled deviant and animalistic, in part because of West African agriculture and people's proximity to wildlife. From a white colonialist perspective, killing, caging, or objectifying Black people seemed reasonable as they were not considered fully human. Akin to wildlife, Black people were believed to be inherently violent, uncivilized people who required taming. The use of Black bodies for breeding and regenerative labor colored white Europeans' image of Africans as hypersexual deviants, further justifying their sexual objectification. For example, in the 1800s, Saartjie (Sarah) Baartman, a South African slave, was sent to London to be exhibited as part of a "freak show." She was displayed in a cage where onlookers paid to touch her large buttocks and gawk at her physiology. In America, the subhuman status of Black people was eventually formalized in Article 1, Section 2 of the 1787 US Constitution, qualifying enslaved Africans as three-fifths of a person (Anderson et al., 2018).

In modern US culture, enduring racial stereotypes fuel the perception of Black women and men as savage and hypersexual, making Black people vulnerable to ongoing sexual debasement and fetishization (Holmes, 2016). Anti-Black imagery in cinema and television portrays Black women as innately promiscuous compared to the controlled, respectful, and modest depictions of white women. Meanwhile, Black men are often stereotyped to have unusually large penises with hypermasculine features of untamed aggression, portraying them as violent, sex-crazed criminals (Hutchinson, 1997). In pornography, Black men are often featured for their anatomy with labels such as *Big Black Cock*, or *BBC*, a reference to breeding qualities promoted during slave auction blocks. Similarly, Black women with exaggerated physical features are promoted to reinforce a narrative of child-bearing and promiscuity and to fan the enduring obsession with the Black aesthetic. Racial fetishism, or the preoccupation of cultural and/or racial characteristics, particularly for Black people, is rooted in the exploitative breeding patterns of enslaved Africans and maintained through colonial imperialist ideologies embedded in Western social systems (Collins, 2004). Likewise, the ideology of Black inferiority further regulates gender embodiment and sexual expression of racialized bodies through implicit and explicit social messaging. To some degree, the hypersexual myths of Black men and women have been retained in the media as cultural norms, impeding the ability of Black people to exercise agency over their sexual expression (DeFrancisco & Palczewski, 2007; Doss, 2013; Meyer, 2003).

Although anti-Black imagery is prominent in global mass media, Black feminists argue that the reappropriation of Black imagery is empowering and necessary to resist subjugation. Through the medium of hip-hop, for example, African American artists have reclaimed their assertiveness through words like *bitch*, *savage*, *freak*, and *ho*, historically disapproving terms used to reduce Black women to sexual objects (Collins, 2004). Similarly, Black-owned adult production company Royal Fetish Films is challenging the adult film industry by creating inclusive, ethical, and safe spaces for BIPOC performers (Song, 2020). The condition of sexual liberation, however, can only be facilitated under the conditions of cultural awareness. Through an acknowledgment that Black people have a complicated relationship with their bodies due to white colonialism and through conscious engagement with one's body, Black people may deliberately generate more love, pleasure, agency, and personal power within social interactions (Lorde, 1978). Cruz (2016) furthers advocates for the reclamation of body autonomy, noting that as power dynamics materialize in social interactions, seeking opportunities to push and play with boundaries is a way for people of color to practice transgressing oppressive systems. Through an awareness of one's capacity for feeling and bonding, BIPOC individuals may use BDSM as a stage for reclamation and further identify other areas of their life where a similar fulfillment can be achieved.

Following the release of the film *Fifty Shades of Grey*, Luna Malbroux (2016) confronted the notion of Black people's participation in BDSM in a blog post entitled "When You Want to Be into BDSM, but It's Too Soon Because You're Black." Although the column mentions the presence of BDSM in traditional African culture and the early Black leather scene post–World War II, Malbroux contends with a popular assumption that BDSM is inaccessible to Black people because of historical oppression and marginal social status. BDSM practice can appear counterintuitive when Hollywood depictions of subjugation in films such as *Roots, Amistad, Birth of a Nation*, and *Twelve Years a Slave* expose Black people to images of enslaved persons being held captive and assaulted by their white masters. Some activities popular in BDSM practice such as restraining body parts, using whips for impact, or obeying verbal directives may feel antithetical to Black people. In his theory of race-based traumatic stress, Robert T. Carter (2007) concludes that experiences of race-based discrimination, including present-day violence against Black people, result in mental injuries or sensitivities that challenge the notion of safety within interracial interactions. Kobi Kambon (2012) described how the crack of a single-tail whip, a popular implement in BDSM, can conjure generational reactivity stored in the memory systems of Black bodies. As braided leather whips were a regular implement used to punish and terrorize Africans into submission, cultural and contextual considerations must be taken into account prior to using this tool with—or in the presence of—Black Americans in particular. Malbroux (2016) further notes that the presence of oppressive imagery and memories may interfere with fantasy role play. For example, a Black person may find it difficult to participate in a police–civilian role play as they concurrently work to process the deaths of George Floyd, Eric Garner, Sandra Bland, and other victims of police brutality. Even so, a similar scenario in which a Black person chooses their role, actions, and outcomes may find a police–civilian role play empowering and reparative.

The ethics of BDSM practice identify consent, context, and mutuality as necessary features of informed play, distinguishing power-exchange practices in BDSM from actual violence or coercion (Weinberg, 2006). In theory, BDSM activities are situated rather than generalized and carried out under a shared, bilateral agreement between all persons involved in a scene or relational dynamic. However, marginal social status (i.e., race, gender, sexual identity) often undermines personal agency, resulting in limited choices that may impact one's sense of safety in the relationship or ability to provide meaningful consent within unequal power dynamics (Bauer, 2014). Historic narratives and racial privilege, driven by social imbalances between white and Black people, present an inherent contextual barrier to mutuality. In BDSM play, racial inequity can influence one's ability to make decisions about which roles to play and who to play with, creating a discernible gap in negotiation protocol. For racial and sexual minorities with limited social power, communicating needs about boundaries within the power-laden practice of BDSM can be complicated and hazardous. Little analytic attention has been given to how cultural context shapes interactional identities, power dynamics, and embodied meaning within BDSM cultural networks, particularly as it relates to Black practitioners. The inclusion of Black practitioners in BDSM discourse is necessary to further examine the compounding effect of social systems, such as race, on BDSM practice.

Methods

The following study explored how Black practitioners enact roles, regulate boundaries, and preserve their agency in BDSM practice. The narratives of 13 Black BDSM practitioners were examined to gain insight into their lived experiences as they relate to kink, racial identity, partner selection, negotiation, decision-making, and racial fetishism play. Primary recruitment for this study took place at the 2019 Sex Down South Conference held in Atlanta, Georgia. The city of Atlanta is the second largest majority Black metropolitan area in the United States and boasts the second highest LGBTQ percentage in the southern United States. The Sex Down South Conference, cofounded by Marla Renee Stewart and Tia Marie Mosley, is a space designed for sex educators, mental health counselors, professional kinksters, and sexual enthusiasts. With an emphasis on Black sexuality and centering marginalized voices, the conference was an ideal site to learn more about the Black BDSM community. The conference consists of interactive educational sessions, BDSM demonstrations, after-hour shows, and a play space.

Participants

Black BDSM practitioners were recruited for this study using a set of criteria based on their self-reported identities. Estimates of individuals who practice

BDSM are varied, and even more ambiguous is the available data on non-white BDSM practitioners. Langdridge and Butt (2004) assert that all sexual practices involve power; thus, distinction between BDSM and non-BDSM can be difficult. Furthermore, the implicit or explicit recognition of power differentials in erotic interactions is relative to the participants. To be included in the research sample, participants had to self-identify as Black or African American, criteria that reinforced the single racial focus of the study. Next, participants self-reported that they have engaged in BDSM practice for at least 12 months. Also, participants self-identified with a power role such as *dominant, top, submissive,* or *switch.* Roles within BDSM interactions are variable; a person can identify as a top in one scene and a submissive in a different scene; however, a power position is chosen for each respective scene. The designation of a participant's role identity along the dominant–submissive continuum was used as a criterion for indicating BDSM affiliation. Lastly, participants were given the opportunity to name themselves by choosing their own aliases.

Individuals who expressed interest and met the inclusion criteria were contacted privately and provided information about the research study. Thirteen participants were selected and provided informed consent, detailing the purpose and description of the research study as approved by the University of Central Florida Institutional Review Board. An outline of the data collection procedures was presented along with an expressed intention to contribute an affirming narrative of Black BDSM practitioners. Furthermore, my positionality as both a Black queer cisgender woman and a licensed psychotherapist was important to share with participants as the mental health community continues to debate the social and psychological acceptability of BDSM practice. Prospective participants were informed of the risks and benefits of participation, including their unconditional right to withdraw from the research study at any time, without penalty. As means of safeguarding their identity from the public or institutional colleagues, participants were encouraged to select a separate name from their BDSM stage names. In BDSM, practitioners often use stage names or aliases instead of their legal identities to reflect their unique positionality and communal affiliation. Some of the participants requested that their BDSM stage names be used in order to retain agency over their experiences. Prior to data collection, I confirmed with all participants that the name provided was how they wanted to be referenced in data collection and data reporting, including the publication of results; each participant affirmed their choice.

All 13 participants in this research study self-identified as Black or African American, self-reported active engagement in BDSM practice within the prior 12 months, and self-identified with a power role such as *dominant, top, submissive,* or *switch.* All participants were 18 years of age or older and ranged in experience from 2 to 19 years of BDSM practice. Eight identified a professional aspect to their practice including sex educator, performer, or sex worker. Using their own words, participants were asked to describe their gender and sexual identity. Five participants identified as cisgender man or woman, while the remaining eight identified as non-binary, femme, womyn, womxn, or boi. Regarding sexual identity, 12 participants identified as queer, pansexual, lesbian, or bisexual; and one participant identified as heterosexual.

Interviews were conducted with each participant to learn more about the subjective experiences of Black BDSM practitioners. Of the 13 participants, two practitioners were interviewed as a couple. All other interviews were conducted individually, lasting between 50 and 150 minutes. The semi-structured format of the interview presented lead questions covering topical domains such as power roles, partner selection, and negotiation, followed by probes or questions that allowed for more specific disclosure. For example, one lead question related to negotiation was "Who do you play with in BDSM scenes?" and a secondary question was "How are decisions made?" The interviews were audio-recorded, and the data was organized into four categories aligned with Erving Goffman's (1959) dramaturgical framework. To some degree, we are all "in character," playing out different roles as autonomous individuals, yet deeply influenced by language and symbols used to communicate meaning within social interactions. Goffman posits that we are all performing concurrent, often overlapping, roles according to various identity markers (i.e., age, gender, race, occupation status, etc.), the context or situations we find ourselves in, and the social structures that delineate normative expectations of behavior. As roles are intersectional, Goffman notes that all social interactions include cultural, structural, political, and dramaturgical characteristics. As such, role-taking and performative actions in BDSM play take on contextual and reflexive meanings when converged with race, gender, and sexual identity (Norman, 2020). Within Goffman's social domains, nine themes emerged to synthesize the experiences of Black BDSM practitioners. Three themes specifically, role enactment, racial fetishism, and negotiation, highlight how racial identity engages with power dynamics in BDSM practice.

Results

Role Enactment

During each interview, Black practitioners were asked to share the power roles they assume during BDSM interactions. The role-play experience in BDSM presents an opportunity to explore and push boundaries, and some practitioners shared that BDSM helps them express and/or reconcile parts of themselves deemed otherwise flawed. When asked about her entry into BDSM, Evanye, a 35-year-old queer switch, described BDSM practice as "an awakening within my sexual self" and emphasized the importance of having a practice that makes her feel comfortable expressing all parts of herself without judgment. Similarly, Trey, a 31-year-old queer dominant, describes BDSM as an opportunity to embody the fullness of his identity:

> I recognize that I got pleasure from being perceived as very sweet and very innocent in some settings, but very controlling and dominant in others. [Kink] allows me to live out my full spectrum of expression. For me, it created this duality. Kind of like drag. So, having that space to be able to take my drag off and on. One, it's been really pleasurable. But two, it's also been very comforting, in the sense of being able to express everything I need to express, that I may not be able to express in other spaces.

Generally, Davita, a 28-year-old bisexual switch, describes herself as "very independent." She holds a corporate job that requires pragmatism and analytic strengths but disclosed how BDSM provides a space to practice submission in a liberating and intellectual way:

> For me, submission and BDSM is about allowing myself to release control. It's very stimulating. So, when he is [biting and spanking] me, I feel energy there. And if there is trauma there, I ask myself, "What is this trauma associated with?" I'm not just getting my ass beat. I'm processing my life and processing our relationship. It activates my intellectual side as well, and that turns me on. To me, it's a very holistic experience.

Black BDSM practitioners place value in the ability to embrace and engage themselves in both dominant and submissive dynamics of BDSM play. For some, the transgressive nature of the practice allows them to push the boundaries of their erotic expression which previously felt repressed. For others, BDSM presents a container to counter the power structures they live and/or work in daily. Still, how one plays is contingent on the positionality one assumes within the interaction. For Black practitioners, deciding the role they embody has much to do with how they have been socialized to view and feel about themselves. BlakSyn, a 31-year-old non-binary top, discussed how gendered expectations related to power roles can create a conflict between social norms and personal choice:

> I used to identify as a cis man. My masculinity dictated it to me. "Oh, I'm dominant. I'm the man. I should be dominant." I saw it depicted in media—when I was watching porn. All I ever saw was men topping. Then, after changing my gender identity [to non-binary], and coming to terms with my orientation, you get a feel for the world around you. You get a feel for the individuals that also participate in this with you. And then you start learning about some of the deeper aspects of kink, and how it can intersect with so many parts of us in our very human experiences. Last year, I began to identify as a "top." It gives me the greatest amount of malleability to call on the different energies that are suited for what I've negotiated with another human being. I identify as a top because that's the position I take. I'm able to call on dominance. I'm able to call on sadism. I'm able to call on humiliation. I'm able to call on discipline, and so many other aspects of kink, as well. Being a top gives me that malleability, both in name and in action.

BlakSyn describes feeling limited in their understanding of dominance when it was solely tied to being a man. Western culture reinforces that a person must be limited to one identity, often assigned by a power structure, or risk being "the other." BlakSyn reports that a more expansive understanding of themselves was embodied when they chose a non-binary identity, giving themselves permission to access the depths of their expression without social boundaries dictating where a man ends and begins. Furthermore, BlakSyn helps us see how roles, such as dominant, can be narrowly defined and symbolic of the limitations communicated through social interactions and cultural conditioning. It appears that relational roles in BDSM account for varied dimensions of one's personality and desired expression, providing practitioners the ability to feel fuller and more authentic in their interactions with others.

All practitioners in this study agreed that BDSM is a useful platform for trying on roles, practicing intimacy, and expressing boundaries. However, some questioned how structurally accessible BDSM is for Black people to explore. Role enactments for Black practitioners of BDSM are not as simple as picking a character and negotiating the details of a scene. Rather, gender and racial narratives influence what roles Black practitioners choose to assume. Beyond that, one must also consider the consequences of embodying certain roles, particularly the submissive stance. The marginal status of Black people, which comes with its own set of vulnerabilities, makes choosing a power role a risk-taking experience on its own. Toya, a 35-year-old non-binary dominant, shared their frustration with masculine expectations based on their stature and appearance:

> There's a lot that comes with being in my body. I get a lot of masculinity attributed to me. I think just being fat and Black and not light-skinned . . . it comes with its own shit. People gatekeep femininity. People gatekeep softness. People gatekeep what it means to be Fem-identifying and/or a woman based on that person's appearance. Growing up, I had my femininity held out of reach by such gatekeepers. My softness—which does exist, held out of reach. It irked me that people just made so many assumptions about me based on how I look. I often question my identity in BDSM, in sexuality, and in relationships. I am an outspoken person, forward thinking. But how much of that was molded by me being thrust into this category just based off how I look? I have an issue with the fact that most people leave no room for me to explore my submissive side. And even if I do look for more masculine-centered [partners], I still get an automatic, "Oh you're dominant, you run the show." It makes me question my identity a lot. How much of this is me just falling into character?

Toya communicated the tragedy of not being able to qualify or name their femininity because their body disqualified them in the normative eyes of others. They also describe how they assumed masculine behaviors to better comply with a Western ideology that says large bodies are less feminine. The gatekeeping of femininity, or the socially imposed criteria of who gets to be seen as feminine or a woman, creates an enduring dilemma for Toya. When a person is relegated—against their will—as "the other," they are invariably denied access to the modes of expression that feel right to them. This leads Toya to question the validity of their identities as authentic or socially imposed.

In her interview, Jet Setting Jasmine™ emphasized how the inflation of masculine and feminine stereotypes has contributed to the misuse of Black bodies and the crippling of healthy sexual expression. More specifically, she asserts that the hypermasculinity programmed and/or stereotyped to Black masculine-presenting people has made submissive practices such as listening or being receptive nearly inaccessible—not because they don't want to try things associated with a submissive stance but because the aggressive stereotypes attached to Black men and their sexuality may result in shame and psychological wounding if they choose to depart from that character. BlakSyn shared a similar sentiment regarding Black cisgender men in BDSM:

> You don't see a lot of Black male submissives. You don't. It's not a thing. And when I do see Dominants in the Black community, they are this caricature of hyper-masculinity. "I'm the man. And I've got to do the thing." That was me back when I was a youngster and believing those same exact things. The exploration of sexuality amongst Black folks is stunted, for whatever reason.

Cultural norms and stereotypes may challenge the notion of consensual role enactment for Black BDSM practitioners. Black people must ask themselves how much of their role has been impressed upon them, at what cost, and to what degree dominant and/or submissive embodiments, in any way, threaten their Blackness.

Racial Fetishism

Prior to engaging in power play, it is essential that BDSM practitioners have an awareness of the embedded nature of whiteness and racial supremacy in everyday discourse and interactions. Historically, white people have managed the majority of the BDSM community, establishing protocols that align with their needs and expectations. And while shared language and interpretation are necessary, it would be unfair to ask racial minorities with limited social power to adopt frameworks that inadvertently keep them subjugated.

When asked to elaborate on Black people's accessibly to kink spaces, BlakSyn asserted the following:

> Black people have a history of experiencing gatekeeping at the hands of white people. And when you spend so long looking at media that does not reflect your experiences, then you're more inclined to believe [BDSM] is not something for you.

The mechanics of BDSM thus cannot be realized or beneficial if the players act from a lens of cultural superiority or exclusivity. European imperialism set a standard of predominance, mastery, and control over resources, information, and standards of appropriateness. Western values of dichotomy, competition, separateness, independence, and individuality in cooperation with the categorization and valuation of people and objects lead to continued stratification of racial groups and discriminatory behavior (Kambon, 2012). The classification of European ideology as superior in comparison to the perceived savagery of other ethnic groups cannot be overstated. For example, a history of colonialism has taught white people to take up space; meanwhile, Black people are expected to "know their place" or assume a subjugated position. The means and context of power play must be understood from a political lens that recognizes the consequences of racial dominance, including systems that profit directly from the exploitation of Black bodies. Thus, racial dichotomies and subsequent marginalization must be discerned as inherent fragilities within the strength and safety of the BDSM container. In the absence of boundaries rooted in racial consciousness, Black practitioners become vulnerable to racial fetishism and exploitation.

Analogous to "age play" in BDSM contexts, race may be one of the most unspoken power dynamics to explore yet one of the easiest to exploit. The sensitivity of racial dynamics arouses both contention and confession, creating a need for shame to be confronted and avowed. In her work *The Color of Kink*, Ariane Cruz (2016) refers to the consensual eroticism of race as "the dark side of desire." Race play, as an inherently grotesque practice, challenges the participants and witnesses to confront racial stereotypes from a complicated stance of historical discomfort and "unspeakable pleasure." The controversial nature of racial subordination and domination in BDSM play, however, lies in the disagreement of its intention and generated outcomes. Black BDSM practitioners interviewed in this study discussed how differences in objectives around fetishism can result in malignant harm. Trey shared the following:

> When I'm playing with non-Black folks, especially white folks, I have those conversations [about race]. I'm very mindful that I can be having a certain fantasy and they can be having another fantasy. The history of fetishizing Black men, stereotypes like Black thugs or big black cock (BBC), stuff like that is very unnerving. And, to me, it is a form of violence. An experience happened to me recently, where I was talking to somebody who said they were into the thugs . . . they like the "thug personality." I was very much weirded out by that point because I'm like, "You're just really talking about a bunch of stereotypes that I'm not feeling." And they continued with sharing how in the past they called Black guys "colored boy." At this point, I was like, "I'm going to end this conversation right here. I want to end this conversation right here." They got pissed off, and then they started calling me a nigger.

Trey experienced a literal progression of implicit bias to explicit racism while negotiating BDSM play with a white man. He acknowledges a sensitivity to racial stereotypes that objectify Black bodies and verbally expressed his disapproval. In this case, when Trey set a boundary, the white person became offended, leading to an explosive projection of his racist attitudes. Encountering implicit or explicit bias generates anxiety and weakens agreement within a relational dynamic. For example, after being called the n-word, Trey labeled that person dangerous and someone who may cause him harm; when a white person calls a Black people the n-word, it is meant to degrade. It is not meant to empower. Thus, it is more difficult for a disempowered person to decide of their own volition. When decision-making power is diminished, a person becomes more vulnerable to exploitation.

Consensual role enactments, such as fetishism, are challenged when Black practitioners encounter racist attitudes or the sexual debasement of their bodies in BDSM spaces. Many practitioners interviewed discussed how the hypersexualization of Black bodies and racial stereotypes create a unique vulnerability when navigating BDSM power structures. In order to minimize the risk of exploitation, they must assess for racial bias in an already layered negotiation process. Beyond race play itself, some argue that BDSM in the Black community is counterintuitive to subverting systems of dominance that perpetuate social inequity. When asked about transactional race-based play, Toya likened their work with interracial partners as a form of reparations:

> Mentally it's hard to wrap my mind around paid domination for Black people. You know what I'm saying? I was out here to beat on white boys. They loved it. They ate that shit up. But the resentment was real for me; that came from my core. I'm not a Mistress unless you're a white man. My level of domination depends on who you are. I know there are some Black people who enjoy humiliation, but I'm not the Mistress for you.

Toya expresses that past and present racial inequities play a role in how they choose who to work with in BDSM spaces. They use the power-laden platform of BDSM to take back or recuperate personal agency which historically has been inaccessible to them. In the United States, federal reparations have never been issued to African Americans whose family members were slaves, so it's reasonable for Toya to demand time, space, and resources from white men as an attempt to recuperate their stolen identity. Cruz (2016) mentions that it is often unclear if participation in race-based play is meant to reproduce or subvert racial stereotypes. However, she argues that either or both outcomes can be pleasurable in their own right. Jet Setting Jasmine™ summarized the explicit and implicit struggle Black practitioners contemplate when considering the embodiment of submission in power play:

> Our community, our bodies have not been our own for as long as we've been on this continent. Our bodies are still fetishized. Our bodies are stereotyped to the point that it's dangerous for us. Our bodies are mimicked. They are appropriated. The power dynamic that happens in BDSM—giving, relinquishing power—is a really big thing, when you live in a world that has set you up to be powerless. So, when we are in these spaces for pleasure, and we're considering giving up power, we don't just ask ourselves, "Should I let this person?" We go through generations of, "Is this okay?"

Negotiation

Historical trauma connected to dominance and violence creates a sensitivity to power that situates the experiences of marginalized people as distinct, communal, and contentious (Haraway, 1989). The participants in this study shared a keen awareness of their racial identity in BDSM spaces, as Shakti Bliss outlined, "When I step into a dungeon, I don't get to *not* be Black. I'm Black wherever I go, and that is something I deal with in every space that I navigate." The color-coded system of racial hierarchy is embedded in all human interactions. To downplay or ignore a quality such as race would require the erasure of historical context critical to the makeup of humanity—an act of denial that could render relational consent incomplete or void (Bauer, 2014; Bloomer, 2019). Sentiments such as, "I don't see color, I see the person" are a gross disregard for the complexity of racialized power that we all move through. Furthermore, so-called color blindness overlooks the role of European colonialism in racial oppression and the ongoing posturing of racial privilege.

Even with thorough preparation, practitioners in this study disclosed that at times they may encounter unexpected responses or outcomes during play. It is possible to consent to an activity (e.g., spanking); however, the sensation caused by the activity (e.g., the physical contact or sound of being spanked) can result in an unpleasant memory or cause a negative reaction. Black practitioners shared that prompt and compassionate responses help minimize the dramatic and lasting impact of triggers. But in some cases, practitioners shared that a trigger can be activated by the context of the environment rather than the sensation itself. Shakti Bliss recalls a jarring experience with a white dominant:

> I kind of played around a little bit with whips, but not enough to know a lot about my own self-awareness around them. So, I wanted to try getting whipped. I think I got two lashes before I was like, "Oh, this is making me uncomfortable because you're a white dude whipping me in the middle of a dungeon in Florida." There was a lot that then came into my brain. I was in that blissed out removed space that kink gets to put us in, right? That's why we all love it, because we get to play a character and we get to feel outside of ourselves. And it was just a quick moment of me being like, "Oh, I'm not even uncomfortable with the pain. I'm not even worried about how this is going to feel. I feel awkward because you are an older white dude whipping me, a Black girl, in the middle of a fucking dungeon full of white people. And that is not going to happen today."

Syre, a 29-year-old queer domme, shared a similar experience of physical reactivity during a scene with a white partner:

The first time I was suspended, a white man suspended me. And for like the rest of the month my head hurt—my body hurt. It took a lot of reflection, and a lot of clearing to be like, "I can't take that energy." I don't feel like a lot of white people in these kink spaces are cognizant of that. If I don't feel safe, I'm not going to be able to open myself up to explore.

For these BDSM practitioners, triggers were experienced sensationally and symbolically.

Racism, or the conditional belief of racial supremacy, is often considered an open wound of American culture, which persists in its failure to face the reality of its brutal history (Riley, 2018). Thus, the denial of racial identity as historically significant serves only as a protective device for the oppressor, creating distance between deeply rooted shame and indignation. Furthermore, compartmentalizing race is akin to minimizing the role of other identity features such as age, gender, or ability. Black BDSM practitioners in this study emphasized the importance of accounting for all identity markers, including race, to minimize blind spots and enhance emotional safety. As a person-centered practice, BDSM requires the thoughtful consideration of the entire person as part of ethical scene negotiation. Critical consent, therefore, begins with the explicit recognition that race plays a role in the relational dynamic itself, not necessarily as a problem but as a reality (Bauer, 2014).

Central to Goffman's theory of impression management is understanding how individuals regulate and preserve agency within any social interaction (Goffman, 1963). The interplay of dominance and submission acts as a conscious and unconscious communicative device used to defend and maintain power positionality. From a pragmatic stance, impression management is not necessarily problematic as it can be useful in establishing protocol and maintaining boundaries in power relationships. However, holding a fixed perspective (i.e., racial superiority) may contribute to stigmatizing individuals and groups in order to uphold a power position. This subconscious practice of regulating and reinforcing the status quo can lead to marginalized people feeling inherently disempowered in social relationships. As stated previously, the oppressor often reinforces a position of dominance through the denial of his subjugate. And the prejudicial perspective of white superiority could deny racial minorities access to their own relational power (Lenhardt, 2004).

The concept of consent can be generalized as the practice of giving permission or expressing agreement; however, the application of this idea in social interactions is layered and complex (Bloomer, 2019). As a marginalized group, Black people are often asked to do things or engage in interactions they don't necessarily consent to or want to participate in. For example, marginalized people are targets of microaggressions or subtle, hostile indignities that occur in everyday settings (Sue et al., 2007). Meanwhile, state-sanctioned violence makes minorities vulnerable to being overpoliced, discriminated against, exploited, verbally and physically assaulted, and defenseless in death (Pulido, 2017). Furthermore, continuous exposure to race-based violence is related to minority stress and traumatic responses (Polanco-Roman et al., 2016). Thus, the consequences of holding minority status persist throughout various social contexts. From a dramaturgical perspective, skin color is a fixed part of our daily costuming that accompanies us wherever we go and dictates how others interact with us (Tyler, 2018). Considering the social stigmas and disparities experienced while having Black skin, is it reasonable to assume that the experience of being Black may interfere with one's ability to generate power or preserve agency within social interactions?

Conclusion

Black BDSM practitioners in this study shared how their racial and gender identity most often dictated their power roles, partner selection, the dynamics of negotiation, and perceived safety within the physical spaces of BDSM. Some practitioners clarified that, whereas BDSM helps them access multiple dimensions of themselves, they are not always keen to playing with white people in BDSM spaces. Cruz (2016) postulates that because Black people's history of racialized violence has been perpetual in many ways, consent can become more complicated when negotiating dynamics of dominance and submission. However, she asserts that when Black people recognize the power of consent, not only is consent possible but it can also be pleasurable and satisfying. The conscious and deliberate centering of racial identity in power relationships and BDSM protocol can enhance trust and relational bonding.

Jet Setting Jasmine and Marla Stewart have ascended as cultural leaders for the Black BDSM community. They design culturally sensitive BDSM spaces intended to neutralize power dynamics and provide a safe space for Black people who want to learn more about BDSM practice. The most distinguishing feature of their play spaces is that they do not host BDSM events in traditional dungeon spaces. Other participants who identify as BDSM educators echoed a similar approach, hosting BDSM events and workshops for people of color in housing collectives, private homes, basements, swingers' clubs, art galleries, bookstores, and specialized conferences such as Sex Down South. Jet Setting Jasmine asserts that BDSM spaces founded on limited knowledge of people of color put the safety and comfort of Black practitioners at risk:

> Safety is paramount. Like if you and I are having a play session, or a group of us are having a play session, we always talk about physical safety, psychological safety, and emotional safety. This is not just a physical exchange. It's an energetic exchange. It's an emotional exchange. [In BDSM] you experience changes in your body chemistry. You may feel something that you didn't feel before. We must take extra time to warm people up emotionally to a space. We must account for that. We can't just walk in and get to beating on folk.

Jet Setting Jasmine affirms that an approach to BDSM informed by racial trauma will lead to enhanced safety and quality of care between practitioners. She advocates for Black people to have ample space to become familiar with their bodies and their emotional needs. She further implies that individuals who engage in power play without consideration for race-based traumatic stress and its impact on the mind and body demonstrate a flagrant disregard for personhood.

From a mental health perspective, the physical, energetic, and emotional elements of BDSM are necessary to assist Black people in acknowledging their complexities, reclaiming their bodies, and preserving agency. The reclamation enhances decision-making powers, allowing Black people to feel secure in exploring their sexualities. Furthermore, the potential for somatic and relational bonding through culturally responsive BDSM can position marginalized people to make decisions that align with their desires rather than behaving from a place of constraint. BDSM for Black people is personal, political, and pleasurable. Shakti Bliss describes her participation in BDSM as a necessary journey:

> It's an inward journey of getting to know yourself. I am still doing that. I spent years building up this armor, like years. Piece by piece; shined it,

hardened it. It was perfect. It was beautiful armor and it kept everything out. I was safe and I was accomplished because that is how you survive trauma. We have this generational work that has been, it's in our blood. It's in our DNA. And it's about how to work with our everyday life and let go of the imposter syndrome. Let go of feeling like we need to prove to other people that we're good enough. Let go of the survival tactics that we have had to build around white supremacy and just allowing yourself to exist and feel resourced so that whatever crosses your path you feel ready. And you do not have to feel like you're in defense mode all the time.

Above all, the BDSM practitioners in this study described a liberating quality to their practice. Black practitioners not only get to name themselves but find that BDSM also gives them a space to articulate their preferences, dislikes, and limitations. It is important for Black people to relearn to effectively communicate what they want and don't want in real time and to access their own energy when they need to employ better boundaries. The reclamation of agency enhances decision-making power, allowing Black people to feel secure in their bodies and identities. Rather than making decisions from a place of constraint, BDSM helps marginalized people make decisions that align with their desires and increase their capacity for intimacy. For Black people, power play offers a container for unapologetic strength and determination, which alone is a symbol of righteous rebellion.

References

Anderson, J. R., Holland, E., Heldreth, C., & Johnson, S. P. (2018). Revisiting the Jezebel stereotype: The impact of target race on sexual objectification. *Psychology of Women Quarterly, 42*(4), 461–476. https://doi.org/10.1177/0361684318791543

Bauer, R. (2014). *Queer BDSM intimacies: Critical consent and pushing boundaries.* Palgrave Macmillan.

Bloomer, M. L. (2019). *Exploring the framework of consent and negotiation in the BDSM community for broader application within corporate environments* [Doctoral dissertation, Prescott College]. ProQuest. https://www.proquest.com/openview/13bc385ed 2f76ee0f1e5e97c43cb4d88/1?pq-origsite=gscholar&cbl=18750&diss=y

Bogues, A. (2012). And what about the human?: Freedom, human emancipation, and the radical imagination. *Boundary 2, 39*(3), 29–46. https://doi.org/10.1215/01903659-1730608

Carter, R. T. (2007). Racism and psychological and emotional injury: Recognizing and assessing race-based traumatic stress. *The Counseling Psychologist, 35*(1), 13–105. https://doi.org/10.1177/0011000006292033

Collins, P. H. (2004). *Black sexual politics: African Americans, gender, and the new racism.* Routledge.

Cruz, A. (2016). *The color of kink: Black women, BDSM, and pornography.* New York University Press.

DeFrancisco, V. P., & Palczewski, C. H. (2007). Gendered/sexed bodies. In T. R. Armstrong (Ed.), *Communicating gender diversity: A critical approach* (pp. 81–106). SAGE Publications. https://doi.org/10.4135/9781483329284.n4

Doss, A. (2013). Black bodies, white spaces: Understanding the construction of white identity through the objectification and lynching of Black bodies. *Black Diaspora Review, 3*(2), 14–17. https://aaads.indiana.edu/research/publications/black-bodies-white-spaces.html

Goffman, E. (1959). *The presentation of self in everyday life.* Doubleday.

Goffman, E. (1963). *Stigma: Notes on the management of spoiled identity.* Prentice-Hall.

Haraway, D. (1989). Situated knowledges: The science question in feminism and the privilege of partial perspective. *Feminist Studies, 14*(3), 575–599. https://doi.org/10.2307/3178066

Holmes, C. M. (2016). The colonial roots of the racial fetishization of Black women. *Black & Gold, 2*(1), Article 2. https://openworks.wooster.edu/cgi/viewcontent.cgi?article=1026&context=blackandgold

hooks, b. (1995). *Killing rage: Ending racism.* Henry Holt and Company.

Hutchinson, E. O. (1997). *The assassination of the Black male image.* Simon & Schuster.

Kambon, K. K. (2012). *African/Black psychology in the American context: An African-centered approach.* Nubian Nation Publications.

Langdridge, D., & Butt, T. (2004). A hermeneutic phenomenological investigation of the construction of sadomasochistic identities. *Sexualities, 7,* 31–53. https://doi.org/10.1177/1363460704040137

Lenhardt, R. A. (2004). Understanding the mark: Race, stigma, and equality in context. *New York University Law Review, 79,* 803. https://ir.lawnet.fordham.edu/faculty_scholarship/458/

Lorde, A. (1978). *Uses of the erotic: The erotic as power.* Freedom.

Malbroux, L. (2016, March 16). When you want to be into BDSM but it's too soon because you're Black. *Splinter.* https://splinternews.com/when-you-want-to-be-into-bdsm-but-its-too-soon-because-1793855556

Meyer, I. H. (2003). Prejudice, social stress, and mental health in lesbian, gay, and bisexual populations: Conceptual issues and research evidence. *Psychological Bulletin, 129,* 674–697. https://doi.org/10.1037/0033-2909.129.5.674

Nittle, N. K. (2019). The U.S. government's role in sterilizing women of color. *ThoughtCo.* https://www.thoughtco.com/u-s-governments-role-sterilizing-women-of-color-2834600

Norman, A. (2020). *A critical microethnographic examination of power exchange, role identity and agency with Black BDSM practitioners* [Doctoral dissertation, University of Central Florida]. *STARS.* https://stars.library.ucf.edu/cgi/viewcontent.cgi?article=1259&context=etd2020

Polanco-Roman, L., Danies, A., & Anglin, D. M. (2016). Racial discrimination as race-based trauma, coping strategies, and dissociative symptoms among emerging adults. *Psychological Trauma: Theory, Research, Practice, and Policy, 8*(5), 609–617. https://doi.org/10.1037/tra0000125

Pulido, L. (2017). Geographies of race and ethnicity II: Environmental racism, racial cap-italism and state-sanctioned violence. *Progress in Human Geography*, *41*(4), 524–533. https://doi.org/10.1177/0309132516646495

Riley, R. (2018, February 8). Column: Why America can't get over slavery, its greatest shame. *USA Today*. https://www.usatoday.com/story/news/nation-now/2018/02/08/column-why-america-cant-get-over-slavery-its-greatest-shame/1000524001/

Song, S. (2020, November 5). Meet the couple fighting porn's race problem. *Paper*. https://www.papermag.com/royal-fetish-porn-race-problem-2648632642.html?rebelltitem=1#rebelltitem1

Sue, D. W., Capodilupo, C. M., Torino, G. C., Bucceri, J. M., Holder, A., Nadal, K. L., & Esquilin, M. (2007). Racial microaggressions in everyday life: Implications for clinical practice. *American Psychologist*, *62*(4), 271–286. https://doi.org/10.1037/0003-066X.62.4.271

Tyler, I. (2018). Resituating Erving Goffman: From stigma power to black power. *The Sociological Review*, *66*(4), 744–765. https://doi.org/10.1177/0038026118777450

Weinberg, T. S. (2006). Sadomasochism and the social sciences: A review of the socio-logical and social psychological literature. *Journal of Homosexuality*, *50*(2–3), 17–40. https://doi.org/10.1300/J082v50n02_02

13

Survivors of Sexual Victimization and the Negotiation of BDSM Play

Karen Holt

Introduction

This chapter explores the meanings and experiences of sexual victimization among those who identify as BDSM participants in a kink community in the Midwest region of the United States. I explore the ways in which sexual, erotic, and intimate behaviors can serve functions beyond pleasure, such as attempts toward restoration and healing (Barker et al., 2007; Bauer, 2014; Hammers, 2014; Ortmann & Sprott, 2013). While engagement in BDSM is unrelated to mental illness, trauma, or victimization, those who do report histories of sexual victimization may have unique BDSM experiences and construct their practices differently, drawing more from therapeutic narratives. For these individuals, BDSM can be both traumatic and therapeutic (Thomas, 2020). Additionally, heteronormative, non-BDSM discourses surrounding consent and boundary violations may fail to capture the complex practices and experiences of these individuals.

Thus, the focus of this chapter is to explore how a history of sexual victimization affects BDSM play and the ways in which these individuals understand, define, and experience BDSM. I draw from the literature on sexual victimization, constructions of consent, and BDSM as therapy and trauma play to examine the cases of five individuals who identified as members of a BDSM community and survivors of sexual victimization. These cases represent a small but important minority as these participants reported more instances of harm and boundary violations than those who did not share this history. By hearing the stories of these individuals, we can provide accounts of how forms of erotic practice are used by the participants to make sense of their experiences. Implications of the research for practice and treatment as well as future avenues for exploration are discussed.

Karen Holt, *Survivors of Sexual Victimization and the Negotiation of BDSM Play* In: *The Power of BDSM*.
Edited by: Brandy L. Simula, Robin Bauer, and Liam Wignall, Oxford University Press. © Oxford University Press 2023.
DOI: 10.1093/oso/9780197658598.003.0014

Constructions of BDSM as Pathology and Trauma

Behaviors which fall under the umbrella term *BDSM* have traditionally been framed by the psychological and medical disciplines as indicative of a psychological abnormality or sexual deficit (Richters et al., 2008). These behaviors were theorized to represent distinct desires and motivations rooted deeply within the individual, often as a symptom of maladjustment, sickness, disease, abuse, or trauma (Cross & Matheson, 2006; Taylor & Ussher, 2001). BDSM participants were constructed as "damaged" or as possible risks to society who warranted social or legal regulation (Richters et al., 2008). Early studies supported these notions through studies which employed flawed methodology (clinical and forensic samples; non-empirical, hypothetical discourse; and single-case studies) to assert that psychopathology underlies all BDSM interests and behaviors, even those expressed safely and consensually (Connelly, 2006; Dunkley & Brotto, 2020).

The medical practice of diagnostic labeling established the persistent stigmatizing of individuals based on sexual interests and desires (Reiersol & Skeid, 2006). For example, the American Psychiatric Association's (APA's) *Diagnostic and Statistical Manual of Mental Disorders*, fifth edition (2013), includes BDSM practices such as sadism and masochism, which can be diagnosable disorders. This has facilitated the negative public perceptions and social stigma associated with these behaviors (Yost, 2010). Despite the APA's vague criteria of "non-consensual" behavior explicitly stated in the diagnoses, consensual BDSM remains associated with mental disorder and mental illness (Williams, 2006).

BDSM as the Re-enactment of Trauma

Specifically, the psychodynamic approach attempted to explain BDSM as compensation for previous victimization, abuse, or trauma. Sigmund Freud, one the founders of psychoanalysis, discussed the concept of repetition compulsion and specifically applied it to those who engaged in masochistic behaviors or those who enjoyed more submissive roles and receiving pain, sensation, or humiliation. Repetition compulsion involved the repeating or reliving of events, endless loops in which individuals tried to gain control and mastery by replicating traumatic events in controlled situations (Freud, 1923/1961, 1920/1975). The assertion was that BDSM play was essentially recreating the trauma and placing the person in situations where trauma can reoccur. This approach was especially concerned with linkage—to find an underlying cause, typically some early experience, that could explain the current "pathological" behaviors (Nordling et al., 2000).

While these early discourses of pathology still permeate public perceptions of BDSM, extant and contemporary research exists which demonstrates that BDSM is a diverse erotic or sexual activity enjoyed by a minority of the population who suffer no more emotional, psychological, or mental distress than the non-participants who engage in "normative" or "vanilla" sexual behavior (Cross & Matheson, 2006; Richters et al., 2008). Those who engage in BDSM are well adjusted, and the prevalence of mental illness mirrors that of the general population (Alison et al., 2001; Cross & Matheson, 2006; Sandnabba, et al., 2002; Williams, 2006). Additionally, BDSM interest is not indicative of past victimization or trauma. Estimates of sexual victimization among BDSM participants are similar to those among the general population, with about 23% of women and 8% of men reporting that they have experienced sexual abuse in their lifetime (Nordling et al., 2000). Despite these findings, BDSM is still a marginalized and stigmatized practice (Tomazos et al., 2017).

BDSM as Therapeutic

Yet despite the pathological framing of these activities, evidence suggests that there are associated health benefits which can contribute to well-being. Studies of sex work and erotic practices have demonstrated that clients often find these services therapeutic and frame these practices as beneficial forms of both touch or talk therapy (Bernstein, 2007; Lindemann, 2011). Play can lead to fluctuations and changes in hormone levels associated with mood and feelings of well-being (Sagarin et al., 2009). There are physiological responses to BDSM play which are emblematic of catharsis, such as altered states of consciousness (subspace) consistent with the feel of a "natural high" or feelings of temporary escape from self-awareness (Baumeister, 2010; Pitagora, 2017; Williams, 2006).

The term *therapy* was once defined narrowly in psychological discourse. Over time, it has been conceptualized more broadly to include a range of activities, including those which may have been previously framed as deviant and pathological and stigmatized by the dominant culture (Lindemann,

2011). BDSM practices can have positive effects on both physiological and psychological states. BDSM play facilitates psychological and physical confrontation; exploration of repression, emotion, or trauma within a controlled setting; and overall improved psychological functioning (Andrieu et al., 2019; Lindemann, 2011). For some participants, BDSM represents a unique opportunity to engage in healthy and beneficial practice which can improve psychological functioning.

Empowerment is a key element in trauma work, and BDSM may allow for participants who have experienced past victimization to regain a sense of control. Werder (2017) described how the steps of trauma work and BDSM scenes are similar in structure—the focus of both includes skill-building, controlled exposure, and integration of skills into daily life. Masochism specifically has been explored as a means to cope with trauma (Gavin, 2010). In fact, trauma play, or intentionally and consensually engaging in BDSM activities which individuals connect to their past trauma, to "play" with one's past trauma or abuse, has been one way in which participants explore harms and move toward healing (Thomas, 2020). These activities can be integral to gaining control over the self, the body, and the past (Hammers, 2014; Lindemann, 2011). For those who are survivors of sexual victimization, BDSM can be used as a way to challenge somatic dissociation or to become more connected to oneself, one's body, and the environment while also forcing others to bear witness (Hammers, 2014). As Hammers (2019) explains,

> These reenactments of lived trauma are performative scenes of consensual violence where the critical role of fantasy is front and center. This is a reworking, a working out, of trauma, as S/M transfigures the unbearable suffering of violence—sexual and/or gender trauma—into something more bearable. (pp. 491–492)

Although despite the therapeutic elements of trauma play, it can also be traumatic in some cases (Thomas, 2020).

This qualitative study sought to answer this fundamental research question: How do individuals with a history of sexual victimization understand, define, and experience BDSM play? The goal was to further an understanding of the experience of sexual victimization and how it affects future interactions among those who participate in BDSM.

Method

The Sample

The cases included in this analysis were drawn from data collected for a larger study of over 150 hours of ethnographic observations and 21 semi-structured interviews with individuals active in BDSM scenes in the Midwestern region of the United States, specifically the metropolitan areas of Lansing, Michigan; Detroit, Michigan; Chicago, Illinois; St. Louis, Missouri; and Indianapolis, Indiana. These locations were selected because most BDSM research has focused on the East and West coasts due to their social closeness and the size of their BDSM scenes (see Lindemann, 2010). Thus, the Midwestern region provided fruitful ground for investigation, and despite the differences in size of communities, the results are consistent with these locations.

A purposive sample of participants was recruited using snowball sampling. Inclusion criteria for the study were that participants had to be at least 18 years of age, must have been active in the BDSM lifestyle for at least 6 months, and must have participated in BDSM activities with at least one other individual (in order to have had some interactions with individuals during BDSM play). The study was an investigation of how participants experienced and defined notions of harm, which included questions about victimization. For the present study, cases were selected based on disclosure of victimization ($n = 7$).

Seven of the 21 interview participants (31.8% of the sample) reported that they had histories of victimization that occurred in childhood or young adulthood. Five were cisgender women, (71.4%; $n = 5$) and two were cisgender men. All participants were white. Of these participants, two were abused by non-family members and one was abused by someone outside of the family in a BDSM setting. Four participants were abused by family members in the non-BDSM setting of the home. Although this is a small number of individuals reporting from a purposive sample of BDSM participants, the percentage of individuals with a background of sexual victimization is consistent with the literature on sexual victimization as more women often report being victimized as children or youth, with the abuse perpetrated by someone with whom they had a relationship (Mancini, 2014).

For the purposes of this study, only cisgender women were included in the analysis. The two individuals who identified as men did not discuss their victimization other than to report it had occurred. The analysis revealed several themes which described the meaning of BDSM for these participants. These included situating experience, identifying triggers, recreating and playing with triggers, and weakened boundaries.

Ethnographic Observations

Participant ethnographic methodology was utilized to establish relationships with the participants in their own spaces, to observe and describe social actions, to interact and participate in their pratices, and to learn about their norms and values (Gobo, 2008). I attended BDSM-related events advertised online, which included educational workshops and events, play parties, dungeons, and bars. All participants were given an informed consent document which stated the nature and purpose of the observation as well as their protections as participants. Observations focused on the physical setting, activities, the human and social environment, formal and informal interactions, and nonverbal communications. Informal discussions with participants at these events were especially salient and provided context for what was being observed. No recordings of any kind were made during an event so as to avoid any intrusive data collection. All detailed field notes were recorded after leaving the premises. Attending these various events yielded over 150 hours of observational data.

Semi-structured Interviews

Semi-structured qualitative interviews were conducted, either in person, by phone, or via Skype, to gain insight into participants' beliefs and experiences. Prospective interview participants were identified through either public events organized for local BDSM scenes, threads on a social media website for those interested in kink called FetLife which described the study and provided the contact information for the researcher, and snowball sampling where interviewees recruited people they knew.

All individuals interested in participation were given the researcher's email address and asked to initiate contact. They were provided a brief description of the study or directed to a blog that was created for the study that they could access anonymously. Once individuals read the description of the study, a 1- to 2-hour interview was scheduled. Depending on the location of the participant, the interview took place either in person, via Skype, by telephone, or through email messages. Although face-to-face interviews allow for more interactions with participants, interviewing via computer can increase both the participant's feeling of anonymity and the quality of reports (see Tournegeau & Smith, 1996). Thus, the interviewee chose which form of interview they felt most comfortable completing. In the transcription of the interviews and in subsequent publications, aliases were used for all participants so as to protect their confidentiality.

Qualitative Analysis

The analysis was facilitated through the use of the qualitative software program ATLAS.ti, which has tools to explore large amounts of rich data in a systematic way, allowing for the fundamental process of qualitative coding (Corbin & Strauss, 1990; Friese, 2013). Several key steps comprised the coding process. First, multiple readings of the interviews, field notes, and memos were performed. This allowed for the identification of relevant first-level codes, which are "tags or labels for assigning units of meaning to the descriptive or inferential information compiled during a study" (Huberman & Miles, 1994, p. 56). Coding decisions were focused and guided by the central research question and goal of the study (Auerbach & Silverstein, 2003; Saladana, 2009): How do individuals with a history of victimization understand, define, and experience BDSM play?

Codes were theory-driven, meaning derived from the extant theoretical research on BDSM, sexual victimization, and consent. Additionally, codes were data-driven, or derived directly from the raw data; organized into small units; and used to draw meaningful inferences. Initial or open coding, where important words or groups of words are identified and labeled, was conducted through line-by-line coding, or coding on the level of sentence, and what is termed *level of meaning*, which included paragraphs or the entire narrative (DeCuir-Gunby et al., 2010). Research memos were constructed to explore the data, examine relationships, and develop second-level axial codes, which establish relationships between first-level codes and the data. Axial codes were used to develop categories, or groups of related codes.

Saturation of the data was obtained when no new codes emerged from the data, and all cases were explained using existing categories (Birk &

Mills, 2011). Categories were selectively coded by identifying core qualitative variables and developing them into meaningful themes. Triangulation of the data included the use of interview data, observations, fieldwork, field notes, and research memos (Boeri, 2007; Nichter et al., 2004). These multiple sources and methods allowed for comparison of findings, rigorous analysis, and increased validity (Miles et al., 2014).

Results

Situating Experience

Participants felt the need to make sense of their BDSM activities to understand how they related to their sexual victimization. This appeared to play an important role in constructing personal narratives which situated their experience within their identity.

For example, Cindy worried about the motivations behind her BDSM participation as she did not want them to be a direct result of the trauma she experienced as a child. She explained,

> I'm a rape survivor. I was emotionally abused as a child. I think that a lot of us have those kinds of thoughts—like, oh gee, I wonder if I'm just trying to relive this, or if I'm trying to work through it in unhealthy ways.

This uncertainty of why she engaged in BDSM and her need to situate her behavior within her identity and personal story were sources of concern. Cindy maintained that she believed BDSM was a healthy way to explore power dynamics, although she was keenly aware that this was related to her traumatic experiences. For her, situating her experiences into a coherent narrative was crucial to her identity.

Another participant, Danielle, was a cisgender woman submissive who became interested in BDSM as an adult after a failed heterosexual marriage. Danielle was vehement that her BDSM activities were unrelated to her sexual victimization, which was perpetrated by her grandfather when she was a young girl. Despite her claims that BDSM was unrelated to her trauma, she situated her experience in a way that directly linked her abuse with her desire to relinquish control through submission. She described how she came to identify as submissive:

It's a struggle because I've had to be in control over everything all my life. As a child I grew up in a very abusive childhood and I was in charge. I was my mother's best friend. Very inappropriately. I had to be in charge and I've had to be in control for so long, so it's nice not to be. That mechanism that kept me healthy and sane growing up in an abusive environment no longer serves me. It's nice just to completely let go and trust. I do feel like I lose control all the time. In a good way.

Danielle viewed BDSM as a mechanism to separate herself from her past and her history of victimization. While young Danielle was forced to control all aspects of her life to survive, adult Danielle rejected control and gladly submitted to her partner. She situated her experience as being a catalyst for change and healing. She denied that her BDSM activities or predilections were in any way related to her history of childhood abuse, rather viewing BDSM as a pleasurable activity which attracted her because of the power dynamics. As she explained, "I don't believe that I am interested in the dominance and submission and the pain and all of the activities we do because of the childhood I had. I don't think it's related." For her, the element of control is related to an abusive past, which made BDSM activities attractive; but the abuse and BDSM participation were situated as separate.

Making sense of their sexual victimization and the role it played in BDSM behaviors by situating their experiences was a crucial part of participant identity. For the participants, the stories which they constructed were a way to define and understand themselves and create coherence and meaning (McAdams, 2001). This meaning informed future actions, relationships, and interactions.

Identifying Triggers

For participants who have a history of sexual victimization, the concept of a trigger is an important facet of interaction. A *trigger* is anything that brings the person back to the trauma they have suffered. It can be the result of a physical act or sensation or an emotional response to an interaction. This concept is related to scripting and emotional memory. Scripts provide blueprints for behavior—they specify with whom people should have sex, when and where they should have sex, what kind of sex they should have, and the reasons for having sex (Laumann et al., 1994). Scripting involves past narratives regarding experiences that individuals have had that are employed in current situations. These scripts inform and affect interactions. Related to the idea of scripting is emotional memory, which involves the re-creation and regeneration of the feelings experienced during traumatic experiences, which are then projected onto present events (Benedetti, 1998). For cisgender women in the sample who have experienced sexual victimization, these scripts colored their BDSM experiences.

For these women, there were general behaviors that were identified as triggers which they listed as hard limits. Some of these included age play, which is a form of role playing in which participants play as different ages (this was especially harmful for those whose victimization occurred as children) and consensual non-consent, where consent is given prior to play but actors might say no or actively resist during the interaction as part of the play. Mutually satisfying consensual non-consent play is dependent on boundaries and the notion that these activities constitute play. For those with a history of victimization, this type of play can elicit thoughts and feelings associated with their abuse or abusers. Others identified triggers that were specific to their abuse incidents. For example, Dawn described her experience with blindfolds:

> When I was a teenager, for three years, from 12 to 15 I was being abused by one specific person. Every so often he would blindfold me and tie me up. And he would have other people pay to come in and use me. So I always associated being blindfolded with being used by somebody who I didn't know and I didn't know what they were going to do with me. Being blindfolded, yeah, it absolutely terrifies me.

Many struggled to identify triggers so that they could be avoided, but for some this was a formidable task. Annie, a cisgender woman who was a bottom, explained,

> Playing with me can be like playing in a minefield. I was emotionally, physically, and sexually abused as a child. I don't always know what will trigger me and what won't. A lot of my triggers are related to my kinks. I've listed my triggers in my limits, but I just don't know them all.

For Annie, it was important to make sure that partners were clear regarding her limits; however, the issue was that her triggers were elusive in nature.

They were not static and stable across time, acts, and partners. The ability to identify triggers was active work that she engaged in consistently.

Participants reported that it is impossible to identify everything that could possibly remind them of the experience of being abused. Additionally, once they were triggered, it was challenging to deal with the emotional experience. Sarah, a cisgender woman who identified as a bottom, described,

> I was playing with a guy for the third or so time that day, and I got triggered and had a flashback to a very unpleasant experience with my rapist. I safeworded, and everyone was really wonderful and supportive, but there's not really a good fix for that.

While she was able to recognize immediately that she had been triggered and used her safe word to end the scene, dealing with the emotional aftermath was difficult.

Identifying when they have been triggered was also a challenge as some participants expressed that the emotional processing of a trigger can be slow and may not have an immediate effect. Blue explained,

> Usually if I don't know what the trigger is it's the first time something's triggered me. I'm completely oblivious to what it is, sometimes for several days. So it can be quite a difficult process and sometimes it doesn't all happen at once, it happens in little intervals and I don't realize I've triggered sometimes. And it gets very messy and very complicated.

She went on to give an example of how difficult it is to describe the triggering process to potential partners:

> The last guy I was with, I think he assumed that I would just use a safeword. I was trying to explain to him that sometimes it's a bit more complicated than that. Because sometimes I don't realize that I actually need to use a safeword. And sometimes I don't know that I'm triggered. I'll start to trigger and I'll trigger very slowly or gently and I don't know that I'm triggering.

Sarah emphasized the unpredictable nature of triggers despite planning and precautions. She explained, "The last scene I had was very nice up until I was suddenly triggered. There was rope, some light impact play, some general lovely feeling of physical dominance, and then it all went to hell in a hand-basket."

Annie described playing with partners as a never-ending learning process which consists of trial and error:

> So every person I'm with, in every relationship, I seem to uncover triggers which I've had to overcome. But it seems to be coming easier now than it was a couple of years ago. Hopefully, I'll continue to manage them better and better each time.

For her, through the process of identifying triggers, although painful and unpleasant at the time they occurred, brought more self-knowledge and strengthened her ability for self-care.

Re-creating and Playing with Triggers

Several participants expressed purposeful engagements with their triggers. This was a way in which they could safely explore them within a controlled setting. They expressed that BDSM allowed for avenues of exploration that may be difficult in a non-BDSM relationship. Annie expressed,

> For me, BDSM is way, amongst other things, to allow me to express and explore some things that I probably wouldn't be able to in a vanilla sex life. How could I turn to a vanilla man and explain that I want to be tied up and essentially raped and pretending to be a kid at the time. You can't do that in a vanilla sex life. It just doesn't happen. So I guess maybe a lot of people get into BDSM, not necessarily into the lifestyle completely but they get into different aspects of it as a form of catharsis. You know, to exorcise some of the things that have happened.

She recounted when she had developed and created a scene for a girlfriend who had experienced a brutal rape:

> We'd been playing together for about six months and we really knew each other and liked each other and trusted each other. So I set up a situation where she thought she was being raped. I put a blindfold on her,

noise cancelling headphones on her, and I put a ball gag in her mouth. She couldn't have used a safe word because she'd had the ball gag but I was very comfortable with her body language, I knew that I would be able to tell if she needed to use a safe word. And through the noise cancelling headphones, she couldn't hear what was going on very well. I used an Mp3 on my laptop to simulate the sound of a man in the room and used a sex toy to simulate a penis. So essentially she was put into this position—the door was opened and closed, she heard the door close, and then she just heard this Mp3 of a man start up and then she feels someone behind her.

Annie felt that she had created a safe space in which to explore her girlfriend's victimization and engage in trauma work:

What I'd actually done was I'd brought something up to the surface that she'd been suppressing for a very, very long time. And it gave her the opportunity to have a breakdown over it, talk about it with a degree of safety and in a calm way and she was really appreciative.

Annie also re-created scenes from her own victimization:

People I talk to can't understand why it is that I essentially look to re-create some of my worst experiences. And I explain to people that it's a way of distancing my current sensual activities from the things that were done to me in the past. And it gives me the opportunity to take this horrible thing, to isolate it, cut it away, and put it in a little black box and then to bring that box into my current life, and put it into something good and enjoy it. And it kind of destroys it ultimately. It's almost like digging out this horrible thing in my past and turning it into something positive that I can enjoy and explore with someone I love. It's, essentially, in my own mind at least, it's psychologically raping the rapist. It's about taking the power back. I speak to a lot of people in my, in my sort of position or with my sort of history, who to one extent or another say exactly the same thing.

BDSM allowed her to make sense of her experiences and to regain the sense of control that her abusers had stolen from her. It was an avenue for catharsis.

Danielle described how, under the right conditions and with the right person, identified triggers can be enjoyable practices:

If I am with somebody who I trust then being blindfolded gives me this thrill, this rush. A little bit like having sex and somebody's downstairs and could come up at any time or could hear you. It's a similar thrill but it's much more intense. But sometimes, if the person I'm with doesn't touch me enough, doesn't talk to me enough then sometimes I'll forget who I'm with and I'll trigger. But as long as it's done well and it's handled properly it can be really, really thrilling.

Others expressed that their triggers commingle with sexual excitement. Caroline, a submissive cisgender woman, explained, "I'm one of those weird people who a lot of my triggers are also my turn-ons but I have to be really secure with the person I'm with." For some, playing with these triggers was an exciting and arousing experience. In these cases, sexual scripts were used and incorporated to experience pleasure. The interactions had more aspects of edge play (play that pushes the boundaries or limits of participants) than trauma play as they were motivated by excitement and fun rather than past victimization (Thomas, 2020).

Weakened Boundaries

Despite the controlled nature of their play, participants acknowledged that it could be difficult to engage in necessary self-care and protective actions. Participants described that they often struggled to maintain their personal boundaries during play. They experienced difficulty with communication when triggers occurred unexpectedly. Blue described that her victimization history complicated her ability to play safely. She explained that she often had difficulty advocating for herself: "Sometimes I'll feel unable to use a safeword because I feel like if I do so, I'm a failure." She was hesitant to express her needs and assert herself and felt a sense of guilt for experiencing triggers. She felt that this difficulty in boundary-setting and maintenance was inextricably linked to her abuse.

Annie had similar experiences:

I know that BDSM is all about consent and everyone walking away from it happy. I know that logically. But I spent my formative years of sex being in a position where I wasn't allowed to say no or where I was punished for saying no. I would feel bad about the prospect of saying no. You feel like it's your purpose to serve them and if you say no to them or try to put any restrictions on them then you're doing something wrong. You're messing up.

Thus, in some cases participants felt that their sexual victimization experience made it difficult to advocate for themselves and that this often weakened the boundaries they attempted to draw. There was a sense of guilt and fear that accompanied saying no or stopping a scene that was unique for each participant. It is important to note that all the participants recognized that they needed to improve their communication and to better assert themselves.

Discussion

Contemporary social science has demonstrated that BDSM is a sexually diverse practice which can have positive psychological effects, including a sense of empowerment, for those who participate (Andrieu et al., 2019). For the participants who reported a history of sexual victimization, BDSM was a way in which to situate their experiences, regain a sense of control, and rebuild trust and worth. While participants differed in their responses when asked about the role of sexual victimization in shaping their BDSM practices and identity, all reported that this part of their life history shaped their experiences in some ways. The participants in this study were engaged in some of the same trauma work as non-participants of BDSM—particularly in identifying triggers, paying attention to psychological and physical signs of triggers, and engaging in self-care (in their cases, often through aftercare) (Smith & Segal, 2020).

Trauma play occurs when adults consensually engage in BDSM behaviors which are connected to past trauma or abuse, where the individual is aware of this association (Thomas, 2020). BDSM allowed for these participants to confront their trauma, whether directly through trauma play, generally through other play, or through dealing with issues of power and control, in a safer and more structured.

The complex nature of trauma and histories of victimization among these participants resulted in triggers and weakened boundaries which sometimes complicated satisfying play. Triggers caused participants to recall and rely on early scripts of victimization, which affected their ability to advocate for themselves. Harmful prior scripts and emotional memory associated with their abuse often re-emerged when engaging in BDSM activities, which occasionally resulted in healthy, consensual activity becoming a negative experience for the participant. Participants had to actively work to identify, master, and overcome these triggers.

The concept of consent has been rooted in heteronormative assumptions of the yes-means-yes/no-means-no axiom (Edenfield, 2019). This framing has rarely been questioned or contested (Bauer, 2014). Recent work has proposed that, rather than conceptualizing consent as black or white, it can be understood as a gray concept, or as an intersubjectivity where some behaviors are experienced as boundary violations and others are not (Fanghanel, 2020). Rather than a dichotomous choice discussed at the beginning of an interaction, queer notions of consent involve ongoing negotiations where individuals discuss and evaluate their own power, privilege, and desires in a more inclusive and nuanced approach (Barker, 2013; Bauer, 2014, 2020; Edenfield, 2019; Livingston, 2015). Consensual BDSM behaviors do not always conform to the espoused formalized consent models of more "mainstream" sexual practices and interactions (Weiss, 2011). Practitioners also engage in what is termed *consensual non-consent*, where they create scenes and play that appear violent, abusive, or anti-feminist, especially to those unfamiliar with BDSM culture and practice (Deckha, 2011; Tsaros, 2013). For participants with a history of sexual victimization, these frameworks of consent better elucidate the unique dynamics of BDSM play. Consent is a process, one rife with pitfalls and challenges which can shift and change depending on the situation. It is impossible for an individual to comprehensively predict all the activities that may require negotiation and even renegotiation, especially for those with unique needs (Beres & MacDonald, 2015). Rather than rely solely on the participant for a declaration of consent prior to play, consent must be constantly negotiated and should be a collaborative process. To better protect participants from abuse, it is critical to understand and situate the responsibility of consent among BDSM practitioners Thus, it is critical to think about consent not as an individual choice but at the community level with varied and intersecting social power dynamics and differences involved (Barker, 2013; Bauer, 2014).

When the dominant culture denies that BDSM can be a healthy form of sexual expression and instead situates it as abuse and violence, it creates more barriers for those who experience abuse to access support and resources, especially agents of social control such as law enforcement (Pitagora, 2016). Thus, BDSM provided an outlet for those for whom therapy may not have been an option, whether due to fear of stigma or a lack of resources. Yet

BDSM practice alone is not a panacea for trauma or abuse; other resources are necessary for healing (Hammers, 2019).

There has been a growing awareness of the need for kink-centered therapy. For example, the Kink and Polyam Aware Chicago Therapists acknowledge and celebrate gender and sexual diversity and offer training and education to therapists on working with diverse groups and individuals. As more kink-friendly resources become available, participants can not only work through trauma in their own BDSM practices but feel supported by professionals who can assist them through the healing and self-exploration process. While several of the participants reported seeing therapists, none were trained in BDSM or kink, and participants were hesitant to discuss their lifestyles.

Limitations

The present study was limited in several ways. First, the sample size was small, although this is not uncommon among BDSM research due to the history of stigmatization and marginalization of participants and practices (Beres & MacDonald, 2015; Pitagora, 2017). This sample was drawn from the Midwestern United States. Thus, in areas where there are more established and larger BDSM scenes, such as New York City or San Francisco, communities may be more diverse and more accessible and may have access to more kink-friendly resources.

While the larger sample for the study included more diversity in terms of race, gender, and sexual identity, only white cisgender women openly discussed their sexual victimization. All identified as heterosexual or bisexual. The positionality of the researcher may have played a role as her own identification as "straight" meant that she was less familiar with gay, lesbian, trans, and queer kink spaces. These spaces are also less visible and accessible than others in the kink community and are more consistent with what has been considered mainstreamed kink (Barker & Gill, 2012; Weiss, 2006). As such, this analysis was unable to explore the ways in which those who identify as LGBTQIA+ with a history of sexual victimization experience and make sense of their BDSM engagement. Additionally, the lack of diversity in race and ethnicity limits the experience to only white females, and future work should explore issues of intersectionality, consent, and BDSM experience. The sample was also comprised of submissives, bottoms, and switches. Thus, it is unclear how other BDSM identities with a history of sexual victimization may frame and understand their engagement. These voices are critical as much of BDSM practice reproduces and maintains the prevailing power dynamics of class, ethnicity, gender, and sexuality (Fanghanel, 2020). Some research has focused on queer BDSM experiences (Bauer, 2014, 2020), which is critical to understanding the diverse experiences among practitioners. This is especially important as transgender persons are more likely to report consent violations than cisgender males or females (Wright et al., 2015).

Despite these limitations, this work contributes to the existing literature on how heterosexual cisgender women with histories of sexual victimization negotiate consent. The results support more recent research which demonstrates the therapeutic benefits of BDSM and rejects the pathological framing of these practices (Andrieu et al., 2019; Wismeijer & van Assen, 2013). Participants did not understand their victimization to have a causal role in their BDSM engagement, as previous research has argued (Blum, 1991; Holtzman & Kulish, 2012). Rather, they found the practice intrinsic and enjoyable (Labreque et al., 2020). In addition, it served the function of exploring the trauma they experienced. Rather than simply re-creating sexual victimization, participants employed BDSM to achieve mindfulness, regain control, and rebuild and reclaim themselves and their power (Sagarin et al., 2009; Wismeijer & van Assen, 2013). This was a dynamic and ongoing process, one which participants navigated through building knowledge, skills, and resilience. It is both therapeutic and traumatic, both healing and hurting (Thomas, 2020). For these women, empowerment through erotic practice serves a critical function in identity work and boundary-setting as they attempt to navigate their BDSM interactions.

References

Alison, L., Santtila, P., Sandnabba, N. K., & Nordling, N. (2001). Sadomasochistically oriented behavior: Diversity in practice and meaning. *Archives of Sexual Behavior*, 30(1), 1–12. https://doi.org/10.1023/A:1026438422383

American Psychiatric Association. (2013). *Diagnostic and statistical manual of mental disorders: DSM-5* (5th ed.).

Andrieu, B., LaHuerta, C., & Luy, A. (2019). Consenting to constraint: BDSM therapy after the DSM-5. *L'Évolution Psychiatrique*, 84, 17–30. https://doi.org/10.1016/j.evopsy.2019.02.005

Barker, M., Gupta, C., & Iantaffi, A. (2007). The power of play: The potentials and pitfalls in healing narratives of BDSM. In D. Langdridge, M. Barker (Eds.), Safe, Sane and Consensual: Contemporary Perspectives on Sadomasochism (pp. 197–216). New York: Palgrave Macmillan.

Barker, M. (2013). Consent is a grey area? A comparison of understandings of consent in *Fifty Shades of Grey* and on the BDSM blogosphere. *Sexualities, 16*(8), 896–914. https://doi.org/10.1177%2F1363460713508881

Barker, M., & Gill, R. (2012). Sexual subjectification and *Bitchy Jones's Diary. Psychology and Sexuality, 3*(1), 26–40. https://doi.org/10.1080/19419899.2011.627693

Bauer, R. (2014). *Queer BDSM intimacies: Critical consent and pushing boundaries.* Palgrave Macmillan.

Bauer, R. (2020). Queering consent: Negotiating critical consent in les-bi-trans-queer BDSM contexts. *Sexualities, 24*(5–6), 767–783. https://doi.org/10.1177%2F1363460720973902

Baumeister, R. (2010). Masochism as escape from self. *Journal of Sex Research, 25*(1), 28–59. https://doi.org/10.1080/00224498809551444

Benedetti, J. (1998). *Stanislavski and the actor: The method of physical action.* Taylor and Francis.

Beres, M. A., & MacDonald, J. E. (2015). Talking about sexual consent. Heterosexual women and BDSM. *Australian Feminist Studies, 30*(86), 418–432. https://doi.org/10.1080/08164649.2016.1158692

Bernstein, E. (2007). *Temporarily yours: Intimacy, authenticity, and the commerce of sex.* University of Chicago Press.

Blum, H. P. (1991). Sadomasochism in the psychoanalytic process, within and beyond the pleasure principle: Discussion. *Journal of the American Psychoanalytic Association, 39*(2), 431–450. https://psycnet.apa.org/doi/10.1177/000306519103900207

Connelly, P. (2006). Psychological functioning of bondage/domination/sadomasochism (BDSM) practitioners. *Journal of Psychology & Human Sexuality, 18*(1), 79–120. https://doi.org/10.1300/J056v18n01_05

Cross, P., & Matheson, K. (2006). Understanding sadomasochism. *Journal of Homosexuality, 50*(2), 133–166.

Deckha, M. (2011). Pain as culture: A postcolonial feminist approach to S/M and women's agency. *Sexualities, 14*(2), 129–150. https://doi.org/10.1177%2F1363460711399032

Dunkley, C. R., & Brotto, L. A. (2020). The role of consent in the context of BDSM. *Sexual Abuse, 32*(6), 657–678. https://doi.org/10.1177%2F1079063219842847

Edenfield, A. (2019). Queering consent: Design and sexual consent messaging. *Communication Design Quarterly, 7*(2), 50–62. http://sigdoc.acm.org/cdq/queering-consent-design-and-sexual-consent-messaging/

Freud, S. (1961). The economic problems in masochism. In J. Strachey (Ed. and Trans.), *The standard edition of the complete psychological work of Sigmund Freud* (Vol. 19, pp. 159–170). Hogarth Press. (Original work published 1923)

Freud, S. (1975). Beyond the pleasure principle. In J. Strachey (Ed. and Trans.), *The standard edition of the complete psychological work of Sigmund Freud* (Vol. 18, pp. 20–45). Hogarth Press. (Original work published 1920)

Friese, S. (2013). *Atas.ti 7 user manual.* Scientific Software Development.

Gavin, B. (2010). No pain, no gain: Masochism as a response to early trauma and implications for therapy. *Psychodynamic Practice, 16*(2), 183–200. https://doi.org/10.1080/14753631003688134

Gobo, G. (2008). *Doing ethnography.* Sage.

Hammers, C. (2014). Corporeality, sadomasochism and sexual trauma. Body & Society, *20*(2), 68–90.

Holtzman, D., & Kulish, N. (Eds.). (2012). *The clinical problem of masochism.* Rowman & Littlefield.

Huberman, A. M., & Miles, M. B. (1994). Data management and analysis methods. In N. K. Denzin & Y.S Lincoln (Eds.), *Handbook of qualitative research* (pp. 428–444). Sage Publications, Inc.

Labrecque, F., Potz, A., LaRouche, E., & Joyal, C. C. (2020). What is so appealing about being spanked, flogged, dominated or restrained? Answers from practitioners of sexual masochism/submission. *The Journal of Sex Research, 58*(4), 409–423. https://doi.org/10.1080/00224499.2020.1767025

Laumann, E. O., Gagnon, G. H., & Michaels, S. (1994). *The social organization of sexuality: Sexual practices in the United States.* Chicago University Press.

Lindemann, D. (2010). Will the real dominatrix please stand up: Artistic purity and professionalism in the S&M dungeon. *Sociological Forum, 25*(3), 588–606. https://doi.org/10.1111/j.1573-7861.2010.01197.x

Lindemann, D. (2011). BDSM as therapy? *Sexualities, 14*(2), 151–172. https://doi.org/10.1177%2F1363460711399038

Livingston, K. A. (2015). *The queer art & rhetoric of consent: Theories, practices, pedagogies* [Doctoral dissertation]. Michigan State University.

McAdams, D. P. (2001). The psychology of life stories. *Review of General Psychology, 5*(2), 100–122. https://doi.org/10.1037%2F1089-2680.5.2.100

Mancini, C. (2014). *Sex crime, offenders, and society.* Carolina Academic Press.

Miles, M. B., Huberman, A. M., & Saldana, J. (2014). *Qualitative data analysis: A methods source book* (3rd ed.). Sage.

Nordling, N., Sandnabba, N. K., & Santilla, P. (2000). The prevalence and effect of self-reported childhood sexual abuse among sadomasochistically oriented males and females. *Journal of Child Sexual Abuse, 9*(1), 53–63.

Ortmann, D. M., & Sprott, R. A. (2013). *Sexual outsiders: Understanding BDSM sexualities and communities.* Rowman & Littlefield.

Pitagora, D. (2016). Intimate partner violence in sadomasochistic relationships. *Sexual and Relationship Therapy, 31*(1), 95–108. https://doi.org/10.1080/14681994.2015.1102219

Pitagora, D. (2017). No pain, no gain? Therapeutic and relational benefits of subspace in BDSM contexts. *Journal of Positive Sexuality, 3*(3), 44–54.

Reiersol, O., & Skeid, S. (2006). The ICD diagnoses of fetishism and sadomasochism. *Journal of Homosexuality, 50*(2–3), 243–262.

Richters, J., de Visser, R., Rissel, C., Grulich, A., & Smith, A. (2008). Demographic and psychosocial features of participants in bondage and discipline, sadomasochism, or dominance or submission: Data from a national survey. *Journal of Sexual Medicine, 5,* 1660–1668. https://doi.org/10.1111/j.1743-6109.2008.00795.x

Sagarin, B. J., Cutler, B., Cutler, N., Lawler-Sagarin, K. A., & Matuszewish, L. (2009). Hormonal changes and couple-bonding in consensual BDSM. *Archives of Sexual Behavior, 38,* 186–200. https://doi.org/10.1007/s10508-008-9374-5

Sandnabba, N. K., Santilla, P., Alison, L., & Nording, N. (2002). Demographics, sexual behaviour, family background, and abuse experiences of practitioners of sadomasochistic sex: A review of recent research. *Sexual and Relationship Therapy, 17,* 39–55. https://doi.org/10.1080/14681990220108018

Smith, M., & Segal, J. (2020). *Recovering from rape and sexual trauma*. HelpGuide. Retrieved April 20, 2020, from https://www.helpguide.org/articles/ptsd-trauma/rec overing-from-rape-and-sexual-trauma.htm

Taylor, G. W., & Ussher, J. M. (2001). Making sense of S&M: A discourse analytic account. *Sexualities, 4*(3), 293–314. https://doi.org/10.1177%2F136346001004003002

Thomas, J. N. (2020). BDSM as trauma play: An autoethnographic investigation. *Sexualities, 23*(5–6), 917–933. https://doi.org/10.1177%2F1363460719861800

Tomazos, K., O'Gorman, K., & MacLaren, A. (2017). From leisure to tourism: How BDSM demonstrates the transition of deviant pursuits to mainstream products. *Tourism Management, 60*, 30–41. http://dx.doi.org/10.1016/j.tourman.2016.10.018

Tournegeau, R., & Smith, T. W. (1996). Asking sensitive questions: The impact of data collection mode, question format, and question context. *Public Opinion Quarterly, 60*, 275–304.

Tsaros, A. (2013). Consensual non-consent: Comparing EL James's *Fifty Shades of Grey* and Pauline Réage's *Story of O*. *Sexualities, 16*(8), 864–879. https://doi.org/ 10.1177%2F1363460713508903

Weiss, M. (2006). Mainstreaming kink: The politics of BDSM representations in U.S. popular media. In P. Kleinplatz & C. Moser (Eds.), *SM: Powerful pleasures* (pp. 103–132). Haworth Press.

Weiss, M. (2011). *Techniques of pleasure. BDSM and the circuit of sexuality*. Duke University Press.

Werder, C. (2017, November 20). Kink and trust: How some trauma survivors find healing through BDSM. *GO Magazine*. Retrieved April 20, 2020 from http://gomag. com/article/healing-through-bdsm/

Williams, D. J. (2006). Different (painful¡) strokes for different folks: An overview of sexual sadomasochism (SM) and its diversity. *Sexual Addiction and Compulsivity, 13*, 333–346. https://doi.org/10.1080/10720160601011240

Wismeijer, A. A. J., & van Assen, M. A. L. M. (2013). Psychological characteristics of BDSM practitioners. *Journal of Sex Medicine, 10*, 1943–1952. https://doi.org/10.1111/ jsm.12192

Wright, S., Stambaugh, R. J., & Cox, D. (2015). Consent violations survey (Tech report). National Coalition for Sexual Freedom. Retrieved April 20, 2020 from https://ncsfree dom.org/wp-content/uploads/2019/12/Consent-Violations-Survey.pdf

Yost, M. R. (2010). Development and validation of the attitudes about sadomasochism scale. Journal of Sex Research, *47*, 79–91.

14

From Pain to Healing

Kink and Communication in Sexual Assault Recovery

Valerie Rubinsky, Angela Cooke-Jackson, and Alejandre Rodriguez

Introduction

While a plethora of scholarship on BDSM[1] investigates its potential to do harm or manifest underlying problems (Gemberling et al., 2015; Krueger, 2010; Moser, 2009; Sprott, 2020; among others), other research has explored the potential for BDSM sexual activity or BDSM sexual partner communication to heal. One recent research study suggests that some women who survived sexual trauma in childhood are able to gain a sense of agency and empowerment through relational, interpersonal, and community healing that allows them to embrace a whole sexual self (Hitter et al., 2017, p. 266). For some people who have survived rape or sexual assault, BDSM play may produce a means of individuation, a reclamation of bodily experience after a trauma that often produces disassociation from the body as a means of coping (Hammers, 2013, 2019).

We suggest in this chapter that a key process in the potential for BDSM to heal or harm is grounded in its communicative nature. This chapter explores specific BDSM communication practices with the intention to frame them as potential tools and means to reclaim sexual agency for some people who are recovering from sexual trauma. Grounded in communication practices that emerge from a number of sexual identity communities, including boundary-setting and the use of safe words, we argue that these community communication practices may facilitate healing amid sexual activity that sometimes, even consensually, hurts. This chapter will draw on data from a survey on sexual and reproductive health among women and people of diverse genders, utilizing qualitative data analyses of open-ended survey data. We begin by

Valerie Rubinsky, Angela Cooke-Jackson, and Alejandre Rodriguez, *From Pain to Healing* In: *The Power of BDSM*.
Edited by: Brandy L. Simula, Robin Bauer, and Liam Wignall, Oxford University Press. © Oxford University Press 2023.
DOI: 10.1093/oso/9780197658598.003.0015

briefly reviewing the literature on trauma play and re-creation and its inter-section with sexual communication. For this chapter, the authors consider the term *communication* to entail all of the verbal and nonverbal meaning-making processes that occur between or among people. In other words, the communication process considers any meaningful interactional behavior between or among people and the context(s) in which it is embedded.

BDSM and Healing

A recent body of literature on the intersection of healing from various traumas and BDSM does exist. For example, a recent special issue of the *Journal of Humanistic Psychology* explored the topic of reimagining kink and BDSM through transformation, growth, and healing (Sprott, 2020, para 1). Sprott (2020) argued that kink presents opportunities for healing and self-actualization. Thematic to discussions of healing and BDSM are considerations of agency. Consent is often discussed in the language of agency or, by some, as the mechanism for obtaining agency in an interac-tion (Langdridge, 2007; Pitagora, 2017, p. 49). As we will explore further in this chapter, consent is a complicated process embedded in multiple layers of meaning-making. First, we will discuss trauma play and re-creation and where we see communicated consent as informing this process.

Trauma Play, Trauma Re-creation, and Communication

A small but concrete subset of both survivors of sexual trauma and practitioners of BDSM who are interested in consensual non-consent, or other kinds of rape and trauma play, may utilize play scenes as a way to reim-agine, rework, or reclaim their traumatic experiences (Hammers, 2013, 2019; Thomas, 2020). Hammers' ethnographic and interview study with survivors who engage in trauma reenactments notes,

> These are reenactments as opposed to replications, as this is not a repetition
> of an original trauma—as if that were possible. Rather, these reenactments
> of lived trauma are performative scenes of consensual violence where the
> critical role of fantasy is front and center. This is a reworking, a working out
> of trauma as S/M transfigures the unbearable suffering of violence—sexual

and/or gender trauma—into something more bearable. (Hammers, 2019, pp. 491–492)

Hammers (2013, 2019) has argued that certain erotic practices transcend language and that, when enabled by certain necessary social conditions for engaging safely, can reconfigure embodied trauma. Similarly, Thomas' (2020) ethnographic investigation into trauma play describes the practice as intentionally participating in a BDSM activity or scene that in some way plays with a person's previous experiences of trauma. Thomas (2020) calls for more research into the practice and the mechanisms through which healing may or may not occur. We suggest that communication is at the center of such mechanisms.

Thematic to these innovative understandings of trauma play is the notion that, perhaps contrary to common understanding, subspace can be particularly empowering (Meeker et al., 2020, p. 1594; Pitagora, 2017). Outside of specifically traumatic re-creations, people who have survived sexual assault may participate in BDSM activities and can find comfort in role-based activities. Indeed, research suggests that many people find empowerment in the intense embodiment of submissive roles (Baker, 2018; Newmahr, 2008, 2010; Pitagora, 2017); the notions of trust, safety, and respect that can accompany particular experiences in subspace (Cinquino, 2020); as well as the physiological reduction of stress in certain cases (Pitagora, 2017, p. 51). Research on professional dominatrices finds that many view themselves as providing a therapeutic service (Lindemann, 2011). As we will elaborate on in the following section, an important distinction in the positive experiences associated with BDSM and traumatic experiences that may manifest similarly is rooted in the meaning-making processes surrounding consent (Pitagora, 2017, p. 49).

A Communicology Approach to Sexuality: Communication as a Tool for Understanding

Although rarely the focus of communication studies scholarship, we suggest that the conditions under which trauma play, or other BDSM activities, may be beneficial to some sexual assault survivors are largely communicative. Beyond the concession that sexual activity and relational closeness are communicative phenomena (Manning, 2014, p. 263), conditions for safe play, such as establishing boundaries and safe words, are verbal communication behaviors (Rubinsky, 2018, 2020). While the particular effects of embodiment might transcend verbal language (Hammers, 2013, p. 68), embodiment is a form of non-verbal communication; and we suggest that the circumstances that necessitate safe play are grounded firmly in communication as a meaning-making process (Rubinsky, 2018). A holistic approach to connecting the experiences of sexual and personal well-being to communicating sex and sexuality may be found in Manning's (2014) holistic communicology of sexuality. Manning (2014, p. 271) reminds us that communication constitutes relationships and of the connections between communication as constitutive and relational and overall well-being. Manning's communicology approach is discipline-specific (i.e., similar to sociological or psychological approaches to the examination of a phenomenon, a communicology approach centers on the discipline of communication as a perspective) but aims to provide a framework broad enough to be useful outside the discipline as well (2014, p. 263). Manning's perspective draws on a view of communication that is constitutive (2014, p. 270), that is, focused not on the process of information transmission but on the process of meaning-making in interactions. The communicology approach positions communication, especially interpersonal communication, as a part of any holistic understanding of sexuality because communication, according to this view, constitutes relationships (Manning, 2014, p. 271). Specifically, Manning calls for more research into the ways that different cultural groups "Create meaning and social structures and healthy sexual practices via communication" (Manning, 2014, p. 278).

While scholars outside of the discipline of communication studies critique the notions of consent as purely communicative (Bauer, 2020), and even those within the discipline acknowledge the limitations and utility of strictly verbal understandings of consent amid an increasingly complicated sexual landscape even for vanilla relationships (Hanebutt, 2021, p. 101), we suggest that a perspective of consent as communicative embraces definitions of communication that expand beyond an understanding of it as only language. A disciplinary perspective on communication often considers all interactional behaviors to have message value and therefore to be communication (Watzlawick et al., 1967). Communication is a process that also consists of the contexts the message is embedded within as this is a component of the meaning-making process (Watzlawick et al., 1967). For example, a difference of power or status impacts the meaning of a verbal or non-verbal message, comprising a component of the communication process. An understanding of communication as a meaning-making process thus both considers the messages themselves and the context(s) in which they are embedded. This is the perspective from which we approach the remainder of the chapter. However, we acknowledge that others may disagree that factors such as social hierarchy, structural barriers, or the personal will fall under the purview of communication.

As others have noted, consent conversations in BDSM are complicated and can even sometimes be erotic (Barker, 2013, pp. 896, 904). Communication encompasses both language and other concrete, verbal aspects of meaning-making such as a safe words (Beres & MacDonald, 2015; Kaak, 2016, p. 50) or obtaining verbal consent as aspects of BDSM (Pitagora, 2013, p. 33) but also includes listening (Pitagora, 2013); non-verbal communication such as touch, reacting to non-verbal cues, and use of space (Floyd et al., 2009); and combinations of both verbal and non-verbal communication to provide safety, clarity, or comfort. In one study, Kaak (2016) examined the specific conversational phases of consent negotiation processes in BDSM. Importantly, Kaak notes that navigating these conversations requires a degree of "social proficiency" to ensure "that the locally produced understandings of certain terms can be agreed upon" (p. 50). In contrast, a communicology perspective might describe Kaak's understanding of social proficiency as communication competence, specifically interpersonal communication competence, which is understood as one's ability to engage in meaning-making activities that are personally effective and socially appropriate (Hecht, 1978). Kaak (2016, p. 50) found that those with greater proficiency are able to help those with lesser proficiencies navigate these conversations.

A plethora of previous research outside the scope of this chapter argues that consent plays an important role in understanding BDSM interactions, but consent may also manifest in ways that differ from mainstream understandings of "yes means yes" in the context of BDSM interactions (Fanghanel, 2020, p. 269; Hanebutt, 2021; Pitagora, 2013). An understanding of communication as a collaborative meaning-making process enables us to explore both the instances of safety that emerge in language and those that manifest in listening, touch, or even a look. This nuance is especially important in the context of BDSM, where, dependent upon the perspectives of those involved, language can take on wholly different meanings (Pitagora, 2017, p. 45). For instance, Pitagora (2013, p. 34) discusses that one means through which BDSM practitioners accomplish consent and shared meaning, especially those who might prefer rape play or other forms of trauma play, is through the negotiation of specific scripts. While this negotiation in practice may take verbal and non-verbal means, the emphasis is on shared meaning-making, a communication activity.

Identity, Community, and Trauma

Of course, while this chapter explores the mechanisms through which certain individuals who have experienced sexual trauma and who participate in BDSM might facilitate healing through communication practices, the BDSM community is not immune from non-consensual encounters or being the source of one's sexual assault or relational trauma experience. The National Coalition for Sexual Freedom's Consent Survey in 2012 found that 33% of those within a power exchange context indicated that their pre-negotiated limit had been violated or safe word ignored during a BDSM encounter (Wright et al., 2012), indicating that the prevalence of this is not sparse. Pitagora (2016, p. 95) notes that individuals who are members of the BDSM community and experience sexual violence within the context of those relationships may face an intersectionality of stigmatization, especially in cases where consensual dominance/submission activities become conflated with abuse.

Another perspective can be found in Holt (2015b), who describes the embedded protective and predatory processes facilitated by BDSM. Holt suggests that protective elements are largely comprised of more explicit, verbal scripting of consent, verbal negotiations, wide support systems, communicating needs and boundaries verbally and explicitly, and emphasizing transparency and responsibility. The support systems embedded in safe communities may facilitate learning of healing practices, a subject the present study will further explore. Holt (2015a) has also emphasized that boundary violations do occur even in negotiated encounters. Similarly, Fanghanel's (2020, p. 269) recent research on BDSM consent narratives highlights that boundary violations occur within the community and that unequal power relations and hierarchies are embedded within contexts that necessitate obtaining consent, making the process anything but straightforward.

One of the authors of this chapter, Alejandre Rodriguez, brings forth a perspective that comes from personal experience as a survivor of childhood sexual abuse with clinically diagnosed post-traumatic stress disorder (PTSD) and from doing in-group research on LGBT populations about the communication of intimacy within non-normative committed relationships. Gleaming from community knowledge and trauma-informed research, Rodriguez recommends a trauma-informed lens on BDSM, which may be a more meaningful way forward for the communities that need healing from sexual assault. Rodriguez (personal communication) laments at the prevalence of sexual trauma among transgender people: "I seldom meet a transgender person who did not confess to me about their sexual trauma upon first meeting, it is deeply embedded in our identities and as a part of the transgender community." Diverse sexual and gender minority populations within the BDSM community bring an intersection of experiences and sometimes trauma to their own meaning-making processes. Of course, Rodriguez's experience and that of participants from their own research studies is not representative of all transgender and gender-non-conforming people. While transgender people experience sexual assault at a higher rate than the general population (US Department of Justice, 2014), we do not suggest it is a universal experience.

In summary, previous scholarship on the role of trauma play and other forms of consensual non-consent and trauma re-creation focus on embodiment, feminist ethics, and affect. We also explore the role of communication as meaning-making in understanding consent. These important insights shed light on often very private processes, but the present study extends them to focus on the specific communication behaviors involved in healing or harm that may come with BDSM play for people who have survived sexual assault and where community practices can inform communication behaviors.

Methods

Sample

Participants included a subset of volunteers from a larger study who identified, to some degree, as practitioners of BDSM ($n = 39$), with six of those participants also identifying as polyamorous. Ages ranged from 18 to 44 ($M = 26.54$, $SD = 6.53$). Most participants were white ($n = 29$, 78.4%), while others were Asian or Pacific Islander ($n = 4$, 10.8%), Hispanic or Latinx

(n = 2, 5.4%), or of two or more races (n = 2, 5.4%). About half of participants identified as cisgender women (n = 19, 47.5%) with the rest identifying as transgender women (n = 4, 10.8%), transgender men (n = 6, 16.2%), genderqueer (n = 1, 2.7%), non-binary (n = 4, 10.8%), or otherwise under the transgender or gender-non-conforming umbrella (n = 3, 8.1%). In terms of sexual orientation, participants mostly identified as bisexual (n = 17, 45.95), as well as gay or lesbian (n = 13.5%), heterosexual (n = 5, 13.5%), pansexual (n = 4, 10.8%), asexual spectrum (n = 3, 8.1%), or otherwise under the LGBQ umbrella (n = 3, 8.1%). This was an internet survey. Geographic location of participants was not collected, but the questionnaire and responses were all in English. It should be noted that not all participants consistently provided demographic information (e.g., some participants wrote their age but left out their gender or sexual orientation, some indicated their gender but not their race). As a result, we did not consider these identities specifically as a component of our analysis.

Recruitment and Procedure

The data presented in this chapter is a subset of a larger online survey, hosted on Qualtrics.com, that asked for women and people of diverse genders to respond to questions about their sexual and reproductive health communication. The questionnaire took approximately 45 minutes to complete, and participants had the option to include an email address to be entered into a raffle to win one of 50 Amazon gift cards worth $10 for participation. Participants were recruited from various social media sites, including the US-based researchers' Facebook, Instagram, and Twitter pages; the /sample size, /women, and /lgbt subreddit forums on Reddit.com; and other web spaces. The subset presented in this chapter includes participants who identified that they are part of the BDSM communities, with several participants who were also polyamorous.

If respondents volunteered to participate, they were directed to an online consent form where they were informed of their rights as a research participant and could read a short description of the study's aims and goals. If they consented to participate, they were then taken to the survey. The open-ended survey questions addressed in this chapter asked participants if they believed there were any practices affiliated with the BDSM community that have helped them or others recover from sexual trauma and, if so, to describe them. In addition, they were asked how, if applicable, they learned of those practices. No quantitative questions were included. All responses address how, if at all, affiliation with BDSM practices, identity, or community have helped them or others they know recover from sexual trauma and how, if applicable, they learned of those practices.

Data Analysis

To address the research question, we utilized Owen's thematic analysis (Owen, 1984) as a guide to analyze the qualitative data. The first author read through the data twice and created a loose codebook based on in vivo themes, primarily preserving participant language. Next, the first author used Owen's conditions to thematize the codes, using repetition, recurrence, or forcefulness as a condition for a theme (Owen, 1984). All three authors read the themes with the entire data set, and the findings reflect 100% agreement between all authors. The findings represent the research team's interpretation of participant responses to the questions asked. See below, "Limitations and Future Research," for considerations about this methodology and sample.

Findings and Discussion

Sixty-six open-ended survey responses addressed their perceptions of practices affiliated with the BDSM community and their association to sexual trauma recovery, as well as how, if at all, they learned about that information. Participants describe (1) safety and control as elements of BDSM that enable recovery, (2) the centrality of communication to BDSM, and (3) performing and reclaiming spaces of trauma as communication tools embedded in kinky communities. Four participants also identified that no practices affiliated with BDSM were useful for anyone in sexual assault recovery, and three suggested that the community was actively harmful to their recovery. Many participants spoke from their own experience as an individual who had experienced sexual assault, rape, or other forms of relational trauma. Other participants shared observations of friends, community members, or their general opinions about the relationship and sexual practices' potential within BDSM communities. Given the relatively small size of the sample and data, we included both first-hand experiences and second-hand experiences (i.e., those recounted by others). Since all participants had experienced sexual assault in some capacity and answered the question we asked with either first-hand experience or their perspective on general community practices, we interpreted both types of response as addressing the research question. However, we acknowledge that there are differences between those who have experienced it themselves and those who are expressing their opinion on others' experiences.

Safety and Control

First, participants described BDSM practices as enabling them to exert control over sexual situations, thereby increasing their sense of safety. Examples of safe practices include having and practicing use of safe words and being listened to when safe words are utilized or boundaries are communicated. For example, this participant said,

> Yes! It helped a lot in two ways. Sometimes I'm a sub, and will get to experience a controlled loss of control—I always can use my safe word, so I get to experience things in a safe way. I even have practiced just going through and using the safe word every minute or so just to get accustomed to being listened to, to being able to say stop. On the other hand, I'm sometimes the dom, and it gives me a sense of control I've never had before. It allows me to feel in charge of my sexuality and not subject to the whims of someone else. (Participant 8)

Participants identified feeling a sense of control from more submissive and more dominant roles in BDSM play. The above participant highlights the "controlled loss of control," or getting to safely experience a loss of control in a particular environment that feels safe, as well as getting to be in control in a more dominant role that was unlike what they might experience in other relational settings. For another example, one participant echoed, "Yes, feeling like a dominatrix was therapeutic because I felt like I regained control over my sexual life" (Participant 35); and in contrast, another participant noted, "As someone with trauma, being a sub allows for me to know that I have complete control over what I allow to happen to my body" (Participant 12). Thus, both being listened to from more submissive positions and the feelings of control in domination enabled participants to enact control in their sexuality. Similar to previous research (Damm et al., 2018), people find feelings of empowerment in a number of BDSM roles. For those in both dominant and submissive roles, the empowerment came from feeling a sense of control over their sexual lives and bodies.

In addition to speaking generally about control, participants generally discussed feeling safe or that safety was an important concept in BDSM. For example, "The concept of safety in BDSM is so important, and I believe it would transfer well to those with sexual trauma, even outside of the community" (Participant 12). Thus, while control may function as a specific form of safety, others noted that safety itself is an important concept in BDSM. As others have noted (Hammers, 2013), certain conditions, including a sense of safety, are necessary to enable survivors to enjoy and grow from play.

Centering Communication

A more specific means of enacting safety and control in BDSM relationships occurs in communication. Participants largely characterized kink practices as a set of communication tools that enable many healthy relationship practices but may be particularly beneficial to those recovering from sexual or relational trauma. Specifically, participants pointed to boundary-setting, needs communication, negotiation, listening, and consent. Others more generally noted open and honest communication. For example,

> Things such as communication and boundary settings are essential to this community. Without proper communication and boundary settings someone can easily get hurt. Through communication one also gets to not only learn more about their partner, but also about themselves. (Participant 14)

Similarly, another participant noted, "Yes. The ideas of discussing boundaries and really valuing consent (for example safe words) was very helpful" (Participant 16). Thus, boundary-setting and using safe words were of particular importance.

Boundary-setting, then, for these participants functioned as an aspect of BDSM that enabled sexual assault and relational trauma recovery and suggested embodying healthier relational behaviors outside of sexual settings. Boundary-setting is well established as an important practice in both sexual assault recovery (Czerny & Lassiter, 2016) and BDSM play (Kattari, 2015; Pitagora, 2013; Rubinsky, 2018). The present study reinforces that boundary-setting involves a set of communication behaviors that reinforce (or, in its absence, undermine) the safety of a particular encounter and further distinguishes that encounter from traumatic experiences. In other words, it is in communicating safety through mechanisms like boundary-setting, setting and utilizing safe words, needs communication, and both the verbal and non-verbal components of aftercare that not only distinguish trauma play from actual trauma but can make it, for these participants, a space of growth and empowerment that even facilitates reinvigorating a sense of agency important to relational and sexual trauma recovery. While others have argued that embodiment is a component of, constitutive of, or simply is communication (Marvin, 2006), such discussions are outside the scope of this chapter. Instead, we attend to the ways that concrete verbal and non-verbal communication behaviors such as safe words, obtaining verbal consent, checking in, and providing comfort are enacted in communication.

Others described communication behaviors, generally or specifically, that they felt were healthy and conducive to their own or others' recovery from relational trauma or sexual assault. For example, this participant noted, "Yes, absolutely. Due to the nature of BDSM, you have to check in with your partner periodically to make sure they are ok, and you have to talk beforehand about your boundaries and negotiate limits" (Participant 10). For another example,

> My experiences in the BDSM community has [sic] always involved a strong practice of almost aggressively open communication. Even casual partners will sit down and discuss needs, boundaries, and what each expects from the encounter. Consent and physical/emotional safety is [sic] discussed and respected with great enthusiasm. Anyone unwilling to practice this is seen as untrustworthy and possibly dangerous. (Participant 22)

Similarly, another participant wrote, "Needs communication and boundary setting have helped [with sexual assault recovery], as has education about consent, safewords, learning to negotiate consent, and requiring explicit consent at all stages of contact and play" (Participant 34).

In all, participants described a series of communication behaviors (e.g., consent, safe words, boundary-setting, needs communication) as well as general feelings about communication (e.g., be open) that characterize their BDSM encounters as safe. Importantly, participants highlighted not only the verbal processes of communication like explicit negotiation, consent, boundary-setting, and safe words but recalled listening and being listened to as particularly helpful communication behaviors that both facilitate safer encounters generally and their own sexual assault recovery specifically. Being listened to and feeling their words were respected (see Participant 8's excerpt above, in "Safety and Control" and Participant 13's later in "Disassociating and Reclaiming Sex Acts from Trauma") are so drastically different from the experiences of assault that, for some participants, it felt therapeutic (see Participant 12's excerpt above, in "Safety and Control"). Of course, listening and being listened to involve questions of power. In sexual assault, individuals may communicate their refusal and not be respected. When describing what made these experiences safe for them, participants indicated that knowing that if they communicated refusal (e.g., saying stop or using a safe word), they would be listened to. For instance, as with the earlier participant, some practiced using their safe words or communicating refusal, which helped them realize the distinctions between healthy and unhealthy contexts. Another participant (Participant 27) indicated that these both model healthy (or, by comparison to an old relationship, healthier) relationship behaviors as well as provide a toolkit for negotiating and maintaining safe encounters. In addition, some participants echoed that these practices gave them feelings of control and let them feel safe in and reclaim their sexuality after a traumatic encounter or relationship. For example, one participant reflected both the importance of boundary-setting and needs communication and explained why they might be useful, as well as reiterating that feeling in control through certain roles was important after experiencing relational trauma:

> Pre-intimacy boundary-setting and needs communication, after care (These help make a safe space emotionally to let one be open to intimacy and prevent triggering abuse flashbacks, etc. And it helps work through ALL of the emotions attached to intimacy, the good, the bad, and everything else.) safe words, learning proper safe sex practices, learning how to use sex toys (these are learning how to have safe sex again, and helping one learn how to not need a partner to achieve sexual satisfaction), role play/ power dynamic play (I am a casual dominatrix and that has helped me feel in control of my intimate life after my abusive relationship). (Participant 27)

We elaborate on how specific BDSM acts may help dissociate and reclaim specific sex acts from traumatic experiences in the next section.

Disassociating and Reclaiming Sex Acts from Trauma

Although a smaller number of participants, several described either themselves or generally hearing about individuals re-creating or performing sex acts or play scenes similar to their traumatic encounters as a means of sense-making and coping. Similar to Hammers (2013, 2019) and Thomas (2020), participants in the present study echoed that trauma play could be particularly empowering when safe. Consider Weille (2002), Weiss (2011), and Bauer (2014, p. 102) for more, especially in regard to incest play. For example, "yes, sometimes safe loving play in scenes that are somewhat similar to traumatic times can help re-open the mind to the positive possibilities, and not everything needs to be associated to the trauma" (Participant 15).

In addition, participants grappled with what it meant to enjoy types of trauma play and what communication behaviors specifically contribute to making the encounter safe and helpful or triggering:

> Communication and boundaries are really useful for everyone. They probably help survivors feel safer. I have also heard anecdotally that some survivors engage in BDSM practices that re-create their abuse in order to make the memory less painful, however I have not personally known anyone who does this. (Participant 4)

As this participant noted, this was an experience they have heard from others but not experienced themselves.

Participants also echoed that consent, safety, communication, and control enable them to make important distinctions between safe play scenes and unsafe, traumatic encounters. This was particularly important for survivors who may have initially felt guilt over consensual non-consent kinks. For example,

> For me, it's the consent. Being able to have control of a situation similar to my abuse made me feel more in control in general. I always was into BDSM, so there was a lot of conflict between the fact I like non-consent roleplay and fantasies and having been actually raped. I was afraid I somehow gave indication I wanted it, or that I enjoyed it. I orgasmed several times when my ex would rape me. BDSM gave me a way to fantasize and act out those desires without feeling guilty. The community helped me realize that it didn't matter if I gave out subconscious signals, or even if I did enjoy it

sometimes. It's not my fault, because being into rape doesn't actually mean consent doesn't matter, and you can't be raped. (Participant 13)

Thus, participants described using BDSM to disassociate sex acts from trauma, minimize the pain associated with the memories, and, for survivors, exert control and agency in spaces where that was taken from them.

Appropriate BDSM practice requires consent, and consent is given through performance to indicate willful participation in every moment. Communication of cues, safe words, and expected responses to them must be negotiated between partners before practicing either role. Theater directors agree that the secret to treating people with PTSD through performance is to go slow and engage them bit by bit, moment to moment (Van Der Kolk, 2014). The communication of consent, desire, and enjoyment can be the sub's continuous use of *mistress/master* as a way of saying *I'm still playing along and want to continue*. Common safe words like *yellow* and *red* are out of context for sex, so they communicate explicitly *I do not consent*, whereas *stop* or *no* can still be part of play. During impact play, if the dom increases their use of force, a sudden *yellow* communicates a *yield/slow down*; and the dom may be expected to continue the act but with less force than the force that stimulated the safe word. This allows the sub to stay in the moment while exerting control over the situation, enabling them to embrace their own sexual agency and determine if, when, and what is allowed to happen to their body. For example, if a sub were to say "red," the dom may be expected to halt a specific act or stop the role play altogether. This ensures that the sub remains fully in control and always has a choice to end the role play if they desire to do so. Moment-to-moment evaluation of every act ensures that the trauma play is enjoyable and willful and only further establishes trust between partners, bearing in mind that any movement may carry painful memories for survivors' bodies.

BDSM Doesn't Help

Only a handful of participants indicated that BDSM/kink was explicitly unhelpful in their own or others' sexual trauma recovery. Of these, some participants indicated that the community often performs a sense of enlightenment that they do not actually possess, or they had personally unsafe experiences in that community. For example, "Nothing for me yet.

Community mostly unsafe for me, most kinky partners make assumptions even when they say they won't/don't hold themselves accountable to boundaries" (Participant 7), as well as,

> Honestly not really it's kinda fucked me up worse bc I'll say I have xyz boundaries and have partners who consistently cross them, so wtf is the point of acting like ur so much more enlightened cuz ur in the kink/poly community and have sexual discussions if u don't actually follow the shit in those discussions??? (Participant 20)

The present study did not investigate the details of an individual's trauma experiences (or if they stemmed from inside or outside of the BDSM community), which is a limitation. Thus, while most participants in this study identified kink as a tool in recovering from sexual trauma, others did note that it was a part of their trauma or not a particularly safe space for them.

Identity, Community, and Learning Communication Tools

In addition to investigating what communication tools might help individuals in these communities recover from sexual or relational trauma, the present study investigated how, if at all, participants recalled learning about these tools. Some participants described learning about (1) needs fulfillment and other forms of community exposure as acts of healing, but most others identified (2) research and reading, (3) online communities, or (4) general relational experiences.

Needs Fulfillment and Community Exposure

Exposure to the BDSM community through fulfilling particular needs and desires enabled participants to learn about practices that they ultimately found healing. For example,

> I was into BDSM before being raped. Found it through porn and ended up becoming part of the community. After the rapes I learned that some

people in the community used it as a way to help get over their trauma. Kind of like exposure therapy. It's been pretty useful. (Participant 8)

Similarly, this participant noted,

I was interested in BDSM before I was assaulted so mostly I'd say I kind of stumbled upon it as a healing practice. I also briefly dated someone who was a pro dom and also does sexual healing type practices and they introduced me to some things. (Participant 16)

For these participants, BDSM itself and immersion in the community were healing practices that they found through fulfilling personal needs. On a similar note, this participant wrote,

The practice is actually something I'd discovered as my own personal need, and set out looking for sexual practices that fulfilled that. The intricacies of how it works in the BDSM community specifically I learned by talking to more experienced practitioners. (Participant 22)

Thus, some participants did not learn about a specific practice or tool, but rather exposure to the larger community and learning to fulfill their own needs served as forms of healing.

Research, Reading, and Online Communities

Although in typically shorter responses, the vast majority of participants identified "research" or "online" as the means through which they learned practices that could assist themselves or others in sexual assault recovery. For some, these were straightforward: "I did research on BDSM and how to stay safe while doing it" (Participant 10) as well as "Researching on the internet, watching movies and videos, reading articles, identifying myself and embodying the way a dominatrix behaves towards her subs" (Participant 35).

For sexual minorities (e.g., gay/lesbian, bisexual, genderqueer, genderfluid, pansexual) and BDSM communities, finding content in online social media platforms is often described as more comfortable, less judgmental, and more inclusive of unique and different ways to approach sex and sexuality. For many, online spaces allow for more transparency, often embracing nuances of how an individual negotiates their sexuality and sex acts. For instance, one study found that queer focus group members were motivated to use online resources specifically because it felt safer and free of stigma and that the information being shared was interconnected and from multiple perspectives (Flanders et al., 2017).

Echoing previous research that confirms the frequent use of online or technology-mediated communication tools by people who practice BDSM (Rubinsky, 2018, 2020), others in the present study, most of whom were under the LGBTQ umbrella, identified finding community online, reading what others shared in online spaces, or particular online spaces as teaching tools. For example, "Online communities (i.e., fetlife)" (Participant 13), as well as "Internet communities" (Participant 19). These participants elaborated, "Online BDSM communities and safe sexual educational tools for adults like ohjoysextoy.com, and planned parenthood and forums like reddit for kink groups like swingers and the BDSM community" (Participant 27) and "Online; I got to see how people in the communities actually act and interact with each other" (Participant 40). Thus, it seems that many individuals who learned communication practices in BDSM that enabled forms of healing and recovery from sexual or relational trauma learned those practices either through personal research or immersion in online communal spaces. Although not all participants referenced identifying or experiencing affective attachments to the BDSM community, many indicated that community exposure in one way or another influenced these experiences for them. This was especially true of participants who highlighted learning communication tools that were more specific to the BDSM community (e.g., safe words). However, many others specified that a particular online community (or, generally, online communities), rather than a more ambiguous general BDSM community, was where this involvement occurred.

Relational Experience

Lastly, participants described experiences in (mostly healthy) relationships with others who practiced BDSM as how they learned particular tools and practices that aided recovery. For example, "Experience with a healthier relationship" (Participant 11), "with trusting and trusted lovers and doms" (Participant 15), "Partners that care and that I trust as humans" (Participant 25), and "a previous partner introduced me" (Participant 30). While most participants who identified specific partners as their source of learning did not elaborate on how or what specifically they learned, it seems that relational experience may be a means of learning and adopting practices individuals perceive as helpful in recovering from sexual or relational trauma.

Limitations and Future Research

While we believe this exploratory study provides a useful discussion, the methodology limits our ability to draw broad-scale conclusions from a relatively small sample size. In addition, open-ended survey data does not allow us to ask participants follow-up questions where warranted or to make variable analytic connections. Participants responded to a question on their perceptions about the connections between BDSM and sexual assault recovery. Many participants responded with accounts that were not their own. We chose to interpret this as their genuine response to our question, even if it was not initially our intention. Due to this methodological limitation, we cannot draw conclusions about the context(s) of the participants' accounts beyond their response. As noted, many of these responses are hearsay rather than first-hand experience. The excerpts and analysis reflect our research team's reading of their responses; but given the methodology and limited data for this sample of participants, we cannot make wide-scale or generalizable conclusions.

Conclusion

Commonly, although this is perhaps fading, assumptions about BDSM mistakenly define the practice as a selfish and violent kink, which purely enables men's abuse over women's bodies and psyche. This assumption is largely informed by Hollywood and the pornography industry, which are closely associated industries notorious for their profiteering motives and chauvinist values. Counter to these less reliable understandings of BDSM, in his studies on treatment for PTSD, Van Der Kolk (2014) found that trauma can be treated through performances (such as role playing) that inspire imagination and mental flexibility that is lost in trauma survivors who feel stuck in the past. In theater and in trauma, confrontation of the painful realities of life prompts symbolic transformation through action. Love and hate, aggression and surrender, loyalty and betrayal are at play in trauma and in theater. While engaging in BDSM, survivors are physically and psychologically vulnerable for the sake of exploring and enjoying new ways of engaging with their bodies and their partners without becoming overwhelmed. They can allow their bodies to feel a loss of control while remaining engaged and embodying different roles, therefore alleviating physiological reactions to once traumatizing acts—either by subordinating oneself to another or by leading an experience for a vulnerable person, both of which are terrifying for people with post-traumatic stress. Thus, a trauma-informed lens on communication within BDSM practices has the potential to function as a process for treating post-traumatic stress from sexual assault—by activating old sensations and reassembling old information into new non-traumatic experiences where survivors have a sense of agency, engagement, and commitment through ownership of body and mind (Van Der Kolk, 2014).

Consistent with some previous research, community may help foster the necessary communication competencies to enable safe play. Communication behaviors that facilitate safe BDSM play, such as boundary-setting and safe words, are useful sexual assault recovery tools for people who have experienced sexual trauma (Czerny & Lassiter, 2016). For practitioners of BDSM, an expanded sexual and linguistic toolkit (Kattari, 2015, p. 883) for sexual reclamation and empowerment may accompany their experiences in the community or their relationships. Although not everyone who has been sexually assaulted and practices BDSM may find the play therapeutic or have any desire to engage in forms of trauma play, there are communication conditions under which participants in the present study found the practices to enable healing.

Note

1. This chapter uses the terms *kink* and *BDSM* as synonyms.

References

Auerbach, C. F., & Silverstein, L. B. (2003). *Qualitative data: An introduction to coding and analysis*. New York University Press.

Baker, A. C. (2018). Sacred kink: Finding psychological meaning at the intersection of BDSM and spiritual experience. *Sexual and Relationship Therapy*, *33*(4), 440–453. http://doi.org/10.1080/14681994.2016.1205185

Barker, M. (2013). Consent is a grey area? A comparison of understandings of consent in Fifty Shades of Grey and on the BDSM blogosphere. *Sexualities, 16*(8), 896–914. http://doi.org/10.1177/1363460713508881

Bauer, R. (2014). *Queer BDSM intimacies: Critical consent and pushing boundaries.* Springer.

Bauer, R. (2020). Queering consent: Negotiating critical consent in les-bi-trans-queer BDSM contexts. *Sexualities, 24*(5–6), 767–783. http://doi.org/10.1177/1363460720973902

Beres, M. A., & MacDonald, J. E. (2015). Talking about sexual consent: Heterosexual women and BDSM. *Australian Feminist Studies, 30*(86), 418–432. http://doi.org/10.1080/08164649.2016.1158692

Birks, M. & Mills, J. (2011). *Grounded theory: A practical guide.* London: Sage Publications.

Boeri, M.W. (2007). Exposing the "Pretty Woman" myth: A qualitative investigation of street-level prostituted women. *Journal of Marriage and Family, 69*(3), 889–890.

Cinquino, V. (2020). *BDSM as performance: The experience of empowerment in the "submissive" role* [Major research paper]. University of Ottawa. Retrieved August 1 2020, from http://hdl.handle.net/10393/40612

Czerny, A. B., & Lassiter, P. S. (2016). Healing from intimate partner violence: An empowerment wheel to guide the recovery journey. *Journal of Creativity in Mental Health, 11*(3–4), 311–324. https://doi.org/10.1080/15401383.2016.1222321

Damm, C., Dentato, M. P., & Busch, N. (2018). Unravelling intersecting identities: Understanding the lives of people who practice BDSM. *Psychology & Sexuality, 9*(1), 21–37. http://doi.org/10.1080/19419899.2017.1410854

DeCuir-Gunby, J. T., Marshall, P. L., & McCulloch, A. W. (2011). Developing and using a codebook for the analysis of interview data: An Example from a professional development research project. *Field Methods, 23*(2), 136–155. https://doiorg.proxy2.cl.msu.edu/10.1177/1525822X10388468

Fanghanel, A. (2020). Asking for it: BDSM sexual practice and the trouble of consent. *Sexualities, 23*(3), 269–286. http://doi.org/10.1177/1363460719828933

Flanders, C. E., LeBreton, M. E., Robinson, M., Bian, J., & Caravaca-Morera, J. A. (2017). Defining bisexuality: Young bisexual and pansexual people's voices. *Journal of Bisexuality, 17*(1), 39–57. http://doi.org/10.1080/15299716.2016.1227016

Floyd, K., Boren, J. P., Hannawa, A. F., Hesse, C., McEwan, B., & Veksler, A. E. (2009). Kissing in marital and cohabiting relationships: Effects on blood lipids, stress, and relationship satisfaction. *Western Journal of Communication, 73*(2), 113–133. http://doi.org/10.1080/10570310902856071

Gemberling, T. M., Cramer, R. J., Wright, S., & Nobles, M. R. (2015). *Psychological functioning and violence victimization and perpetration in BDSM practitioners from the National Coalition for Sexual Freedom* (Technical report). National Coalition for Sexual Freedom. Retrieved August 1, 2020, from https://www.ncsfreedom.org/wp-content/uploads/2019/12/Psychological-Functioning-and-Violence-Victimization-and-Perpetration-in-BDSM-Practitioners.pdf

Hammers, C. (2013). Corporeality, sadomasochism and sexual trauma. *Body & Society, 20*(2), 68–90. http://doi.org/10.1177/1357034X13477159

Hammers, C. (2019). Reworking trauma through BDSM. *Signs: Journal of Women in Culture and Society, 44*(2), 491–514. http://doi.org/10.1086/699370

Hanebutt, R. (2021). Beyond the binaries of sexual consent: Developing consent identities through diversification of sexual messaging. In A. Cooke-Jackson & V. Rubinsky (Eds.), *Communicating Intimate Health* (pp. 99–117). Rowman & Littlefield.

Hecht, M. (1978). Measures of communication satisfaction. *Human Communication Research, 4,* 350–368.

Hitter, T. L., Adams, E. M., & Cahill, E. J. (2017). Positive sexual self-schemas of women survivors of childhood sexual abuse. *The Counseling Psychologist, 45*(2), 266–293. http://doi.org/10.1177/0011000017697194

Holt, K. (2015a). Blacklisted: Boundaries, violations, and retaliatory behavior in the BDSM community. *Deviant Behavior, 37*(8), 917–930. http://doi.org/10.1080/01639 625.2016.1156982

Holt, K. M. (2015b). *Negotiating limits: Boundary management in the bondage/discipline/sadomasochism (BDSM) community* [Doctoral dissertation, City University of New York]. CUNY Academic Works. Retrieved August 1, 2020, from https://academ icworks.cuny.edu/gc_etds/976

Kaak, A. (2016). Conversational phases in BDSM pre-scene negotiations. *Journal of Positive Sexuality, 2*(3), 47–52.

Kattari, S. K. (2015). "Getting it": Identity and sexual communication for sexual and gender minorities with physical disabilities. *Sexuality & Culture, 19*(4), 882–899. http://doi.org/10.1007/s12119-015-9298-x

Krueger, R. B. (2010). The DSM diagnostic criteria for sexual masochism. *Archives of Sexual Behavior, 39*(2), 346–356. http://doi.org/10.1007/s10508-010-9613-4

Langdridge, D. (2007). Speaking the unspeakable: S/M and the eroticization of pain. In D. Langdridge & M. Barker (Eds.), *Safe, sane, and consensual: Contemporary perspectives on sadomasochism* (pp. 85–97). Prometheus Books.

Lindemann, D. (2011). BDSM as therapy? *Sexualities, 14*(2), 151–172. http://doi.org/ 10.1177/1363460711399038

Manning, J. (2014). Communication and healthy sexual practices: Toward a holistic communicology of sexuality. In M. H. Eaves (Ed.), *Applications in health communication: Emerging trends* (pp. 263–286). Kendall-Hunt.

Marvin, C. (2006). Communication as embodiment. In G. J. Shepherd, J. St. John, & T. Striphas (Eds.), *Communication as . . . perspectives on theory* (pp. 67–74). Sage.

Meeker, C., McGill, C. M., & Rocco, T. S. (2020). Navigation of feminist and submissive identity by women in the BDSM community: A structured literature review. *Sexuality & Culture, 24,* 1594–1618. http://doi.org/10.1007/s12119-019-09681-9

Moser, C. (2009). When is an unusual sexual interest a mental disorder? *Archives of Sexual Behavior, 38*(3), 323–325. http://doi.org/10.1007/s10508-008-9436-8

Newmahr, S. (2008). Becoming a sadomasochist: Integrating self and other in ethnographic analysis. *Journal of Contemporary Ethnography, 37*(5), 619–643. http://doi.org/ 10.1177/0891241607310626

Newmahr, S. (2010). Power struggles: Pain and authenticity in SM play. *Symbolic Interaction, 33*(3), 389–411. http://doi.org/10.1525/si.2010.33.3.389

Nichter, M., Quintero, G., Nichter, M., Mock, J., & Shakib, S. (2004). Qualitative research: contributions to the study of drug use, drug abuse, and drug use(r)-related interventions. *Substance Use & Misuse, 39*(10-12), 1907–1969. https://doi.org/10.1081/ ja-200033233

Owen, W. F. (1984). Interpretive themes in relational communication. *Quarterly Journal of Speech, 70*(3), 274–287. http://doi.org/10.1080/00335638409383697

Pitagora, D. (2013). Consent vs. coercion: BDSM interactions highlight a fine but immutable line. *The New School Psychology Bulletin, 10*(1), 27–36. Retrieved August 1, 2020, from http://www.nspb.net/index.php/nspb/article/view/180

Pitagora, D. (2016). Intimate partner violence in sadomasochistic relationships. *Sexual and Relationship Therapy, 31*(1), 95–108. http://doi.org/10.1080/14681 994.2015.1102219

Pitagora, D. (2017). No pain, no gain? Therapeutic and relational benefits of subspace in BDSM contexts. *Journal of Positive Sexuality, 3*(3), 44–54.

Rubinsky, V. (2018). "Sometimes it's easier to type things than to say them": Technology in BDSM sexual partner communication. *Sexuality & Culture, 22*(4), 1412–1431. https://doi.org/10.1007/s12119-018-9534-2

Rubinsky, V. (2020). A communicative interdependence perspective of sexual communication and technology in bondage, domination, and sadomasochist relationships. *Communication Quarterly, 68*(4), 375–396. http://doi.org/10.1080/01463 373.2020.1804958

Saldaña, J. (2009). *The coding manual for qualitative researchers.* Sage Publications Ltd.

Sprott, R. A. (2020). Reimagining "kink": Transformation, growth, and healing through BDSM. *Journal of Humanistic Psychology,* Advance online publication. http://doi.org/10.1177/0022167819900036

Thomas, J. N. (2020). BDSM as trauma play: An autoethnographic investigation. *Sexualities, 23*(5–6), 917–933. http://doi.org/10.1177/1363460719861800

U.S. Department of Justice. (2014). Criminal victimization, 2014. *Bureau of Justice Statistics.* https://bjs.ojp.gov/content/pub/pdf/cv14.pdf

Van der Kolk, B. (2014). *The body keeps the score: Mind, brain and body in the transformation of trauma.* Penguin UK.

Watzlawick, P., Beavin, J. H., & Jackson, D. D. (1967). Some tentative axioms of communication In C. D. Mortensen (Ed.), *Pragmatics of human communication: A study of interactional patterns, pathologies, and paradoxes* (pp. 48–71). Taylor & Francis.

Weille, K. L. H. (2002). The psychodynamics of consensual sadomasochistic and dominant–submissive sexual games. *Studies in Gender and Sexuality, 3*(2), 131–160. http://doi.org/10.1080/15240650309349194

Weiss, M. (2011). *Techniques of pleasure. BDSM and the circuit of sexuality.* Duke University Press.

Wright, S., Stambaugh, R. J., & Cox, D. (2012). Consent violations survey (Tech report). National Coalition for Sexual Freedom. Retrieved August 1, 2020, from https://www.ncsfreedom.org/wp-content/uploads/2019/12/Consent-Violations-Survey-Analysis-final.pdf

15

Emotions, Power, and BDSM

The Stance of the Ethnographer

Charlotta Carlström

Introduction

Fieldwork in several BDSM communities in Sweden has not only provided me with invaluable insights into the intricacies of BDSM interactions and identities but also led to methodological and ethical reflections upon ethnographic fieldwork and the complexity of participant observation. Based on years of researching BDSM communities, with diary and field notes, I reflect upon different situations and events which, in various ways, have affected me and given rise to ethical reflections and dilemmas as well as strong emotions. Over the last decade, there have been several ethnographic studies on BDSM in different contexts and across different countries, providing rich empirical data from extensive fieldwork. Examples are Wignall's (2022) ethnography of gay and bisexual male kink subcultures in the United Kingdom, Zambelli's (2017) study of BDSM in Italy, Bauer's (2014) ethnography on women's and queer BDSM spaces and networks in the United States and western Europe, Lindemann's (2012) study of pro-dominatrices in New York City and San Francisco, Newmahr's (2011) ethnography of a community in the northeast United States, Weiss' (2011) ethnography of the San Francisco Bay area community in the United States, and Andrea Beckmann's (2009) study on the BDSM scene in London. While there has been ethnographic research, there hasn't been much in terms of the experiences of the ethnographer. In this chapter, I discuss ethnographic fieldwork within the realm of BDSM, with a focus on the ethnographer.

Charlotta Carlström, *Emotions, Power, and BDSM* In: *The Power of BDSM*. Edited by: Brandy L. Simula, Robin Bauer, and Liam Wignall, Oxford University Press. © Oxford University Press 2023. DOI: 10.1093/oso/9780197658598.003.0016

Reflections on BDSM, the Methods Used, and
the Academic Setting

My ethnographic study is based on several BDSM communities in Sweden. The BDSM scene in Sweden is mainly located in the two largest cities, Stockholm and Gothenburg. In smaller towns and villages, however, private parties, workshops, seminars, and pub evenings are arranged. Interest in BDSM has increased significantly in recent years in Sweden. For example, the membership of Darkside, the largest Swedish BDSM network on the internet, increased from about 40,000 to 270,000 in 10 years. Over a 4-year period, I participated in several gatherings, such as parties, meetings, workshops, and club nights. I also spent time with practitioners in their homes. Furthermore, I conducted 29 interviews with BDSM practitioners. The findings from this ethnography and the accompanying interviews can be found elsewhere (see Carlström, 2016, 2018, 2019, 2021). The criteria for participating in my research was an experience of practicing BDSM and being over the age of 18. I advertised in a sex shop, and through the sex-shop owner, I was invited to meetings once a week, where practitioners exchanged experiences and ideas about exercising BDSM. The chair of the meetings put me in contact with two women who run a BDSM club. Through them I participated in further meetings, club nights, and workshops and recruited additional informants to the study. I also contacted non-profit LGBT organizations working with sexual issues and informed them about my research. On Darkside, I had the opportunity to advertise my project and to search for and keep in touch with informants. I was also able to stay up to date on events and news via its calendar. Interviews were conducted in the cellar of the above-mentioned sex shop, in cafés, at universities, in the interviewees' homes, or at their workplaces.

When conducting fieldwork, it's important to understand and reflect upon one's emotions and responses. I believe that self-examination is called for at every stage in the research process. In line with Coffey (1999), I recognize fieldwork as personal, emotional, and identificatory work. Further, fieldwork deliberately sets out to place the researcher, including their emotional and affective experiences of research and the personal experiences of the research subjects, as central to the research endeavor (Watts, 2008). Being an ethnographer is often a lonely job. During fieldwork, the ethnographer differs from the rest of the group, in their identity as a researcher. Within the academy, the ethnographer differs from their colleagues. Additionally, being an ethnographer in the field of sexuality can be even more lonely as it is often associated with stigma, as I will discuss further in the text. As recommended, for example, by Denzin and Lincoln (1994), one way to deal with the loneliness and to facilitate awareness in the research process is to keep a diary. The boundaries between field notes and diary notes are often blurred, but, compared to field notes, diaries can enable the researcher to write more private and unfiltered thoughts, feelings, and reactions. The diary can be a place in which to evaluate and criticize one's own thoughts and to stimulate reflective thinking about the research. It can also be a way to deal with the strong emotions and reactions (of various kinds), ethical dilemmas, and relational issues that can arise during fieldwork. I started to write a research diary at the beginning of my fieldwork, which helped me not only to remember and process my experiences but also to put into words the emotions that different situations had awoken in me. In addition to diary writing, I have found it of the utmost importance to be able to talk—both spontaneously and in a less well-thought-out manner—about my experiences in the field. However, due to the ethical aspects of my study, I was very careful with whom I talked, confiding only in my life partner and a few very close colleagues.

Focusing on a topic that is still often regarded as deviant and "pathological" has meant that I have had to both explain and defend why it is an important research area both within the academy and in other contexts. In her research on sex work, sociologist Mattley (1998) takes on employment as a phone fantasy worker. She describes how her colleagues ask how she can do that kind of research and say that they would never be able to:

> These questions and comments were usually delivered in such a way as to make it clear to me that, while they could never do "that sort of work", there must be something about me that made it easy for me to do the work. Once again, I was accorded a (dis)courtesy stigma. (Mattley, 1998, p. 154)

I have had similar experiences to Mattley's. Several of my colleagues pointed out that they would find the actions that take place within BDSM difficult and, instead of trying to understand the practices, would be badly affected. There is a great fascination for the topic of BDSM, which has resulted in many questions and discussions. However, there have been times when my colleagues have experienced an uncomfortable atmosphere due to my research subject. For example, after a seminar, one colleague said, "Did you expect such a completely different atmosphere when you presented your research? People became so embarrassed, it's so taboo what you do!" I was surprised because I had not experienced it that way at all and wondered whether I had put up some kind of defense or normalized other people's reactions so that I did not notice them reacting in an uncomfortable way.

My experiences are in line with what Irvine (2014) refers to as "dirty work." She describes how sociologists who study sexuality report challenges to their professional and personal identities. These take the form of snide comments, jokes, assumptions about their sexuality, and challenges to the legitimacy of sexuality research overall. She suggests that the stigma of dirty work is best analyzed as structural inequality in the form of systematic barriers and practices by those with institutional status. Lindemann (2012, p. 15) points out that "ethnographers who research sexually charged topics are unique in that this conflict has the potential to lead to delegitimation within the academic community." I, too, recognize this reasoning. Some people have advised me to tone down my descriptions of BDSM in scholarship applications as they think I would be less likely to obtain a grant if I am too precise about the exact topic of my research. Beckmann (2009) reflects on being singled out due to the choice of research area:

> Even though my "deviance" only went as far as to be conducting research on the topic of consensual SM, a lot of the people in my social environment as well as on the Scene (of consensual SM and Fetishism) in London labelled me anyway. (Beckmann, 2009, p 70)

This experience gave her "insight into the rigidity with which people apply labels and how a label changes the way people interact with an individual once labeled" (p. 71).

Learning to Know the Field and Oneself

An important part of all relationships is giving and receiving trust; so, too, is it in the relationship between the ethnographic researcher and the participant. I think one way to create trust is to be transparent and open. When informants have asked about me (and my interest in BDSM), I have told them that I am a pansexual, cis woman with an interest in and fascination for BDSM, even though I do not see myself as a practitioner and do not belong to any community. Further, learning to know the research field is also about getting to know oneself. To be comfortable in fieldwork, create trust, and build close relationships with research participants requires self-awareness. The researcher needs to be observant of their reactions and feelings toward gatekeepers and other participants as well as to different practices and circumstances in the fieldwork. When I now, retrospectively, read my field and diary notes, I can see clearly that I changed during my fieldwork. The thoughts and feelings that I held initially in the research were tested as the fieldwork progressed, as illustrated in this field note from one of my first visits to a BDSM club:

The sun has set and it will soon be dark. Spring is in the air but it is still cold. I shudder and feel both nervous and expectant when I stand at the locked metal gate. I have just started my fieldwork within Swedish BDSM communities. A man comes from the opposite direction and rings the bell while he greets me. The gate opens and we go down a stone staircase and in through another door. We are met by a doorman. I continue through a long corridor lit by candlelight. The walls are in a dark red tone and on both sides of the corridor there are doors that can be locked from the outside with hasps. In one of the rooms, a woman and two men are preparing for a session. They have an audience of a few people and I stay to watch as well. The woman's upper body is undressed and she is tied with handcuffs to a wall. The men are dressed in suits and, each with a whip, they start hitting the woman's back. They strike every other blow. At first the woman whimpers but, as the sounds she makes grow louder and louder, she cries out in pain. She screams "Please stop" again and again. Her back is red and, in some places, had started to bleed. The men continued to strike. I'm not sure how long it went on but, after a while, it seemed like she was giving up. She was just making a few whimpering noises. I'm starting to feel uncomfortable. Does this really happen with consent? Isn't it an assault? I glance at the other people who are also watching. No one seems to think it's weird or wrong.

Then the session ends. The woman is released from the handcuffs and allowed to sit on a chair with a blanket wrapped around her upper body. She gets something to drink and after a while she starts smiling. She smiles with her whole face and says "Thank you" again and again. She starts to laugh and says that this was the best session she had ever experienced. Euphorically, she recounts what she experienced and how it felt. She said that she was close to "safe wording" but that they knew her limit just before she needed to use the security word. The two men listened attentively and stayed in the room for a long time together. (Field note, June 22, 2012)

I have seen many whipping sessions since that described above but have never again felt any discomfort. As I became more familiar with and knowledgeable about BDSM, the feelings of discomfort I experienced at this first session disappeared. I have come to understand how BDSM and violence are two different things (Dunkley & Brotto, 2020; Fanghanel, 2020). I have learned that people participating in BDSM always consent to what should happen and that there are "safe words" that can be used at any time to stop a session. The common experiences of BDSM create a shared understanding or, with Schütz's words, a "system of knowledge" (1944/2000, p. 223). This system is coherent and clear enough for everyone in the group to interpret and understand. However, there are different rules within various kink communities, and part of being an ethnographer is learning these rules. They can differ between people, events, and communities—as discussed, for example, by Newmahr (2011) and Wignall (2022). I needed to learn about these diverse systems of knowledge, which I accomplished through many hours of conversations and interviews with practitioners and by spending a lot of time in different BDSM communities.

Another aspect that I needed to negotiate in fieldwork is the power dynamics in interactions with BDSM practitioners. Sometimes I felt part of the power shift between people living in 24/7 relationships. For example, an informant, who defines herself as a dominant sadist, said, "I can force him to participate in your study even though he does not want to," referring to her submissive boyfriend. The couple live in a total power exchange (TPE) relationship, and she had previously told me that all their decisions go through her. I thought for a while and responded, "Participation in the study is voluntary but I cannot, of course, control how you decide things in your relationship." This could have led to an ethically problematic situation, but she decided that it probably would not be successful if she forced him to participate. When interviewing couples, the dominant person in the relationship has had the most space, talked the most, and steered the conversation. After an interview with another couple living in a TPE relationship, I wrote the following in my diary:

She talked over his head like he was not there. I had to think about not doing the same and tried to turn to him just as often to let him be involved in the conversation. Sometimes, though, we talked about him anyway. It was clearly she who controlled the conversation and talked the most. When I said that it was my first time interviewing a couple, she said "Yes it will probably be problematic because the submissive is not allowed to talk until he or she is given permission." (Diary note, November 8, 2012)

I have often found it challenging to interview couples, and several times I have reflected on whether I, as an interviewer, am contributing to the imbalance of power. However, even in these situations I have tried to follow the "system of knowledge" principles (Schütz, 1944/2000) by maintaining an empathetic and humble attitude. For example, sometimes when I have directed a question to the submissive partner, they have not had time to respond or finish talking before the dominant partner answered or interrupted. Although a bit frustrated the first few times that it happened, I later allowed it to occur and did not draw attention to it. Instead, I have seen it as an interesting part of the power shift in the relationship. If I had drawn attention to it or actively tried to influence the conversation, I think I would have created a situation that would probably not be comfortable for them. It could have been perceived as blunt and not particularly empathetic to try to disrupt the power (im)balance between them. Usually, the "dilemma" has been solved by additional interviews or has arisen in situations where I have been able to spend more time alone with the submissive partner.

Participating or Observing?

There is a long-standing debate in ethnography over the degree to which the researcher should take part. The role of the observer can vary considerably depending on the context and may have a number of implications, including their incorporation into the field and relations with the respondents, the maintenance of personal boundaries, and the reproduction of gender stereotypes. Inspired by sociologist Loïc Wacquant (2015, p. 5), I have strived to become what he describes as a "vulnerable observer":

> The methodological stipulation here is to dive into the stream of action to the greatest possible depth, rather than watch it from the bank; but to dive and swim along with method and purpose, and not with reckless abandon that would cause us to drown in the bottomless whirlpool of subjectivism.

To "dive to the greatest possible depth" and at the same time to "swim along with method and purpose" implies a balancing act in which the ethnographer needs to be continuously attentive to their own emotions, thoughts, and behaviors. When I started my fieldwork, I decided not to practice BDSM in my role as a researcher; but, as the fieldwork went on, I realized that the boundaries between being an observer and a practitioner were complex and diffuse. Coffey (1999, p. 22) notes that "As a positioned and contexed individual, the ethnographer is undeniably part of the complexities and relations of the field." On several occasions, I had to make decisions regarding the level of my participation and my closeness to the participants. I want to discuss one of these occasions here.

I had been invited to the home of Lena[1] and Kent, who live in a small village in the Swedish countryside. Until a few years ago, they lived as a married couple. Now they are divorced and live in a 24/7 BDSM relationship where Lena is the mistress and Kent is her slave. They invited me to stay overnight and to attend a session. I discuss the invitation with a few colleagues, who question the purpose of my staying overnight and what my attendance at a session could add to my study. They also address the safety aspects, saying "How do you dare? It sounds dangerous, anything can happen!" This made me stop and think, taking the questions seriously. For what reason do I want to go there? What are my motives? I really want and genuinely look forward to a reunion, but is it rather a personal feeling? To satisfy my own desire and curiosity? After some hesitation, I finally decide to go. Kent collected me at the railway station, and we drove back to the house. After food and conversation, we moved into the living room, where Lena has prepared for a session. Later that night I wrote the following in my diary:

> I'm in a bunk bed in Lena and Kent's guest room and it's 2 a.m. I feel completely exhausted but also calm and relaxed. I am happy with the evening and feel a great respect for both Lena and Kent. I am grateful for their hospitality and their willingness to let me partake and be initiated into their lives. They are both relaxed and confident in themselves and what they do. However, I realize that the boundaries between observation and participatory observation are most subtle. During the session, when Kent was tied up, I stood next to him and watched everything that happened, recorded what expressions of pain he showed, asked questions and got to try the whips. When Lena performed CBT [cock and ball torture], I stood next to her to see how she knotted the rope and how to do it and to learn what risks there are. (Diary note, 10 May 2013)

I learned a lot during my (recurrent) visits with Lena and Kent, both about the everyday life in a 24/7 relationship and about specific techniques within BDSM practice—knowledge that I could not have gained in any other way. However, the complexity of participation observation became clear to me. In visiting their home, I became part of their power dynamics. Being an observer involved me in their intimacy, although I did not participate in any BDSM and/or sexual activities per se. Newmahr (2011) describes her path to becoming a BDSM practitioner, observing and then participating in BDSM activities. She uses her own experiences, physical reactions, and emotions as part of her empirical material. Likewise, Bolton (1995) was actively involved in sexual activities in his study of gay networks in Belgium. Not participating in the sexual activities, Bolton argues, would have been to deny his own sexuality. Even though I have not participated in the activities using my own body, I have several times felt like a "sexual actor" since it would have been impossible not to be aware of my own sexuality in the intimate situations that the fieldwork included.

Being with Lena and Kent, I felt a mutual trust, a trust that was crucial to the situation. Bolton (1995, p. 161) highlights the important question that researchers in the field of sexology should ask themselves: "What right do we have to inquire into the sex lives of others, whether in our own culture or in some exotic distant realm, if we insist on our own right to privacy, to remain silent about our own intimate lives?" For me, it has been important to be as open-minded, empathetic, and committed as possible, as well as self-reflexive and attentive to my own attitudes, values, and prejudices in relation to what I experience but without being self-absorbed—to be seen as serious, with a respectful approach, to ask questions without appearing assertive, and with a will to get close and to understand has also been important. I have strived to "blend in" to BDSM communities, to be patient, to take the occasions when they arise, and to show that I am comfortable in the various situations. Further, I think it is important to be able to meet the informants' questions without sacrificing professionalism, integrity, and credibility.

Emotional Ambivalence

It is important to analyze whether the researcher's own emotional frameworks and knowledge help or hinder the research process and whether they can or should be eliminated or controlled. However, with a few

exceptions (Lindemann, 2012; Newmahr, 2008), there is little reflexive attention paid to the ethnographer's emotions within BDSM research. In a fieldwork situation, participants are aware that there is a distanced observer, and
this may affect the whole emotional tone. I have felt many, various emotions
during my fieldwork. I have been confused, excited, tired, happy, exhausted,
and sometimes all at the same time. Together with my informants, I have
both laughed and cried. However, I have tried to never show feelings of disgust or discomfort, even though I also have felt such emotions a few times.
When this happened, I carefully investigated these emotions. One example is
when attending a needle play session. In needle play, needles or other tools
are used on the body for the purpose of enjoying the experience rather than
producing a permanent body decoration. I had a strong feeling of discomfort and was not able to watch—probably because I have a syringe phobia
and easily faint when I see blood. I had to walk away to pull myself together.
Another occasion that really affected me, after which I needed to process
what I had been through, was at a workshop about humiliation. The field
note below is a description of the session.

> A woman is asked to participate in a humiliation session. First, the woman
> is told to keep her hands above her head and to make eye contact with eve-
> ryone in the audience. The leader of the workshop stands behind her. After
> a minute the leader pulls up the T-shirt, so it exposes part of the woman's
> breast. The leader involves the audience by saying "Do you notice that
> she is affected? What physical expression can you see?" Some in the au-
> dience point out that she giggles, becomes red in the face, is ashamed and
> has an increased heart rate. The woman says she has looked at everyone
> in the audience and the leader's voice becomes hard: "Have I told you to
> stop? Continue!" The woman carries on meeting the audience's eyes and the
> leader takes plenty of time, whispering something in her ear and holding
> her in a firm grip by her hair.
>
> After a while the leader takes hold of her T-shirt and makes a hole that
> allows the breast to hang out through the shirt. Then the leader asks for
> assistance to get two plates from the bar, one full of cream, one with choco-
> late pudding. The woman must stand on a towel. The leader then takes her
> hands full and smears her hair, her face, her bared breast. The leader presses
> the chocolate and cream in the woman's mouth until she is no longer able
> to swallow and spits it out. Finally, she presses the chocolate and cream in-
> side the woman's panties between her buttocks. Afterwards, the leader asks

her to take a few steps back, still standing on the towel. The woman is then left there for the rest of the evening, without having washed or put on other clothing.[2] (Field note, May 15, 2013)[3]

During the performance, I had a rush of adrenaline; I was sweating, I blushed, and I felt both allure and disgust at the same time. I also felt a strong connection with the woman on stage and with the audience, of whom I was a part. Afterward, when trying to analyze the performance and my reactions, I could see that many taboos were broken during the session; the woman's T-shirt was torn to expose one breast, parts of her body were undressed, and she was exposed on stage in front of an audience. The gaze connected her body with the other bodies, and the boundaries between her and the audience became blurred. The adrenaline of the scene clearly affected not only me but also the rest of the group. The ability to share these strong emotions and to meet the euphoric smiles of the woman and others in the audience afterward created strong feelings of togetherness. The performance can be understood through Randal Collins' (2005) description of *emotional energy*. Through the energy generated by the common focus directed toward an object, activity, or person, participants become connected to the strong group-dynamic feeling. The ritual created a strong group dynamic that resulted in emotions of affection and community. On social media the day after, several people (as well as the woman on stage) commented on the event in strong and euphoric words, giving the happening a maximum five out of five stars. As a member of the audience that night, I felt—and was part of—the emotional energy. In line with Hochschild (1979), I believe that, in trying to control our own emotional reactions as researchers and separate ourselves from emotional interactions, we risk distorting the data. However, it is very important to be aware of and examine our emotions and how they affect the research. I agree with Newmahr (2008, p. 640):

When ethnographically introspective questions such as "Why did I respond this way? How did I come to feel this way here?" are informed by the social and cultural context of the field, the life stories of the informants and the rituals of the community, these answers have the potential to greatly enrich ethnographic understanding.

For different reasons and in different ways, BDSM gives rise to strong emotions. These feelings often need to be acknowledged, understood, interpreted, and processed—something that also applies to the ethnographer.

To Care

In addition to the strong emotions that have arisen during BDSM sessions, I have experienced feelings of anxiety about, and care for, the informants. Even though the majority of my conversations with informants have been characterized by a positive and great interest in BDSM, a few stories are about abuse and rape and a treatment fraught with misunderstanding and ignorance by professionals. These interviews have at times been very emotional. On a couple of occasions, I have "fallen into" my previous professional role as a social worker, where I often came into contact with women who had been exposed to violence and people with difficult childhood experiences. It then became a balancing act not to let the conversation turn into a therapeutic or advisory one. At one point, I asked the person if she had considered seeking professional therapeutic help. On these occasions or when the person was embarrassed, thinking that what was being told may be too explicit or embarrassing, I have tried to show that I cope with hearing what the person has to say and let the conversation take its time. In one of my diary notes I write the following:

> It's evening and I'm tired. It is an intense and eventful time. I met Natalie today. The interview took two hours and she had many difficult things to tell me. She told me she been raped. When I asked if she had reported it, she said she would never dare to, that people had told her that she had herself to blame for being into BDSM. What she said really upset me. I felt empathy and care for her but at the same time also anger and frustration. I have never felt the need for research on BDSM as strongly as I do now— that the professionals must understand what BDSM means. (Diary note, May 7, 2013)

Stoler (2002) has conducted qualitative research on childhood sexual abuse and notes that emotional needs or responses do not simply disappear because one declares oneself a "researcher." She continues, stating "Ignoring them is unrealistic and deprives us of the opportunity to examine them rationally and take steps to reduce their bias in our work and their impact on our lives and emotional wellbeing" (2002, p. 270). I agree with Stoler, and, in addition to examining the emotions rationally, I have felt that some emotions render a strong motivation and commitment to bring out my research. I have given numerous lectures and presentations about BDSM for professionals in various branches—such as social workers, lawyers, healthcare personnel, therapists, and psychologists. I have also acted as an expert in court in cases involving BDSM. To work to reduce the stigma and exclusion accorded to BDSM and sexual minorities has been an important driving force.

Conclusions

Ethnographic research within the sexual field can be both emotional and intimate. In this chapter, I have discussed ethnographic fieldwork within the realm of BDSM with a focus on the ethnographer's emotions, participation, and etic reflections. The complex relationships between the field, its actors, and the ethnographer are important and salient for all of us who engage in such fieldwork. Ethnographic work requires a high level of personal commitment but also enables a voice to be given to stigmatized populations, prejudices to be revealed, and informants' feelings, lives, situations, dilemmas, and ambitions to be nuanced, though it can sometimes be very exhausting emotionally for the ethnographer. I see fieldwork as a site for identity work; exploring my own emotions, apprehensions, prejudices, and values has helped me to develop as a researcher in several aspects. I agree with Coffey (1999, p. 161) when she states, "Fieldwork is not only about the lives and privacy of others. It is also fundamentally about our own lives, intimate relations and privacy." I hope the chapter will contribute to a deeper methodological understanding concerning the connectedness between the BDSM field and the ethnographer.

Notes

1. All the names of the informants have been replaced by pseudonyms.
2. This scene has been analyzed in the article "BDSM, Interaction Rituals and Open Bodies" (Carlström, 2018).
3. The participant consented to the scene being included in the study.

References

Bauer, R. (2014). *Queer BDSM intimacies: Critical consent and pushing boundaries.* Palgrave Macmillan.

Beckmann, A. (2009). *The social construction of sexuality and perversion: Deconstructing sadomasochism.* Palgrave Macmillan.

Bolton, R. (1995). Tricks, friends, and lovers: Erotic encounters in the field. In D. Kulick & M. Willson (Eds.), *Taboo: Sex, identity and erotic subjectivity in anthropological fieldwork* (pp. 140–167). Routledge.

Carlström, C. (2016). *BDSM: Paradoxernas praktiker* [Unpublished doctoral dissertation]. Malmö University.

Carlström, C. (2018). BDSM, interaction rituals and open bodies. *Sexuality & Culture, 22*(1), 209–219. https://doi.org/10.1007/s12119-017-9461-7

Carlström, C. (2019). BDSM, becoming and the flows of desire. *Culture, Health & Sexuality, 21*(4), 404–415. https://doi.org/10.1080/13691058.2018.1485969

Carlström, C. (2021). Spiritual experiences and altered states of consciousness. Parallels between BDSM and Christianity. *Sexualities, 24*(5–6), 749–766. https://doi.org/10.1177/1363460720964035

Coffey, A. (1999). *The ethnographic self: Fieldwork and the representation of identity.* Sage.

Collins, R. (2005). *Interaction ritual chains.* Princeton University Press.

Denzin, N., & Lincoln, Y. (1994). *Handbook of qualitative research.* Sage.

Dunkley, C. R., & Brotto, L. A. (2020). The role of consent in the context of BDSM. *Sexual Abuse, 32*(6), 657–678. https://doi.org/10.1177%2F1079063219842847

Fanghanel, A. (2020). Asking for it: BDSM sexual practice and the trouble of consent. *Sexualities, 23*(3), 269–286. https://doi.org/10.1177%2F1363460719828933

Hochschild, A. R. (1979). Emotion work, feeling rules, and social structure. *American Journal of Sociology, 85*(3), 551–575. https://doi.org/10.1086/227049

Irvine, J. M. (2014). Is sexuality research "dirty work"? Institutionalized stigma in the production of sexual knowledge. *Sexualities, 17*(5–6), 632–656. https://doi.org/10.1177%2F1363460713516338

Lindemann, D. (2012). *Dominatrix: Gender, eroticism, and control in the dungeon.* University of Chicago Press.

Mattley, C. (1998). (Dis)Courtesy stigma: Fieldwork among phone fantasy workers. In J. Ferrell & M. S. Hamm (Eds.), *Ethnography at the edge: Crime, deviance and field research* (pp. 146–158). Northeastern University Press.

Newmahr, S. (2008). Becoming a sadomasochist: Integrating self and other in ethnographic analysis. *Journal of Contemporary Ethnography, 37*(5), 619–643. https://doi.org/10.1177/0891241607310626

Newmahr, S. (2011). *Playing on the edge: Sadomasochism, risk and intimacy.* Indiana University Press.

Schütz, A. (2000). *Den sociala världens fenomenologi.* Daidalos. (Original work published 1944)

Stoler, L. R. (2002). Researching childhood sexual abuse: Anticipating effects on the researcher. *Feminism & Psychology, 12*(2), 269–274. https://doi.org/10.1177%2F0959353502012002015

Wacquant, L. (2015). For a sociology of flesh and blood. *Qualitative Sociology, 38*(1), 1–11. https://doi.org/10.1007/s11133-014-9291-y

Watts, J. H. (2008). Emotion, empathy and exit: Reflections on doing ethnographic qualitative research on sensitive topics. *Medical Sociology Online, 3*(2), 3–14.

Weiss, M. (2011). *Techniques of pleasure: BDSM and the circuits of sexuality.* Duke University Press.

Wignall, L. (2022). *Kinky in the digital age: Gay men's subcultures and social identities.* Oxford University Press.

Zambelli, L. (2017). Subcultures, narratives and identification: An empirical study of BDSM (bondage, domination and submission, discipline, sadism and masochism) practices in Italy. *Sexuality & Culture, 21*(2), 471–492. https://doi.org/10.1007/s12 119-016-9400-z

Afterword

Thomas S. Weinberg

Introduction

This volume brings together the most recent research in BDSM. While the writers cover a wide range of topics and use a variety of data gathering methods (e.g., ethnography, internet-based, analysis of social media, content analysis, autoethnography, semi-structured interviewing, and case study), there are many interconnections in their work. For example, after reviewing two articles dealing with race in my chapter in this book, I called for more research on people of color in BDSM. However, once I began reading the chapters in this book, I found that several writers were already dealing with different aspects of BDSM and race.

BDSM and Race

In Chapter 3, on rope bondage, Jones interviewed Black people who felt unwanted and unsafe in white-dominated scenes. Similarly, in Chapter 4, on the pup subculture, which advances the work of Wignall and McCormack (2017), Matchett and Berkowitz assert that "our findings reveal that subtle forms of racial inequality permeated the subculture." Norman, in Chapter 12, discusses the dilemma faced by Black practitioners in their choice of roles in BDSM scenes as they are affected by the cultural context. In Chapter 11, Sexsmith discusses feeling discomfort as a white person dominating a person of color in a humiliation scene. In Chapter 8, Stewart writes about Black lesbians and the intersection of various sexual communities. The author notes the spread of kink among Black people and how it has become glamorized by entertainers. In Chapter 7, McCormick examines race, sex, and gender in the Johannesburg, South Africa, BDSM community, finding that while participation by Black BDSMers is growing, there are not many Black participants

Thomas S. Weinberg, *Afterword* In: *The Power of BDSM*. Edited by: Brandy L. Simula, Robin Bauer and Liam Wignall, Oxford University Press. © Oxford University Press 2023. DOI: 10.1093/oso/9780197658598.003.0017 in the larger scene. Public play parties are exclusively white, and there has been no effort to recruit Black BDSMers. So, it seems that while there are some Black participants in BDSM clubs and organizations, Black BDSMers are often structurally excluded and do not feel welcome in these situations.

BDSM and Healing

Some of the contributors in this book emphasize the positive aspects of participation in BDSM, especially its healing potential. In Chapter 14, Rubinsky, Cooke-Jackson, and Rodriquez examine the communication potential of BDSM to heal those who are recovering from sexual trauma. Similarly, in Chapter 13, Holt focuses on how five BDSMers who had been sexually victimized perceived their participation in BDSM play. Holt's respondents used BDSM play to understand what had happened to them and to develop a feeling of control and self-worth.

BDSM Subcultures

This volume includes discussions of a few of the many BDSM subcultures. Matchett and Berkowitz, in Chapter 4, provide a detailed discussion of the pup subculture. In Chapter 3, Jones gives us insight into the rope community; and in Chapter 5, Bauer writes about the complexities of age play. There are, of course, some BDSM subcultures that have been previously explored, like leathersex (Kamel, 1980) and the BDSM lesbian community (Califia, 1979); but there are also others (often based on fetishes) yet to be identified and studied.

Researching BDSM

The chapters on methodology are especially important contributions to our understanding of BDSM. In Chapter 15, Carlström's discussion of ethnography from the ethnographer's point of view was especially valuable. As I was reading the chapter, I kept nodding in recognition at issues like loneliness, dealing with one's emotions and self-examination, ethical and relational issues, courtesy and professional stigmas, power dynamics, and how far to participate were discussed as I had experienced all those concerns in my ethnography of alcohol use in a West Coast gay male community (Weinberg, 1994). Carlström's concern with ethical issues is especially relevant to the ethnographic studies in this volume (e.g., Chapters 3 and 11); ethnographers must be continually aware of how their work may affect the communities and individuals they study.

Another important chapter concerned with research is Chapter 2, where Wignall points out that many researchers use sites "solely as a recruitment tool" for respondents. Instead, Wignall notes that these sites are valuable resources for investigating how the internet is used to create sexual subcultures and communities. Wignall recommends that future recruitment of subjects include, in addition to FetLife, other socio-sexual networking sites (SSNSs); that researchers explore the relationship between online communities and offline interactions; that they look at the significance of online communities to social identities; and that they also study BDSMers who are "immersed in [online] communities."

Lives Outside of BDSM

In Chapter 6, Cardoso, Pascoal, and Quaresma researched the relationship kinksters had with kinky and non-kinky significant others. The researchers identified several challenges and coping strategies, which they organized into several themes: intrapersonal, which referred to the respondents' self-issues, including their kink identities and fear of disclosure; interpersonal, which referred to the individuals' interactions with partners and potential partners; and societal, which referred to how kink is viewed by the larger society, including the media. These different aspects were found to be intertwined, with respondents concerned about negative reactions of partners, internalized "kink-phobia," and societal stigma.

Outside Views of BDSM

Two chapters examine how BDSM is viewed by outsiders. In Chapter 10, Bennett discusses how legal institutions in Australia, England and Wales, Canada, and the United States have traditionally dealt with BDSM. Bennett writes that Western countries have a "criminalizing line" that defines BDSM activities as illegal. That line is severity of injury, but that definition varies across jurisdictions. In a discussion of the negative effects of criminalization of BDSM, Bennett notes that the law is often not enforced. This subjects practitioners to "the shadow of the law," however, since BDSM organizations and practitioners still fear legal repercussions.

In Chapter 9, Graham, Kirakosyan, Fox, and Ruvabalca did a content analysis of how BDSM is represented in a sample of undergraduate sexuality textbooks. The authors emphasized the influence such textbooks have on how students conceptualize sexuality. They found several themes across the books they examined. For example, some of the books relied on the *Diagnostic and Statistical Manual of Mental Disorders*, fifth edition, discussion of BDSM. As a result of their analysis, the authors make several recommendations to improve the discussion of BDSM.

Suggestions for Further Research

There are several areas, suggested by the contributors to this volume, that can be profitably explored to expand our knowledge of BDSM. Some of these topics are relevant to the situation of individuals, while others pertain to the larger BDSM world. For example, on the individual level, in Chapter 6, Cardoso et al. recommend examining in greater depth the types of relationship problems kinksters face and how their partners who are not interested in kink negotiate these relationships. Since Holt's research (Chapter 13) was limited to white females, that author advocates expanding this work to include individuals who identify as LGBTQIA+, as well as those of different racial and ethnic identities. Additionally, Holt calls for investigating the influence of "intersectionality, consent, and BDSM experience."

On the larger BDSM community level, Bauer (Chapter 5) suggests examining age play in communities other than the les-bi-trans-queer subculture. Similarly, Matchett and Berkowitz (Chapter 4) advocate using "an intersectional lens to explore the experiences of heterosexual pups, pups of color, women pups, and transgender pups." Additionally, they call for cross-cultural research on pup communities and longitudinal studies on pups' social–sexual careers. Wignall (Chapter 2) has several ideas for further research, including exploring the relationships between online communities and social identities, looking at the relationship between online and offline interactions, including more SSNSs in recruiting respondents, and studying those who, while signing up to BDSM, are not immersed in those communities.

Stewart (Chapter 8) has an interesting proposal. Noticing that kink is "making its way" into the swinging subculture, as evidenced by the presence at swinging events of dungeons and professional dommes and the growing importance of consent, negotiation, and aftercare, Stewart advocates examining the crossovers of different sexual communities. While Stewart sees this interconnection of the kink and swinging communities as a recent phenomenon, it is not. Back in the mid-1970s, a couple of decades before the advent of the internet, BDSMers connected through what were called contact magazines (e.g., *Amazon, Latent Image, Kinky Contacts*) available in "adult" bookstores (see Weinberg, 1978, 2021). I noted at the time that some of the same people who advertised in the BDSM magazines also advertised in swingers' magazines, sometimes with the same photo and perhaps a slightly different description of their interests.

I have some suggestions for future research in addition to the proposals of this volume's contributors. First, on the individual level, I would like to see more detailed research on the development of a variety of BDSM identities. We do have some work in this area, for example, the research reviewed in my chapter in this book (Chapter 1). However, what I think we need is information on the development of identities as a process. Among the questions that need to be addressed are when, for example, do individuals become aware of feelings that they later identify as BDSM? How does the awareness of different kinks develop? How do people come to define themselves as kinky or BDSM participants, and what part do other individuals and communities play in this process? How do individuals deal with a societal view of their interests as deviant?

On a macro level, I am intrigued by the politics of BDSM organizations, clubs, and communities. Some of the contributors to this volume mention politics implicitly (e.g., Chapters 3 and 6) or more directly (Chapter 12), primarily with reference to race. I am also interested in how communities and organizations are formed, how they differ in their structure and organization, politics as the exercise of power within communities, conflicts within them, hierarchies of prestige and how high status is achieved, the development of norms and traditions within communities, and the criteria used to accept individuals into or exclude them from BDSM communities.

References

Califia, P. (1979). A secret side of lesbian sexuality. *The Advocate, 283*, December 27, 1979.

Kamel, G. W. L. (1980). Leathersex: Meaningful aspects of gay sadomasochism. *Deviant Behavior: An Interdisciplinary Journal, 1*, 171–191.

Weinberg, T. S. (1978). Sadism and masochism: Sociological perspectives. *Bulletin of the American Academy of Psychiatry and the Law, 6*(3), 284–295.

Weinberg, T. S. (1994). *Gay men, drinking, and alcoholism.* Southern Illinois University Press.

Weinberg, T. S. (2021). The beginning of the sociological study of BDSM: A personal reflection. *Sexualities, 24*(5–6), 825–831. https://doi.org/10.1177/1363460720961288

Wignall, L., & McCormack, M. (2017). An exploratory of a new kink activity: "Pup play." *Archives of Sexual Behavior, 46*, 801–811. https://doi.org/10.1007/s10508-015-0636-8

Index

For the benefit of digital users, indexed terms that span two pages (e.g., 52–53) may, on occasion, appear on only one of those pages.

Tables, figures, and boxes are indicated by an italic *t*, *f*, and *b* following the paragraph number.